D1566700

Melanoma Techniques and Protocols

METHODS IN MOLECULAR MEDICINE™

John M. Walker, Series Editor

METHODS IN MOLECULAR MEDICINE™

Melanoma Techniques and Protocols

Molecular Diagnosis, Treatment, and Monitoring

Edited by

Brian J. Nickoloff, MD, PhD

Loyola University Medical Center, Maywood, IL

Foreword by

Leroy Hood, MD, PhD

*President and Director, Institute for Systems Biology
Seattle, WA*

Humana Press ☀ Totowa, New Jersey

RC
280
.M37
M447
2001

Cover illustrations: Clinical appearance of advanced cutaneous melanoma (upper left corner). Microarray demonstrating genes that are overexpressed (red boxes) and underexpressed (green boxes) in melanoma tumor cells relative to normal skin (lower left box). Vaccine approach to treating metastatic melanoma using antigen-pulsed dendritic cells injected either intradermally or intranodally (center box). Histological appearance of cutaneous melanoma with malignant cells arising in epidermis and invading dermis (upper right panel). Quantitative reverse transcriptase/polymerase chain reaction detecting cytokines present in metastatic melanoma lesion (lower right panel). Illustrations courtesy of Dr. Brian J. Nickoloff.

Cover artwork and layout: Heide Bauer and Brian Bonish

Series design: Patricia F. Cleary

For additional copies, pricing for bulk purchases, and/or information about other Humana titles, contact Humana at the above address or at any of the following numbers: Tel: 973-256-1699; Fax: 973-256-8341; E-mail: humana@humanapr.com, or visit our Website at www.humanapress.com

Library of Congress Cataloging in Publication Data

Main entry under title:

Methods in molecular medicine™.

Melanoma: methods and protocols / edited by Brian J. Nickoloff
      p.   cm. —(Methods in molecular medicine; 61)
    Includes bibliographical references and index.
    ISBN 0-89603-684-7 (alk. paper)
    1. Melanoma—Laboratory manuals. I. Nickoloff, Brian J., 1953– II. Series.
    RC280.M37 M447 2001   00-063353
    616.99'477–dc21

Foreword

This book is about melanoma—its biology, immunology, and pathology, as well as the initial use of powerful genomic tools to study its fundamental molecular and genetic characteristics. The study of cancer will be profoundly impacted by the Human Genome Project. I would like to discuss some of these changes. The first draft of the human genome sequence was announced in June 2000, and we have just scratched the surface of the changes it will engender in medicine. A relevant question is what are the long-term effects of the Human Genome Project for medicine? I would argue that there are three, and each of these three point toward the view that systems biology will dominate biology and medicine of the 21st century. First, the Human Genome Project introduced a new type of science—discovery science. Discovery science takes a biological system (e.g., the genome) and defines all of its elements (e.g., the sequences of the 24 human chromosomes). Thus, it creates a rich infrastructure from which the classical hypothesis-driven science can be done more effectively. The effective integration of discovery- and hypothesis-driven science is a key for systems approaches to biology and medicine.

Second, the Human Genome Project has provided a "periodic table of life." This genetics parts list includes the identification of the 40,000 to 80,000 or so human genes and access to the genetic polymorphisms that differentiate most humans from one another (on average, one change every 500 nucleotides). Most of these polymorphisms have no effect on the human phenotype, but a few predispose to late onset diseases such as cancer, cardiovascular disease, and many immunological diseases. Identifying the relevant polymorphisms and understanding their consequences will transform medicine of the 21st century, moving us initially from reactive to predictive medicine, and ultimately to preventive medicine.

Finally, the Human Genome Project has catalyzed a series of paradigm changes in how we view biology and medicine that lead us to conclude that systems approaches will revolutionize biology and medicine of the 21st century.

- Biology is an informational science. This leads to the view biological information is complex and hierarchal (DNA→RNA→protein→protein interactions→informational pathways→informational networks→etc.). The challenge is to capture and integrate information from these different levels so that systems approaches (see below) can be applied.

- High-throughput biological analyses are transforming biology. DNA sequencing, DNA arrays, genotyping, and now proteomics, are examples of high-throughput biology that can gather enormous amounts of information. High-throughput biology is key to systems biology because systems biology requires that all the elements in a biological system be defined before they can be understood.

- Computer science and applied mathematics are critical to capturing, storing, analyzing, graphically displaying, modeling, and transmitting biological information. Powerful new computational tools have been developed over the past 10 years. Being able to handle and analyze most amounts of biologic information is central to systems biology.

- Model organisms are the Rosetta Stones for deciphering biological systems. The Human Genome Project had underscored the striking unity of life; that is, organisms as diverse as fruit flies or humans share many of the same informational pathways and networks. Because systems must be perturbed in order to understand how they function, and because it is generally impossible to experiment on humans, it becomes important to study biological systems in model organisms.

What is systems biology? Let us consider the following metaphor. Suppose you wished to understand how Manhattan functions as a city. You would have to gather information about its infrastructure (roads, buildings, docks, communication channels, etc.), power requirements, the movements of people and animals, the nature of communications, etc. All of these data would have to, in some manner, be integrated and modeled before ultimately predicting the behavior of the city. So it is with systems approaches to biological systems and networks—information must be gathered from the various hierarchal biological levels, integrated, and ultimately modeled mathematically so that both the structure and systems (emergent) properties of the biological system can be predicted.

A cancer such as melanoma arises as a consequence of mutations in particular informational pathways (e.g., cell cycle, DNA repair, developmental, etc.). These mutations either may be inherited (germline) or may arise during the lifetime of the individual (somatic). Two conclusions can be drawn from a systems view of cancer. First, mutations in different informational pathways may give rise to the same general category of tumor (e.g., melanoma). However, the mutations in each distinct pathway will initiate distinct subtypes of tumors. Thus, for each general category of cancer, one must define the distinct subtypes, for they may give rise to tumors with different prognoses (e.g., relatively benign or rapidly metastatic), perhaps ultimately requiring distinct approaches to therapy. This process of identifying the subtypes of a particular tumor is termed stratification.

Second, many tumors progress through additional mutations and become more invasive and malignant as time passes. So, for a given tumor subtype, it is important to know how far progression has advanced.

A systems approach to cancer allows one to identify diagnostic markers for stratification and progression, potential therapeutic targets (generally on the cell surface), and molecules (genes) that may play a direct role in the neoplastic process itself. The idea is to use the high-throughput tools of genomics (DNA sequencing, DNA arrays) or proteomics to examine the changes in gene expression patterns in normal cells and cancer cells and in many different types of cancer cells of the same type (e.g., melanoma). These comparative analyses will reveal the differences (quantitative and qualitative) in gene expression patterns between normal and cancer cells, will facilitate the stratification of cancers of the same general type, and, with the analysis of multiple tumor samples, permit the analysis of changes in gene expression patterns as a particular subtype of tumor progresses. From these subtractive or comparative analyses, diagnostic markers for stratification and progression can be identified. These markers may be secreted (detectable with antibodies), on the cell surface (detectable with antibodies or PCR), or in the cell (detectable by PCR). In a similar view, unique cell surface molecules may be identified on cancer cells that could serve as targets for therapeutic intervention (e.g., immunologic).

Finally, subtractive analyses of the type described above may reveal interesting candidate genes for the neoplastic process. Ultimately, the systems approach will allow these genes (proteins) to be placed in the context of their informational pathways and through an understanding of these pathways, superior therapeutic strategies may be designed.

Systems approaches to cancer are already impacting the field (*1,2*). Throughout *Melanoma Techniques and Protocols: Molecular Diagnosis, Treatment, and Monitoring,* we can see the initial forays of genomics and systems approaches into the study of melanoma. More will be coming very quickly. It appears very likely that systems approaches to diseases will transform the practice of medicine in the early part of the 21st century, moving us irrevocably toward preventive medicine.

Leroy Hood, MD, PhD

1. Golub TR, Slonim DK, Tamayo P, Huard C, Gaasenbeek M, Mesirov JP, Coller H, Loh ML, Downing JR, Caligiuri MA, Bloomfield CD, and Lander ES. (1999) Molecular Classification of Cancer: Class Discovery and Class Prediction by Gene Expression Monitoring. *Science* **286,** *531–536.*
2. Bittner M, Melzer P, Chen Y, Jiang Y, Seftor E, Hendrix M, Trent J. (2000) Molecular Classification of Cutaneous Malignant Melanoma by Gene Expression Profiling. *Nature* **406,** 536–540.

Preface

Finding a cure for melanoma will be dependent on a greater understanding of the complex molecular interactions that begin in the skin, prior to melanoma's ruthless spread and distribution at distant metastatic sites. Melanoma is one of the most virulent forms of cancer that is now at epidemic proportions worldwide. It is increasingly responsible for deaths and loss of livelihood for countless individuals in their second, third, or fourth decades. With the completion of the sequencing of the 3.1 billion nucleotides that comprise the Human Genome Project, it is now possible to intensify efforts at deciphering the biochemical cascade of events in melanoma, beginning with the relevant genes and the proteins they encode. One of the main challenges is not only to come to grips with the rapid pace of technological advances, but to integrate the new tools of modern genomics with a sound biological perspective that has clinical relevance.

The aim of *Melanoma Techniques and Protocols: Molecular Diagnosis, Treatment, and Monitoring* a volume in the *Methods in Molecular Medicine*™ series, is to provide a comprehensive and up-to-date summary of the most important advances in the field pertaining to melanoma. Each author was instructed to provide clear-cut experimental protocols (including detailed "Notes" on points that often are not spelled out in regular publications), to ensure that investigators outside the field could successfully use these techniques in their own laboratories. As can be appreciated by surveying the table of contents, a highly diverse group of authors were enlisted to provide expert reviews in their respective areas including perspectives in clinical medicine, molecular biology, tumor immunology, and pathology. Authors who could write from first-hand experience were selected to ensure that relevant expertise and direct knowledge of the technique and literature were presented for the reader.

This book is divided into four major categories including: Biology, Diagnosis, Treatment, and Monitoring of Patients with Melanoma. For each category, "cutting-edge" techniques are presented, and discussed within a biological context so that the complexities of melanoma may be better understood by each reader who completes the entire book. Though it is true that only modest clinical improvements have been made for melanoma patients, despite the exhilarating progress in the dissection of many molecular mysteries, it is hoped that this book will be seen as providing forward-thinking perspectives and experimental protocols designed to help ensure more rapid clinical breakthroughs. Coupling technology to biology at the molecular level should provide a sound basis for progress, and hope to both patients and investigators grappling with this disease.

I would like to express my gratitude to all of the authors who contributed chapters to this book, and to Professor John Walker for his editorial assistance. This book is dedicated to my wife, Debra, and our daughters, Megan and Kelly.

Brian J. Nickoloff, MD, PhD

Contents

Contributors

FLAVIO ARIENTI • *Unit of Immunohematology, Istituto Nazionale Tumori, Milan, Italy*

JÜRGEN C. BECKER • *Department of Dermatology, School of Medicine, Würzburg, Germany*

FILIBERTO BELLI • *Unit of Colorectal Surgery C, Istituto Nazionale Tumori, Milan, Italy*

CAROLA BERKING • *The Wistar Institute, Philadelphia, PA*

THOMAS L. BROWN • *Department of Microbiology and Immunology, Wright State University School of Medicine, Dayton, OH*

ANDREW CARLSON • *Department of Pathology and Laboratory Medicine, Albany Medical Center, Albany, NY*

ALFRED E. CHANG • *Division of Surgical Oncology, University of Michigan, Ann Arbor, MI*

EDWIN C. CHANG • *Division of Surgical Oncology, University of Michigan, Ann Arbor, MI*

JOSEPH I. CLARK • *Assistant Professor of Medicine, Cardinal Bernardin Cancer Center, Loyola University Medical Center, Maywood, IL*

LIONEL J. COIGNET • *Oncology Institute, Cardinal Bernardin Cancer Center, Loyola University Medical Center, Maywood, IL*

SCOTT R. COOPER • *Department of Pharmacology, Isis Pharmaceuticals, Carlsbad, CA*

NICHOLAS M. DEAN • *Department of Pharmacology, Isis Pharmaceuticals, Carlsbad, CA*

LOUIS DUBERTRET • *Institut de recherche sur la peau, INSERM U312, Hôpital Saint-Louis, Paris, France*

JOS EVEN • *Institut de recherche sur la peau, INSERM U312, Hôpital Saint-Louis, Paris, France*

GABRIEL GACHELIN • *Institut Pasteur, Unité de Biologie Moléculaire de Gène, INSERM U277, Département d'Immunologie, Paris, France*

GIANFRANCESCO GALLINO • *Unit of Colorectal Surgery C, Istituto Nazionale Tumori, Milan, Italy*

MICHEL F. GILLIET • *Department of Dermatology, University of Zurich Medical School, Zurich, Switzerland*

JAMES S. GOYDOS • *Assistant Professor of Surgery, Division of Surgical Oncology, UMDNJ–Robert Wood Johnson Medical School, NJ*

PER GULDBERG • *Department of Tumor Cell Biology, Institute of Cancer Biology, Danish Cancer Society, Copenhagen, Denmark*

MEENHARD HERLYN • *The Wistar Institute, Philadelphia, PA*

DAVID HOGG • *Departments of Medicine and Medical Biophysics, The University of Toronto, Toronto, Ontario, Canada*

W. MARTIN KAST • *Cancer Immunology Program, Cardinal Bernardin Cancer Center, Loyola University Chicago, Maywood, IL*

PHILIPPE KOURILSKY • *Institut Pasteur, Unité de Biologie Moléculaire de Gène, INSERM U277, Département d'Immunologie, Paris, France*

NORMAN LASSAM • *Departments of Medicine and Medical Biophysics, The University of Toronto, Toronto, Ontario, Canada*

PETER P. LEE • *Fred Hutchinson Cancer Research Center, Seattle, WA*

I. CAROLINE LE POOLE • *Department of Pathology, Loyola University, Chicago, IL*

LING LIU • *Departments of Medicine and Medical Biophysics, The University of Toronto, Toronto, Ontario, Canada*

ARABELLA MAZZOCCHI • *Unit of Immunohematology, Istituto Nazionale Tumori, Milan, Italy*

CECILIA MELANI • *Unit of Immunotherapy and Gene Therapy, Istituto Nazionale Tumori, Milan, Italy*

MARTIN C. MIHM • *Department of Dermatopathology, Massachusetts General Hospital, Boston, MA*

PHILIPPE MUSETTE • *Institut de recherche sur la peau, INSERM U312, Hôpital Saint-Louis, Paris, France, and Institut Pasteur, Unité de Biologie Moléculaire de Gène, INSERM U277, Département d'Immunologie, Paris, France*

FRANK O. NESTLE • *Department of Dermatology, University of Zurich Medical School, Zurich, Switzerland*

BRIAN J. NICKOLOFF • *Skin Cancer Research Laboratories, Department of Pathology, Cardinal Bernardin Cancer Center, Loyola University Medical Center, Maywood, IL*

GIORGIO PARMIANI • *Unit of Immunotherapy of Human Tumors, Milan, Italy*

DOUGLAS S. REINTGEN • *Program Leader, Cutaneous Oncology Program, Professor of Surgery, Department of Surgery, H. Lee Moffitt Cancer Center and Research Institute, University of South Florida College of Medicine, Tampa, FL*

ADAM I. RIKER • *Department of Surgery, Loyola University Medical Center, Maywood, IL*

JUNE K. ROBINSON • *Professor of Medicine (Dermatology) and Pathology, Program Leader of the Skin Cancer Clinical Program, Cardinal Bernardin Cancer Center, Loyola University Chicago, Maywood, IL*

MICHAEL P. RUDOLF • *Cancer Immunology Program, Cardinal Bernardin Cancer Center, Loyola University Chicago, Maywood, IL*

DAVID A. SCHMITT • *The Graduate School of Biomedical Sciences, The University of Texas, M. D. Anderson Cancer Center, Houston, TX*

ANDRZEJ SLOMINSKI • *Department of Pathology, Loyola University Medical Center, Maywood, IL*

YAN A. SU • *Department of Oncology, Institute for Molecular and Human Genetics, Lombardi Cancer Center, Georgetown University Medical Center, Washington, DC*

KEISHI TANIGAWA • *Department of Surgery, Tokyo Women's Medical College, Tokyo, Japan*

JENNIFER K. TAYLOR • *Department of Pharmacology, Isis Pharmaceuticals, Carlsbad, CA*

PER THOR STRATEN • *Department of Tumor Cell Biology, Institute of Cancer Biology, Danish Cancer Society, Copenhagen, Denmark*

JEFFREY M. TRENT • *Cancer Genetic Branch, National Human Genome Research Institute, National Institutes of Health, Bethesda, MD*

ADRIAN TUN-KYI • *Department of Dermatology, University of Zurich Medical School, Zurich, Switzerland*

JOEL G. TURNER • *H. Lee Moffitt Cancer Center and Research Center, University of South Florida, Tampa, FL*

STEPHEN E. ULLRICH • *Department of Immunology, The University of Texas, M. D. Anderson Cancer Center, Houston, TX*

MARKWIN P. VELDERS • *Cancer Immunology Program, Cardinal Bernardin Cancer Center, Loyola University Chicago, Maywood, IL*

MARTEN VISSER • *Cancer Immunology Program, Cardinal Bernardin Cancer Center, Loyola University Chicago, Maywood, IL*

JACOBO WORTSMAN • *Department of Medicine, Southern Illinois University, Springfield, IL*

CASSIAN YEE • *Fred Hutchinson Cancer Research Center, Seattle, WA*

HUA YU • *H. Lee Moffitt Cancer Center and Research Center, University of South Florida, Tampa, FL*

JESPER ZEUTHEN • *Department of Tumor Cell Biology, Institute of Cancer Biology, Danish Cancer Society, Copenhagen, Denmark*

I

BIOLOGY

1

The Many Molecular Mysteries of Melanoma

Brian J. Nickoloff

1. Introduction

Melanoma of the skin is one of the most rapidly increasing malignancies in both young and old patients (1,2). Not only is the incidence increasing, but the number of annual deaths from melanoma is also on the rise worldwide (3). In the United States, melanoma will be diagnosed in 43,000 new patients each year and be responsible for 7300 deaths (1 death every 72 min). The capacity of melanoma to develop in young patients is reflected by the rather alarming statistic that it has become one of the top causes of death in both men and women between the ages of 25 and 40 (3). Indeed, among Caucasian females, melanoma is the leading cause of death from malignancy between the ages of 25 and 29 (3). It is expected that by 2002, 1 in 70 Americans will develop melanoma during their lifetime (2). Also, melanoma is second only to adult leukemia as the leader in the number of potential years of life lost, which is significantly greater than for patients with cervical, breast, and colon malignancies (4). Despite the frequent presence of melanoma and major associated health problems around the globe, only recently have clinicians and laboratory-based researchers begun to unravel some of the molecular mysteries of melanoma (5,6). The purpose of *Melanoma: Methods and Protocols*, published as part of the Methods in Molecular Medicine™ series, is to provide an up-to-date review of the many advances that have taken place during the past several years involving the pathophysiology, diagnosis, genetic analysis, and treatment approaches for patients with melanoma (7).

Although the bad news is that the incidence as well as morbidity and mortality rates for melanoma are on the rise, the good news is that our knowledge has tremendously increased across many clinical and scientific disciplines (5–7) The challenge for compiling a valuable multiauthored text containing contem-

From: *Methods in Molecular Medicine, Vol. 61: Melanoma: Methods and Protocols*
Edited by: B. J. Nickoloff © Humana Press Inc., Totowa, NJ

porary viewpoints, scientific facts, clinical treatment protocols, and other discoveries is to select authors who can contribute their ideas and present the state-of-the art techniques from a rather broad-ranging set of perspectives. Thus, this book is written by a quite diverse group of individuals who share several unifying characteristics. First, the authors all are involved in the clinical practice of medicine either directly as surgeons, oncologists, tumor immunologists, or pathologists, or have decided to focus their investigative talents on working closely with these clinicians. Second, and perhaps most relevant for their selection to contribute a chapter in this book, is that they focus on the molecular basis of melanoma. Third, the authors have agreed to include in their respective chapters all relevant literature citations with an emphasis on the most recent available data. Fourth, the authors were encouraged to reduce their experimental procedures to a practical level so that others not familiar with specific techniques could use these important approaches in their own laboratories, hospitals, and cancer centers. Finally, despite the difficulty in translating scientific discoveries into clinical practice, each author was encouraged to select the most medically important advances in their respective areas and highlight the relevance of such findings for clinicians caring for patients with melanoma.

This book provides a rich admixture of clinical perspectives, cutting-edge technological advances, including narrative overviews, as well as specific and detailed laboratory-based protocols. The emphasis on molecular biology throughout reflects the progress made in delineating the genetic basis for melanoma, a forward-thinking approach to rendering molecular-based diagnostic reports, understanding the immunobiology of melanoma, initiating vaccine-based gene therapy to treat patients with melanomas, and using the tools of genomics (i.e., DNA sequencing, cDNA microarray analysis, and proteomics) to facilitate future progress in the field of melanoma.

2. From the Microscope to the Molecular Diagnosis of Melanoma

During the past 15 yr as a practicing dermatopathologist, I have witnessed many changes in the field, particularly regarding pigmented skin lesions. During my initial training in Boston, pathology reports of melanoma focused primarily on the Clark level and Breslow measurements of depths of invasion of the primary cutaneous lesion. In the early and mid-1980s, many academic dermatopathology units were struggling with delineation of accurate and reproducible criteria for potential precursor lesions of melanoma including dysplastic nevi and congenital nevi *(8)*. By examining relatively large databases and using computer-generated multivariant analysis, numerous independent prognostic indicators were put forward to assist the clinician in the management of patients with melanoma *(9)*. Thus, our current pathology reports include the Clark level (defined as level I for *in situ*, Level II for melanomas partially infiltrating papillary dermis, Level III for lesions filling the papillary dermis, Level IV for melanomas extending into reticular dermis, and Level V for melanomas extending into sc fatty tissue), Breslow depth of invasion (expressed in millimeters of thickness from the granular-cell layer in the epidermis to the deepest portion in the dermis), presence or absence of regression, surface ulceration, and microscopic satellitosis, to name a few *(10)*. Although these rather objective measurements provide valuable prognostic information for the patient and physician, there is still a growing awareness and appreciation of the phenotypic complexity and capricious behavior of melanoma. Initially, it appeared that one of the most important determinants of the biologic behavior of melanoma was primary tumor thickness. The first sharp "break point" was set at 0.76 mm in thickness (Breslow measurement) and later changed to 0.85 mm. Thus, it was generally regarded that relatively "thin" melanomas had an extremely high cure rate, and such an anatomic consideration was frequently linked to the lack of vascularization of lesions in the upper dermis that did not grow beyond 1 or 2 mm in diameter before their removal.

However, it has become clear that many other molecular determinants are important to the biologic behavior of melanoma, and the remainder of this chapter is devoted to a brief review of such molecules and the pathways they regulate. A very real problem that remains for the dermatopathologist using only light microscopic criteria is the inability to predict metastatic behavior in relatively "thin" melanomas *(11–14)*. Before delving into the next section, it is important to note that whereas many of the aforementioned "microstaging" criteria are relatively objective and reproducible among dermatopathologists, the classification of certain nevi that may be linked to melanoma such as "dysplastic nevi" has a higher degree of subjectivity *(15)*. Indeed, despite a National Institutes of Health Consensus Panel meeting, and numerous attempts to define suitable histologic criteria, pathologists still are not able to agree consistently on these problematic pigmented legions *(16)*. Given the limitations in rendering meaningful diagnosis when such an element of subjectivity is present, it becomes clear that moving from the microscope to a more molecular-based analysis of melanoma (**Fig. 1**) provides the opportunity to understand better the phenotypic complexity of nevi and melanoma. One of the most important new advances in this area has been the use of molecular staging of the sentinel lymph node in melanoma patients *(17)*.

3. Importance of Sentinel Lymph Node Assessment

As described in more detail in Chapter 17, surgical techniques have greatly advanced in the last decade and provide an opportunity to perform clinical staging of melanoma using the sentinel lymph node (SLN) biopsy *(17)*. It is based on the principle that the sentinel node is the first lymph node a metasta-

MALIGNANT MELANOMA

Moving From:

Microstaging in Skin

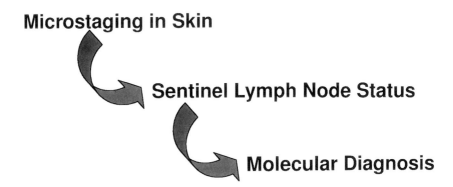

Sentinel Lymph Node Status

Molecular Diagnosis

Fig. 1. Moving from a morphologic to a molecular-based diagnostic approach in melanoma.

sis encounters before entering into other lymph nodes *(18)*. Because SLN biopsy can be performed under local anesthesia, and because it can detect subclinical metastatic disease when assessed using molecular-based techniques, it provides a new method to stage a patient without a period of clinical observation previously requiring a certain period of time to elapse before the detection of palpable lymph nodes could be appreciated by the physician *(19–21)*.

A pathologist can generally detect 1 malignant melanoma cell in a background of 10,000 lymphocytes in a lymph node using routine light microscopy (Fig. 2), but the addition of immunostaining can enhance this detection 10-fold *(17)*. However, using reverse transcriptase polymerase chain reaction (RT-PCR) to detect a simple transcript—e.g., tyrosinase mRNA present in melanoma cells, but not B- or T-lymphocytes—can enhance the detection sensitivity by two to three orders of magnitude over immunostaining results *(17)*. This is not just an academic exercise, because data clearly demonstrate the superior clinical correlation using molecular-based (i.e., RT-PCR) analysis of SLNs, compared to more routinely processed morphology-based visual assessments for patients with malignant melanoma. For example, if an SLN is upstaged (i.e., by routine light microscopic examination, it appears negative for presence of melanoma, but RT-PCR demonstrates the presence of overlooked or rare metastatic melanoma cells), then there is a significantly increased chance of recurrence. The rate of recurrence and overall survival for

H & E Versus RT-PCR

- **Routine light microscopic examination can detect 1 melanoma cell in a background of 10^4 lymphocytes.**

- **Immunohistochemical staining can increase the sensitivity to detect 1 melanoma cell in a background of 10^5 lymphocytes.**

- **Molecular analysis (i.e. RT-PCR) can further increase this sensitivity by 100-1000 fold ! !**

- **Does one melanoma cell make a difference?**
    - **Disease free survival (P = 0.02)**
    - **Overall 10 year survival (P = 0.02)**
  Comparing histologically negative: PCR-SLN vs PCR + SLN.

Fig. 2. The relative sensitivity of detecting a metastatic melanoma cell in a lymph node comparing traditional routine hematoxylin and eosin (H&E) staining with light microscopy vs immunostaining vs a molecular analysis. (Adapted from **ref. *17*.**)

114 patients based on SLN analysis was as follows: histologically positive and RT-PCR positive (34% recurrence rate); histologically negative and RT-PCR negative (2% recurrence rate). But even when histology was negative, a positive RT-PCR detection increased this 2% rate to a 13% rate (more than sixfold higher). It was determined that these differences in recurrence rates and survival were statistically significant (p = 0.02). Indeed, in both univariate and multivariate regression analysis, the histologic and RT-PCR status of the SLNs were the best predictors (**Fig. 3**) of disease-free survival (*17*).

4. Biologic Determinants of Melanoma Behavior

This section provides an analysis of the critical biologic determinants that can supplement the light microscopic and molecular viewpoint, as previously mentioned, with an emphasis on those characteristics that are associated with metastasis. The focus on metastasis is important because despite improvement in clinical diagnosis, surgical techniques, and the use of novel treatments and adjuvant approaches, most melanoma deaths result from metastasis. There is less than a 5% chance of surviving for 5 yr in patients with metastatic melanoma. Indeed, while considerable debate raged for years regarding the appropriate surgical margin, such debate, in my view, focused too much attention on

Molecular Staging of Melanoma

Sentinel lymph node: First node in the regional basis that receives a cutaneous afferent lymphatic from the primary tumor.

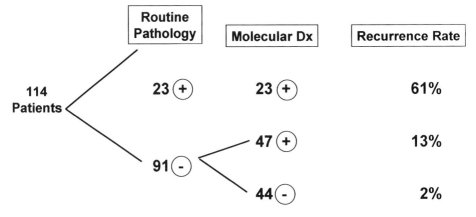

Fig. 3. Molecular staging of melanoma.

the local recurrence rates and not enough on the problem of metastasis. As already mentioned, significant advances have been made so that we can routinely assess, by molecular techniques, the status of the SLN. After all, most patients do not succumb to local recurrence of their melanoma, but they do experience significant morbidity and mortality when their melanoma moves from the skin to extracutaneous sites. None of the randomized double-blind clinical studies of the width of surgical resection of melanoma ever pointed to a statistical significance on long-term survival—only rates of local recurrence.

Having covered these histologic, surgical, and clinical perspectives, we now review some of the molecular determinants that can be useful in understanding and, it is hoped, predicting more reliably the progression of melanoma, including its metastasis beyond the confines of the epidermis and dermis.

Before covering melanoma, it may be instructive first to review the biologic behavior of nevi, because many melanomas develop from such preexisting nevi. Whereas only 1% of individuals are born with nevi (i.e., congenital nevus), almost every individual will develop nevi beginning in adolescence and extending through adulthood. As documented by dermatologists, the number of nevi or moles on each individual actually change over a lifetime, with many nevi coming and going with the passage of time. The molecular factors that prompt a single melanocyte in the basal cell layer of the epidermis in a teenager to change phenotypically into a nevus cell, and then initially proliferate largely in a relatively tightly nested or clustered group to produce a junctional nevus, are not known. Neither is it clear as to the nature of the stimulus that triggers an exodus of the nevus cells from the epidermal compartment into the papillary dermis. However, a few recent molecular clues have emerged that point to the role of basic fibroblast growth factor (bFGF) and its receptor. It appears that nevus cells may use bFGF as a "lifesaver" by promoting the survival of nevomelanocytes as they leave the confines of the epidermis where keratinocytes could supply this essential growth factor in an a paracrine fashion *(22)*. Thus, when nevus cells are in the dermis, they acquire the capacity to produce their own bFGF in an autocrine fashion to ensure their independence of the epidermal-based constraints. As recently discussed, this autocrine switch may represent a double-edged sword, because the acquisition of the ability to produce a potent mitogen, coupled with the constitutive expression of the growth factor receptor, has been demonstrated in several oncologic models to represent an early event in the transformation process *(23)*. Indeed, it has been documented that early stage melanoma cells cannot produce bFGF in abundance compared with late-stage melanoma cells *(24)*. Another relevant molecular change controlling the migration of nevus cells from the epidermis to the dermis are the cadherin-mediated adhesive interactions *(25)*.

A large number of molecular markers have been documented to be correlated to the progression of melanoma. In general, it is possible to classify these changes as resulting from either an increase in the levels relative to normal keratinocytes or nevus cells, or a relative decrease in their expression. There are many examples of so-called gain-of-function molecular markers such as numerous growth factors, cytokines, and their receptors including keratinocyte growth factor, platelet-derived growth factor, stem cell factor, bFGF, and interleukin-1α (IL-1α), IL-2β, IL-6, IL-7, IL-8, IL-10, and IL-12. In addition, melanoma cells express intercellular adhesion molecule-1, MUC-18, integrins (i.e., αVβ3), and proteolytic enzymes (plasminogen activator) or CD95L (Fas ligand). To escape immunosurveillance, melanoma cells may also cease to express other molecules such as class I major histocompatibility complex antigens and CD95 antigen.

Because monoclonal antibodies (MAbs) are available that can detect the presence or absence of many of these molecular markers, one wonders whether pathology reports that include semiqualitative assessments of such molecules could enhance the predictive value of our otherwise routine histologic analysis of primary cutaneous melanomas. After all, we have all had patients with a relatively thin melanoma (i.e., <0.85 mm) who have developed metastatic

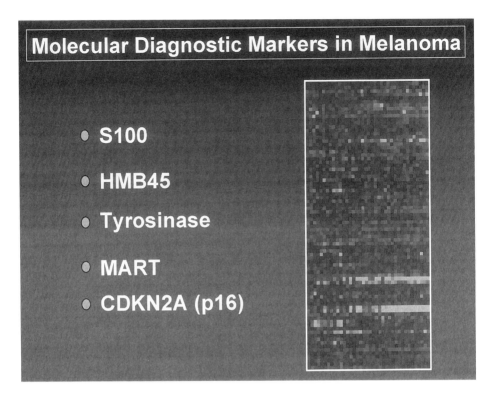

Fig. 4. Forward-looking depiction of sampling a pigmented lesion by needle biopsy followed by array analysis using microchip technology to assess thousands of mRNA transcripts. (Adapted from **refs. *35–38*.**)

lesions that we would not have accurately predicted using conventional microstaging criteria *(12–14)*.

Another important diagnostic dilemma for dermatopathologists is the identification of a metastatic infiltrate in the lymph node or other extracutaneous sites when no primary cutaneous lesion is present. In approx 10% of loss involving metastatic melanoma, no primary site can be identified. If the metastatic cells are producing melanin, there is no difficulty in recognizing the malignancy as melanoma. However, in amelanotic malignant infiltrates, it is necessary to use immunohistochemical analysis to determine whether the tumor is related to melanoma. While ultrastructural studies using electron microscopy can yield insight into the diagnosis by identifying melanomas or premelanomas, several MAbs have permitted assignment of metastatic lesions to the melanoma category (**Fig. 4**). These diagnostic reagents include use of detection of S-100 (highly sensitive, relatively nonspecific), gp100 (i.e., HMB-45), and newer MAbs to detect MART-1 *(26–29)*.

5. Future Directions

Given the limitations in rendering precise and prognostically relevant pathology reports based solely on light microscopic criteria, it is likely that a more molecular-based approach will be forthcoming as the immunobiology and genetic basis of melanoma is better understood. From the practical perspective, determining whether the melanoma cells express the β3 integrin appears to be the single best molecular determinant for distinguishing either benign nevomelanocytes or low-risk melanoma cells in the radial growth phase, from the high-risk melanoma cells in the vertical growth phase of primary melanomas. However, I believe we will rapidly shift our molecular analysis away from expression of single proteins such as β3 integrin, to a more comprehensive analysis that will include examination of the presence and absence of dozens, if not hundreds or thousands, of different transcripts in small biopsy specimens of pigmented skin lesions. Indeed, the Human Genome Project is revolutionizing the practice of biology and medicine in several respects *(30)*. Cancers such as melanoma can be viewed as a systems problem, and using global tools of genomics, the information pathway responsible for conversion of a benign melanocyte to a melanoma cell can be understood *(30)*. As has been shown elegantly by Duggan et al., *(31)* as well as by many others *(32–38)*, assays of genes on various chips can permit the simultaneous analysis of numerous transcripts.

The goal of this next generation of diagnostic tests will be to assign specific "signatures" or to fingerprint a distinctive constellation of both positive and negative transcripts that will have better prognostic value. Not only can this technology assist the pathologist in better cataloguing of various phenotypes of melanoma, but with more experience this approach will also facilitate more customized treatment protocols. For example, there may be considerably greater heterogeneity in the behavior of melanomas besides the current distinction of radial vs vertical growth phases of melanoma. A more prognostically sophisticated classification scheme based on differential transcription profiles may yield several distinctive phenotypes. Within each tumor classification, further distinctions may be made with clinical experience based on therapeutic responsiveness, so that not only will new diagnostic categories be created but also therapeutic decisions based on such molecular analysis will be forthcoming. By examining hundreds, if not thousands, of target molecules, the full range of biologically relevant pathways can be analyzed including molecules that regulate cell-cycle progression, transcription factors, signal transduction, adhesion molecules, cytokine production profiles, growth factors, apoptotic resistance/sensitivity proteins, immunoregulatory cell surface molecules, and chemotactic polypeptides.

It is probable that the next few years will highlight the concomitant use of conventional pathologic analysis with gene assay technology (**Fig. 4**), and I suspect that within the next decade only small-needle biopsies of pigmented lesions will be required and subjected to a molecular analysis without the need of a light microscope. More rapid progress in defining highly accurate and prognostic molecular reports will occur by the active participation of derma-topathologists with our molecular biology–based scientific colleagues. This transitional period will be difficult for classically trained diagnostic pathologists, but it is our obligation to not only support this technological revo-lution, but to provide the necessary quality assurance and critically important correlative light microscopic descriptions to ensure a rapid transition. Perhaps most important we need to prepare the current pathology residents in-training with an appreciation of not only important anatomic-based pattern recognition skills, but the appropriate mentoring and educational experiences and knowledge to facilitate their role in rendering molecular diagnostic profiles of melanoma.

References

1. Hall, H. I., Miller, D. R., Rogers, J. D., and Bewerse, B. B. (1999) Update on the incidence and mortality from melanoma in the United States. *J. Am. Acad. Dermatol.* **40,** 35–42.
2. Parker, S. L., Tong, T., Bolden, S., and Wingo, P. A. (1997) Cancer statistics. *Cancer Clin.* **47,** 5–27.
3. Dennis, L. K. (1999). Analysis of the melanoma epidemic, both apparent and real. *Arch. Dermatol.* **135,** 275–280.
4. Albert, V. A., Koh, H. K., Geller, A. C., Miller, D. R., Prout, M. N., and Lew, R. A. (1990) Years of potential life cost: another indicator of the impact of cutaneous malignant melanoma on society. *J. Am. Acad. Dermatol.* **23,** 308–310.
5. Kamb, A. (1996) Human melanoma genetics. *J. Invest. Dermatol.* **1,** 177–182.
6. Sauter, E. R. and Herlyn, M. (1998). Molecular biology of human melanoma development and progression. *Mol. Carcinogenesis* **23,** 132–143.
7. Rosenberg, S. A. (1992) Karnofsky Memorial Lecture. The immunotherapy and gene therapy of cancer. *J. Clin. Oncol.* **10,** 180–199.
8. Cockerell, C. J. (1993) Atypical melanocytic nevi, in *Cutaneous Medicine and Surgery* (Arndt, K. A., Robinson, J. K., LeBoit, P., Weintraub, B., eds.), WB Saunders, New York, pp. 1571–1575.
9. Morton, D. L., Dartyan, D. G., Wanck, L. A., et al. (1993) Multivariate analysis of the relationship between survival and the microstage of primary melanoma by Clark Level and Breslow thickness. *Cancer* **71,** 3737–3743.
10. Balch, C. M., Murad, T. M., Soong, S.-J., et al. (1978) A multifactorial analysis of melanoma: prognostic histopathological factors comparing Clark's and Breslow's staging methods. *Am. Surg.* **188,** 732–742.

11. Gromet, M. A., Epstein, W. L., and Blois, M. S. (1978) The regressing thin melanoma: a distinctive lesion with metastatic potential. *Cancer* **42,** 2282–2292.
12. Trau, H., Rigel, D. S., and Harris, M. N. (1983) Metastases of thin melanomas. *Cancer* 553–556.
13. Slinghuff, C. L., Vollmer, R. T., Reintgen, D. S., et al. (1988) Lethal "thin" malignant melanoma identifying patients at risk. *Ann. Surg.* **208,** 150–161.
14. Villmer, C., Barilly, C., LeDaussal, V., et al. (1996) Thin melanomas with unusual aggressive behavior: a report of nine cases. *J. Am. Acad. Dermatol.* **34,** 439–444.
15. Prade, M., Sancho-Garnier, H., Cesarini, J. P., et al. (1996) Difficulties encountered in the application of Clark classification and the Breslow thickness measurements in cutaneous malignant melanoma. *Int. J. Cancer* **26,** 159–163.
16. Goldsmith, L. A., Askin, F. B., Chang, A. E., et al. (1992) Diagnosis and treatment of early melanoma. NIH consensus development panel on early melanoma. *JAMA* **268,** 1314–1319.
17. Shivers, S. C., Wang, X., Weigua, L., et al. (1994) Molecular staging of malignant melanoma: correlation with clinical outcome. *JAMA* **280,** 768–774.
18. Wong, J. M., Cagle, L. A., and Morton, D. L. (1991) Lymphatic drainage of skin to a sentinel node in a feline model. *Am. Surg.* **214,** 637–641.
19. Morena, J. G., Cruse, C. M., and Fisher, R. (1992) Detection of hematogenous micrometastases in patients with prostate cancer. *Cancer Res.* **52,** 6110–6112.
20. Naguchi, S., Aihara, T., Motomura, K., et al. (1996) Detection of breast cancer micrometastases in axillary nodes by means of reverse transcriptase-polymerase chain reaction. *Am. J. Pathol.* **148,** 649–656.
21. Wang, X., Heller, R., Van Voorhis, N., et al. (1994) Detection of submicroscopic lymph node metastases with polymerase chain reaction in patients with malignant melanoma. *Ann. Surg.* **220,** 768–774.
22. Alanka, T., Rosenberg, M., and Saksela, O. (1999) FGF expression allows nevus cells to survive in three-dimensional collagen gels under conditions that induce apoptosis in normal human melanonocytes. *J. Invest. Dermatol.* **113,** 111–116.
23. Nickoloff, B. J. (1999) Is FGF a life-saver for nevus cells? *J. Invest. Dermatol.* **113,** 2.
24. Rodeck, U., Melber, K., Kath, R., and Herlyn, M. (1991) Consitutive expression of multiple growth factor genes by melanoma cells but not normal melanocytes. *J. Invest. Dermatol.* **97,** 20–26.
25. Seline, P. C., Norris, D. A., Horikawa, T., Fujita, M., Middleton, M. H., and Morelli, J. G. (1996) Expression of E- and P-cadherin by melanoma cells decreases in progressive melanomas and following ultraviolet irradiation. *J. Invest. Dermatol.* **106,** 1320–1324.
26. Wick, M. R., Swanson, P. E., and Rocamura, A. (1988) Recognition of malignant melanoma by monoclonal antibody HMB-45: an immunohistochemical study of 200 paraffin-embedded cutaneous tumors. *J. Cutan. Pathol.* **15,** 201–207.
27. Ordanez, N. G., Ji, X. L., and Hickey, R. C. (1988) Comparison of HMB-45 monoclonal antibody and S-100 protein in the immunohistochemical diagnosis of melanoma. *Am. J. Clin. Pathol.* **90,** 385–390.

28. Kawakami, Y., Eliyahu, S., Delgado, C. H., Robbins, P. F., Rivoltini, L., Topalini, S. L., Miki, T., and Rosenburg, S. A. (1994) Cloning of the gene coding for a shared human melanoma antigen recognized by autologous T cells infiltrating into tumors. *Proc. Natl. Acad. Sci. USA* **91,** 3515–3519.

29. Kerbel, R. S., Kobayashi, H., Graham, C. H., and Lu, C. (1996) Analysis and significance of the malignant "eclipse" during the progression of primary cutaneous human melanomas. *J. Invest. Dermatol.* **1,** 183–197.

30. Blanchard, A.P. (1996) Sequence to array: probing the genome's secrets. *Nat. Biotech.* **14,** 649.

31. Duggan, D. J., Bittner, M., Chen, Y., Meltzer, P., and Trent, J. M. (1999) Expression profiling using cDNA microarrays. *Nat. Genet.* **21(Suppl 1),** 10–19.

32. Brown, P. O. and Botstein, D. (1999) Exploring the new world of the genome with DNA microarrays. *Nat. Genet.* **21(Suppl.),** 33–37.

33. Nelson, P. S., Ng, W., Schummer, M., True, L. D., Liu, A. Y., Bumgarner, R. E., Fergusson, C., Dimak, A., and Hood, L. (1998) An expressed-sequence-tag data base of the human prostate: sequence analysis of 1168 cDNA clones. *Genomics* **47,** 12–25.

34. Golub, T. R., Slonim, D. K., Tamayoo, P., et al. (1999) Molecular classification of cancer: class discovery and class prediction by gene expression monitoring. *Science* **286,** 531–537.

35. Kammula, U. S., Lee, K.-H., Riker, A., et al. (1999) Functional analysis of antigen-specific T lymphocytes by serial measurement of gene expression in peripheral blood mononuclear cells and tumor specimens. *J. Immunol.* **163,** 6867–6879.

36. Clark, E. A., Golub, T. R., Landen, E. S., and Hynes, R. D. (2000) Genomic analysis of metastasis reveals an essential role for RhoC. *Nature* **406,** 532–535.

37. Bittner, M., Meltzer, P., Chen, Y., et al. (2000) Moleuclar classification of cutaneous malignant melanoma by gene expression: shifting from a continuous spectrum to distinct biologic entities. *Nature* **406,** 536–540.

38. Wang, E., Miller, L., Ohnmacht, G. A., Liu, E., and Marincola, F. M. (2000) High fidelity amplification for gene profiling using cDNA microarrays. *Nature Biotech.* **17,** 457–459.

2

Isolation of Tumor Suppressor Genes in Melanoma by cDNA Microarray

Yan A. Su and Jeffrey M. Trent

1. Introduction

The multistep genetic alterations thought to involve both oncogenes and tumor suppressor genes that are causally related to melanocytic transformation remain largely undetermined *(1)*. Mapping of alterations to chromosome 6 indicates that multiple genetic loci on 6q contribute causally to the development and progression of malignant melanoma *(1)*. This notion is also supported by the introduction of chromosome 6 in malignant melanoma cell lines suppressing either their tumorigenicity *(2)* or metastasis *(3,4)*. However, the suppressor genes involved have yet to be identified.

Human melanoma cell lines UACC903, UACC903(+6), and SRS3 were derived from two steps of genetic manipulation *(2,5)*. Specifically, the parental malignant melanoma cell line UACC903 was derived from a primary melanoma specimen and displays anchorage-independent growth and rapid population doubling in plastic culture *(2)*. The UACC903(+6) cell line was generated by introduction of a *neo*-tagged human chromosome 6 into the parental cell line via a microcell-mediated chromosome transfer *(2)*. Phenotypically, the chromosome 6–mediated suppressed cell line UACC903(+6) is anchorage dependent and slower in growth than the parental cell line UACC903 *(2)*. The SRS3 cell line was induced from the UACC903(+6) cell line by retroviral transduction *(5)*. The phenotypic features of SRS3 are similar to those of its grandparental cell line UACC903. These three cell lines are genetically linked and phenotypically display readily distinguishable growth features. They provide us with the unique cellular resource for the successful identification of tumor suppressor genes by DNA microarrays *(6)*.

From: *Methods in Molecular Medicine, Vol. 61: Melanoma: Methods and Protocols*
Edited by: B. J. Nickoloff © Humana Press Inc., Totowa, NJ

The DNA microarrays allow the simultaneous detection of RNA levels of thousands of genes *(7,8)*. Briefly, cDNA templates for genes of interest are amplified from plasmid clones carrying human genes by polymerase chain reaction (PCR) using the vector sequence-specific primers. Following purification and quality control, aliquots of cDNA (1–16 ng) are printed on poly-lysine-coated glass microscope slides using a computer-controlled, high-speed robot. Total RNA from both the test and reference samples are labeled with either Cy3-dUTP or Cy5-dUTP using a single round of reverse transcription from oligo-(dT) primers. Equal amounts of the labeled DNA are combined and allowed to hybridize under stringent conditions to the probes on the array. Laser excitation of the incorporated fluorescence yields an emission with characteristic spectra, which are measured using a laser scanner. The scanned images are pseudo-colored and merged for comparison of a normalized ratio between the labeled Cy3-dUTP and Cy5-dUTP DNA hybridized to the clones on the array. Information about the clones, including gene name, clone identifier, intensity values, intensity ratios, normalization constant, and confidence intervals, is attached to each clone. The normalized intensity ratios from a single hybridization experiment are interpreted as follows. The significant deviations in the ratio from 1 (no change) are indicative of increased (>1) or decreased (<1) levels of gene expression relative to the reference sample. This technology has greatly facilitated studies of genomewide gene expression in various cancers *(6,8–17)*. Applying this technology, we have measured the relative expression levels of thousands of genes among the cell lines UACC903, UACC903(+6), and SRS3 and have identified tumor suppressor genes *(6)*. In this chapter, we describe this technology as a general method for isolation of tumor suppressor genes.

2. Materials

1. Tissue culture dish (60-mm) with grid (cat. no. 83.1801.001; Sarstedt, Newton, NC).
2. PCR plates (96-well) (cat. no. T-3031-21; ISC BioExpress, Kaysville, UT).
3. SeqPlaque low-melting agarose (cat. no. 50101; FMC BioProducts, Rockland, ME).
4. Bio-Spin 6 chromatography column (cat. no. 732-6002; Bio-Rad, Hercules, CA).
5. Cleaning solution: 400 mL of ddH$_2$O, 100 g of NaOH (cat. no. S-0899; Sigma, St. Louis, MO), 600 mL 95% ethanol (190 proof; Warner-Graham, Cockeysville, MD).
6. Cot1 DNA, 10 mg/mL (cat. no. 15279-011; Life Technologies, Rockville, MD).
7. Cover slips (22 × 55 mm) (cat. no. 125485E; Fisher, Pittsburgh, PA).
8. Cy3-dUTP (1 m*M*) (cat. no. NEL578; NEN, Boston, MA).
9. Cy5-dUTP (1 m*M*) (cat. no. NEL579; NEN).
10. ddH$_2$O: deionized water repurified by Barnstead E-pure System (Chesapeake Instruments, Columbia, MD).

11. Diethylpyrocarbonate (DEPC)-treated ddH_2O: 1 mL of diethylpyrocarbazole (cat. no. D-5758; Sigma) and 1 L of ddH_2O; mix well, leave at room temperature overnight, and autoclave for 20 min.

12. dNTP (100 mM each) (cat. no. 27-2035-02; Amersham Pharmacia Biotech, Piscataway, NJ).

13. dNTP with low dTTP (10X): contains 5 mM dATP, dGTP, and dCTP; 2 mM dTTP.

14. 0.1 M Dithiothreitol (cat. no. 18064-014; Life Technologies).

15. 0.5 M EDTA, pH 8.0 (cat. no. 360-500; Biofluids, Rockville, MD).

16. 100% Ethanol (200 proof; Warner-Graham).

17. Ethanol/acetate precipitation mixture: 247 mL of 100% ethanol and 13 mL of 3 M sodium acetate (pH 6.0).

18. 5X First-strand buffer (cat. no. 18064-014; Life Technologies).

19. Glass slide racks (cat. no. 900200; Wheaton Science, Millville, NJ).

20. Gold Seal slides (cat. no. 3011; Gold Seal Products, Portsmouth, NH).

21. Hybridization bottles (35 × 150 mm) (cat. no. 052-002; Biometra, Tampa, FL).

22. KH_2PO_4 (cat. no. P-0662; Sigma).

23. Microcon 100 (cat. no. 42412; Millipore, Bedford, MA).

24. Microcon 30 column (cat. no. 42409; Millipore).

25. MicroHyb hybridization solution (cat. no. HYB125.GF; Research Genetics, Huntsville, AL).

26. 1 M Na borate buffer: 61.83 g of boric acid (Sigma, Cat. No. B0394), 750 mL ddH_2O, adjust pH to 8.0 with 10 N NaOH (cat. no. S-0899; Sigma), add ddH_2O to 1 L, autoclave for 20 min, cool to room temperature, and filter through with a 0.22-mm filter.

27. Oligo dT primer (1 µg/µL of 10–20mer mixture) (cat. no. POLYT.GF; Research Genetics).

28. pcDNA3 (Invitrogen, Carlsbad, CA).

29. Poly dA (cat. no. POLYA.GF; Research Genetics).

30. Poly-L-lysine solution: 70 mL of poly-L-lysine (0.1% [w/v]) (cat. no. P8920; Sigma), 70 mL of tissue culture phosphate-buffered saline (PBS), and 560 mL ddH_2O.

31. Primers for PCR amplification of cDNA inserts (cat. no. GF200.primer; Research Genetics) including forward primer (5′-ctgcaaggcgattaagttgggtaac-3′) and reverse primer (5′-gtgagcggataacaatttcacacaggaaacagc-3′).

32. RNAsin (40 U/µL) (cat. no. 799025; Boehringer Mannheim, Indianapolis, IL).

33. RNeasy Midi Kit 50 (cat. no. 75144; Quiagen, Valencia, CA).

34. Sodium dodecyl sulfate (SDS) (cat. no. L5750; Sigma).

35. Sequence-verified human cDNA clones (cat. no. 042600; Research Genetics).

36. Succinic anhydride blocking solution: 6 g of succinic anhydride (cat. no. 23969-0; Aldrich, Milwaukee, WI), 325 mL of 1-methyl-2-pyrrolidinone (cat. no. 32863-4; Aldrich), and 25 mL of 1 M Na borate buffer (pH 8.0).

37. Superbroth (cat. no. 08-406-001; Advanced Biotech, Columbia, MD).

38. Superscript II reverse transcriptase (200 U/µL) (cat. no. 18064-014; Life Technologies).

39. *Taq* polymerase with PCR buffer and 50 mM Mg^{2+} (cat. no. 10342-020; Life Technologies).

40. TE buffer: 10 mM Tris and 1 mM EDTA, pH 7.5.
41. TE$_L$ buffer: 10 mM Tris-HCl and 0.1 mM EDTA, pH 8.0.
42. AGTC kit (cat. no. 91528; Edge BioSystems, Gaithersburg, MD).
43. Tissue culture PBS: 8.00 g of NaCl (cat. no. S9625; Sigma), 0.20 g of KCl (cat. no. P-3911; Sigma), and 1.44 g Na$_2$HPO$_4$ (cat. no. S-0876; Sigma); add ddH$_2$O up to 1 L, autoclave for 20 min, cool to room temperature, and filter through a 0.22-μm filter (cat. no. 430517; Corning Costar, Corning, NY).
44. Tris base (cat. no. BP152-1; Fisher).
45. 1 M Tris-HCl, pH 7.5 (cat. no. 351-007-10; Quality Biological, Gaithersburg, MD).
46. Trizol reagent (cat. no. 15596-026; Life Technologies).
47. U-bottomed and 96-well plates (cat. no. 3799; Costar).
48. V-bottomed 96-well plates (cat. no. 3894; Costar).
49. Yeast tRNA (cat. no. R-8759; Sigma).
50. α^{33}P-dCTP (cat. no. AH9905; Amersham Pharmacia Biotech).
51. 2X RPMI medium (cat. no. 402G-777; Biofluids, Rockville, MD).
52. Fetal bovine serum (FBS) (cat. no. 10437-028; Life Technologies).

3. Methods

3.1. Extraction of Plasmid DNA from Cultured Bacteria

3.1.1. Day 1

1. Add 100 μL of Superbroth with 200 μg/mL of ampicillin in the wells of U-bottomed 96-well plates. Label the A1 corner.
2. Place the frozen 96-well plates holding the cDNA library at room temperature.
3. Spin the thawed plates at 1000 rpm for 2 min in a centrifuge (Sorvall Super T21).
4. Fill a container with 200 proof alcohol. Dip the 96-pin inoculation block in the alcohol. Flame the pins using a lit gas burner.
5. Allow the inoculation block to cool. Dip the pins in the library plate. Inoculate the LB plate (be sure to match the A1 corners of two plates). Reflame the inoculation block. After the flames are extinguished, return the inoculation block to the alcohol bath.
6. Repeat as necessary for each plate that you need to inoculate.
7. Reseal the library plates and return to –80°C.
8. Place the inoculated plates into a "zip-lock" bag containing a moistened paper towel. Inoculate the bag at 37°C overnight.

3.1.2. Day 2

1. Label the A1 corner of the 96-well AGTC culture blocks. Fill each well with 1 mL of Superbroth with 200 μg/mL of ampicillin.
2. Inoculate the culture blocks with the 96-pin inoculation block as in **Subheading 3.1.1., step 4**. Incubate the culture at 37°C and 200 rpm overnight in an Innova 4300 (New Brunswick Scientific, Edison, NJ).

3.1.3. Day 3 (Using the AGTC Kit)

1. Place the lysis buffer at 37°C. Fill the receiver plates with 350 μL of 100% ethanol. Label the receiver plates and place the filter plates on top.
2. Spin the 96-well AGTC culture blocks containing the bacteria at 3000 rpm for 7 min. Decant the supernatant immediately. Invert briefly and tap on a clean paper towel to remove the remaining droplets.
3. Add 100 μL of resuspension buffer with 1% RNase (v/v) to each well. Mix thoroughly using the Vortex Genie II Mixer (cat. no. 12-812; Fisher) with the 96-well plate insert (cat. no. 12-812D; Fisher). Add 100 μL of lysis buffer and mix well by tilting the block. Incubate at room temperature for 5 min.
4. Add 100 μL of precipitation buffer and then 100 μL of neutralization buffer. Seal the plates with the sealers from the AGTC kit. Vortex the plates.
5. Transfer the mixture immediately to the labeled filter/receiver plates prepared in **step 1**. Tape the stacks together without the lids.
6. Spin the stacked plates at 3000 rpm for 12 min in the centrifuge (Sorvall Super T21).
7. Remove the filter block. Decant the liquid in the receiver block. Touch off on clean paper.
8. Add 500 μL of 70% ETOH to each well. Decant immediately. Touch off excess drops on a clean paper towel.
9. Place the plates in a drawer with the lids off and cover with clean paper towels and allow to dry overnight.

3.1.4. Day 4

1. Add 200 μL of TE_L buffer to each well. Place the plates at 4°C overnight to allow the DNA to dissolve in the solution.
2. Randomly select 10 samples from each plate to measure the concentrations using a spectrophotometer (Beckman DU640). The concentrations are 100–300 ng/μL.

3.2. PCR Amplification of cDNA Inserts from Plasmid DNA

3.2.1. Day 1

1. Make up the PCR mixture (scale up the volume as necessary) as given in **Table 1**.
2. Add 79 μL of the PCR mixture to each well of 96-well PCR plates and then 1 μL of DNA templates (100–300 ng).
3. Carry out PCR cycles at 95°C for 5 min; 35 cycles of 94°C for 30 s, 55°C for 30 s, and 72°C for 90 s; 72°C for 10 min. Store at 4°C.
4. Fill each well of the V-bottomed 96-well plates with 160 μL of the alcohol/acetate mixture. Label each plate appropriately (library, plate number, date).
5. Transfer the PCR products from **step 3** to the equivalent wells containing the alcohol/acetate mixture.
6. Keep the plates overnight at –20°C.

Table 1
TK

Reagent	Stock solution	Final concentration	1 Reaction (µL)	100 Reactions (µL)
PCR buffer	10X	1X	8	800
dATP	100 m*M*	0.2 m*M*	0.16	16
dTTP	100 m*M*	0.2 m*M*	0.16	16
dGTP	100 m*M*	0.2 m*M*	0.16	16
dCTP	100 m*M*	0.2 m*M*	0.16	16
Forward primer	1 m*M*	0.4 µ*M*	0.032	3.2
Reverse primer	1 m*M*	0.4 µ*M*	0.032	3.2
Taq polymerase	5 U/µL	0.03 U/µl	0.5	50
ddH$_2$O			70.79	7079.6
Total			80	8000

3.2.2. Day 2

1. Keep the plates at room temperature for 5 min.
2. Spin the plates at 3200 rpm for 60 min. Decant the supernatant and add 70% ethanol.
3. Turn on the ImmunoWash 1575 (cat. no. 170-7009; Bio-Rad). Open the cover. Prime the system twice following the manufacturer's instructions. Select "Run" and then "Remove ETOH." Remove the ETOH and reprime. Select "Run" and then "Add ETOH" to add ETOH.
4. Spin the plates at 3200 rpm for 60 min. Remove ETOH with the ImmunoWash 1575.
5. Place the plates in a drawer, cover with clean paper towels, and allow the plates to dry overnight.

3.2.3. Day 3

1. Add 30 µL of 3X saline sodium citrate (SSC) to each well of the plates. Seal the plates with foil sealer. Keep the plates at 60°C for 2 h and room temperature for 2 h to dissolve the DNA. On average, the concentrations of these DNA samples are >200 ng/µL. Randomly select six clones from each plate to run 1% agarose gel to visualize the sizes of the clones.
2. Store the plates at –20°C.

3.3. Coating Slides with Poly-L-lysine

1. Place Gold Seal slides in a glass slide rack (10 slides/rack) in a glass tank.
2. Add 250 mL of cleaning solution. Shake the glass tank at room temperature for 2 h on an Environ Shaker (model 3527-5; Lab-Line, Melrose Park, IL).
3. Rinse the slides with ddH$_2$O five times, 2–5 min each time.

4. Transfer the slides into a new slide tank with 250 mL of poly-L-lysine solution.
5. Shake at room temperature for 1 h. Rinse the slides for 1 min with ddH$_2$O once.
6. Spin the slides at 1000 rpm for 2 min in the centrifuge (Sorvall Super T21).
7. Place the slides in the slide rack within a dust-free drawer at room temperature overnight.
8. Transfer the slides into a clean slide box. Age the slides for 2 wk at room temperature.

3.4. Printing cDNA Clones on Treated Slides

1. Turn on GMS 417 Arrayer (Affymetrix) and the PC controlling the arrayer. Run GMS 417 Arrayer software.
2. Click the "Setup" button. Select "Microplates Preference." Select 96-well plates. Enter "3" for microplates per group and "1" for hits per dot. Click the "OK" button.
3. Click the "Setup" button. Select "Slides Preference." Select the type of slides to print. Click the "OK" button.
4. Click the "Microplates" button. Select "Auto Generate Microplate" button. Click the "Array" button. Enter the number of 96-well plates with genes to be printed. As many as 72 plates (6912 genes) can be printed on a single slide by using pins with 150-μ diameters.
5. Prime the pumps of the GMS 417 Arrayer by clicking the "Prime Pumps" button.
6. If necessary, adjust the levels of the ring and the pin by following the manufacturer's instruction in the user handbook.
7. Wash the pin and ring by clicking the "Wash Pin Head" button.
8. Place 42 of the prepared glass slides on the slide holders in the GMS 417 Arrayer.
9. Transfer 25 μL of prepared DNA samples into V-bottomed 96-well plates.
10. Place three 96-well plates on the plate holders in the GMS 417 Arrayer and close the door.
11. Start to print by clicking the "START" button.
12. Change the 96-well plates when all three plates are printed. Repeat changing until all the plates of genes are printed.
13. Age the printed slides for 1 wk at room temperature.
14. Create one spreadsheet of 96 genes for each 96-well plate printed. Each spreadsheet contains Row (A–H), Column (1–12), Clone ID, and gene title. This spreadsheet will be used to generate the Array List file to analyze arrayed images later. *See* **Table 2** from example of 14 genes on Plate 1 printed.

3.5. Succinic Anhydride Blocking

1. Place the printed slides in the UV crosslinker (Life Technologies).
2. UV crosslink DNA on the slides at a dosage of 450 mJ.
3. Place the slides in a glass slide rack (10 slides/rack).
4. Place the slide rack in the glass tank with 250 mL of the succinic anhydride blocking solution. Shake at room temperature for 25 min on the Environ Shaker at 75 rpm.

Table 2
Example of 14 Genes on Plate 1

Row	Column	Clone ID	Title of Gene
A	1	136798	Fibronectin 1
A	2	34449	Expressed sequence tags
A	3	141953	CD36 antigen
A	4	271478	Max-interacting protein 1
A	5	24415	Tumor suppressor gene p53
A	6	131268	Growth factor receptor-bound protein 14
A	7	138345	Protein tyrosine phosphatase type IVA
A	8	140352	Colony-stimulating factor 2 receptor, alpha
A	9	155145	Matrix metalloproteinase 19
A	10	161172	Growth arrest–specific homeo box
A	11	49496	Programmed cell death 8
A	12	50893	Expressed sequence tags
B	1	172726	Neurexin II
B	2	259291	Integrin, beta 5

5. Transfer the slides immediately into boiling ddH_2O in a beaker on a stirrer/hot plate (cat. no. 43-2904-50; PGC Scientific). Turn off the heat, and incubate for 2 min.
6. Transfer the slide rack in the slide tank with 100% ethanol for 1 min.
7. Spin the slides at 1000 rpm for 2 min in a Sorvall Super T21 centrifuge.
8. Keep the slides at room temperature in a clean slide box overnight.

3.6. Purification of Total RNA from Cultured Cells

3.6.1 RNA Extraction (using Trizol Reagent)

1. Decant the medium in two culture flasks (175 cm²) containing 90% confluent cells. Wash the cells with 15 mL of PBS once. Add 17.5 mL of Trizol reagent to each flask.
2. Transfer the cell lysate to a 50-mL Oak Ridge centrifuge tube (cat. no. 3119-0050; Nalge Nunc, Rochester, NY). Add 0.2 mL of chloroform/mL of Trizol reagent used. Mix well and incubate at room temperature for 5 min.
3. Spin the tubes at 12,000*g* for 15 min at 4°C in a centrifuge (Sorvall RC5B).
4. Transfer the aqueous phase solution to three fresh tubes (cat. no. 352059; Falcon, Becton Dickinson, Franklin Lakes, NJ). Add 0.9 mL of isopropyl alcohol to each milliliter of aqueous solution collected. Mix well and incubate at room temperature for 10 min.
5. Spin the tubes at 12,000*g* for 10 min at 4°C. Remove the supernatant. Wash the RNA pellet once with 75% ethanol. Air-dry the pellet at room temperature for 10 min.

6. Dissolve the pellet into 200 µL of DEPC-treated ddH$_2$O. Measure the concentration of RNA and adjust the concentration to 0.5 mg/mL.

3.6.2. RNA Purification (using RNeasy Midi Kit 50)

1. Mix 1 mL (500 µg) of the extracted RNA with 3.8 mL of Buffer RLT. Mix well.
2. Add 2.8 mL of 100% ethanol. Mix well.
3. Transfer the sample to one Rneasy Midi spin column. Spin at 5000g for 2 min.
4. Apply 2.5 mL of Buffer RPE. Spin at 5000g for 5 min.
5. Transfer the column to a new collection tube.
6. Add 250 µL of DEPC-treated ddH$_2$O. Spin at 5000g for 5 min. Repeat the elution once.
7. Transfer the samples to a Microcon 100 with collection tubes. Spin at 500g for 12 min.
8. Invert the Microcon 100 and place them into new collection tubes. Spin at 3000 rpm for 3 min to collect purified RNA samples.
9. Measure the concentrations of RNA. Adjust the concentration to 10 µg/µL with DEPC-treated ddH$_2$O.

3.7. Labeling First-Strand cDNA with Cy3- and Cy5-dUTP (using MicroMax Kit)

1. Mix the following in a tube: 5 µL of RNA (10 µg/µL), 2 µL of unlabeled control RNA, 2 µL of DNTP/primer mix, 4 µL of DEPC-treated ddH$_2$O.
2. Incubate for 10 min at 65°C. Cool for 5 min at room temperature.
3. Add 4 µL of Cy3-dUTP to one sample. Add 2 µL of Cy5-dUTP and 2 µL of DEPC-treated ddH$_2$O to the other sample. Warm to 42°C for 3 min.
4. Add 2.5 µL of 10X RT reaction buffer and 2 µL of AMV RT/Rnase inhibitor mix to each tube. Mix well, and quick spin.
5. Incubate for 1 h at 42°C. Cool to 4°C for 10 min.
6. Add 2.5 µL of 0.5 M EDTA and 2.5 µL of 1 N NaOH to each tube.
7. Incubate for 30 min at 65°C. Cool to 4°C for 5 min.
8. Add 6.2 µL of 1 M Tris-HCl (pH 7.5) to each tube.
9. Add 500 µL of 10 mM Tris-HCl (pH 7.5) to the Microcon 100. Spin for 10 min at 500g.
10. Add 200 µL of 10 mM Tris-HCl (pH 7.5) to the Microcon 100. Add Cy3-dUTP-labeled cDNA and Cy5-dUTP-labeled cDNA into the Microcon 100.
11. Spin at 500g for 4 min. Check the volume in the Microcon 100. Repeat the spin until the sample volume reaches about 25 µL.
12. Add 500 µL of 10 mM Tris (pH 7.5). Repeat the spin until the sample volume reaches about 25 µL.
13. Invert the Microcon 100 and place them into a new collection tube. Spin at 500g for 5 min to collect the labeled cDNA sample.
14. Dry the sample in a SpeedVac Concentrator (Savant).

15. Completely dissolve the sample in 20 µL of hybridization buffer by heating at 50°C for 10 min.

3.8. Microarray Hybridization

1. Overlay a cover slip onto a microarrayed glass slide.
2. Heat the labeled sample at 90°C for 2 min to denature the DNA. Cool for 5 min at room temperature. Quick spin.
3. Pipet all 20 µL of the sample onto the edge of the cover slip and allow the material to be drawn underneath the cover slip by capillary action.
4. Pipet 400 µL of 2X SSC onto a 10-cm^2 dust-free tissue (e.g., small KimWipe) and place in a 50-mL conical tube.
5. Place the microarrayed glass slide over the tissue and seal the cap tightly.
6. Ensure that the slide is level and stable in a 65°C incubator. Allow the hybridization to proceed overnight.
7. Wash the slide in 0.5X SSC and 0.01% SDS until the cover slip falls off.
8. Wash in 0.5X SSC and 0.01% SDS for 15 min.
9. Wash in 0.06X SSC and 0.01% SDS for 15 min.
10. Wash in 0.06X SSC for 15 min.
11. Spin the slide at 1000 rpm for 2 min in a centrifuge (Sorvall Super T21).

3.9. Scanning and Analyzing Microarray Images (using GenePix 4000A)

1. Turn on the GenePix 4000A Microarray Scanner (Axon Instruments, Foster City, CA). Turn on the computer of the scanner, and run the GenePix software.
2. Slide the door of the GenePix 4000A open. Lift the locking latch to unlock and open the door of the slide holder. Insert a microarray slide with the arrays facing down into the holder. Close the door and lock the latch. Slide the door of the GenePix 4000A closed.
3. Click the "Preview Scan" button to acquire rapidly a rough representation (40 µm/pixel) of the microarray.
4. Click the "View Scan Area" button to draw a region to be scanned. Select the "Zoom" button and zoom in the region.
5. Click the "Hardware Settings" button. By increasing or decreasing the current voltage, each of the photomultiplier tubes can be set such that only a few pixels are saturating in each image and the peak of the green histogram overlaps quite closely with the peak of the red histogram.
6. Click the "High Resolution Scan" button to acquire a high resolution (10 µm/pixel) of the selected microarray image with the selected photomultiplier tubes.
7. Click the "Save Images" button to save the images as 16-bit multiimage TIFF files with a file name you select.
8. Click the "New Blocks" button. For "Blocks," enter the row and column numbers for total blocks that are 2 and 2 for the GMS 417 Arrayer 2 × 2 pins. Specify the distance between the blocks. For "Features," enter the row and column num-

bers for total features (printed spots) within each block. Specify the distance between two spots and the size of the spots. For "Feature Layout," select rectangular.

9. Align the features within a single block precisely on the image by zooming, moving, resizing and rotating the blocks on the computer screen.

10. Double-click the block that has been aligned to open the "Block Properties" dialog box. Select the "Apply to all" to align all blocks.

11. Click "Feature Mode." Click a feature indicator that is not aligned precisely. Move it by clicking arrows. Resize it by pressing "Control Key" and clicking arrows.

12. Click "Save/Loading Settings" to save the image with the settings.

13. Click "Array List Generator." Add each spreadsheet generated at **Subheading 3.4, step 14** in the same order as printing, i.e., from Plate 1, Plate 2, Plate 3, to the last plate printed.

14. Click "Create Array List." Save the Array List file.

15. Click the "Load Array List" button. Open the Array List file.

16. Click the "Analyze" button. The results (gene title, clone ID, intensities, ratios, and others) analyzed and computed from the raw images of each printed gene are displayed and can be saved as a tab-delimited text file using the "Save As" button.

17. From these results, differentially expressed genes are readily identified. If necessary, one can perform Northern analysis to confirm the differential expression of genes interested.

18. If analyses such as clustering, construction of two-dimensional classification trees (dendogram), and principal components are needed, investigators should consult a statistician or a bioinformatic expert.

3.10. Database Search

1. Go to Netscape.
2. Go to www.nhgri.nih.gov/DIR/LCG/arraydb/cgi/query_clone_sets.cgi.
3. Type one of the items such as gene title, clone ID, accession number, plate number, or cluster number that you need to search. Click the "Submit" button.
4. Click on the gene title to find bioinformation under UniGene Cluster for ESTs or Gene Card, PubMed, GeneBank, Genomes, LocusLink, OMIM, Proteins, and Structures for a known gene.
5. The database search allows one to see the current bioinformation of genes interested.

3.11. Transfection (using Cell-Porator [cat. no. 71600-019, 11609-013; Life Technologies])

1. Clone a DNA fragment containing an interested coding region into mammalian expression vector pcDNA3.1 (cat. no. V790-20; Invitrogen) by using standard molecular cloning methods *(18)*.
2. Harvest human cells cultured in an appropriate medium to 70% confluence.
3. Mix 5 µL of plasmid DNA (1 µg/µL) with 5×10^6 cells in 0.5-mL serum-free culture medium in a 0.4-cm gap electroporation chamber (cat. no. 11601-028; Life Technologies). Keep the chamber on ice for 10 min.

4. Add ice water between the safety chamber and the chamber rack of the Cell-Porator.
5. Place the electroporation chamber into the chamber rack.
6. Set up the conditions at 500 V/cm, low Ω, and 330 μF capacitance.
7. Start the electroporation by clicking the "Start" button.
8. Remove the chamber from the chamber rack and place on ice for 10 min.
9. Transfer the electorporated cells on 100-mm tissue culture dishes (2.5×10^6 cells/dish). Add 10 mL of culture medium. Incubate at 37°C with 5% CO_2 overnight.
10. Change the fresh medium with 600 μg/mL of G418 on the next day to select for the transfected cells.

3.12. Soft Agar Assay

1. Bottom SeqPlaque low-melting agarose: Mix 0.9 g of agarose with 34 mL of ddH$_2$O in a 125-mL bottle. Autoclave for 20 min. Keep the bottle in a 45°C water bath for 45 min.
2. Medium for bottom agarose. Mix 10 mL of FBS, 45 mL of 2X culture medium, 0.6 mL of G418 (100 mg/mL), and 10.4 mL of ddH$_2$O for a total of 66 mL. Filter through a 0.22-μ Sterile Filter System (cat. no. 430767; Corning Costar) and warm in a 45°C water bath for 45 min.
3. Mix the medium with the bottom agarose very well. Pool 5 mL to each 60-mm dish. Store the dishes at 4°C overnight.
4. Top SeqPlaque low-melting agarose: Mix 0.35 g of agarose with 20 mL of ddH$_2$O in a 125-mL bottle. Autoclave for 20 min. Keep the bottle in a 45°C water bath for 45 min.
5. Medium for top agarose: Mix 10 mL of FBS, 45 mL of 2X culture medium, 0.6 mL of G418 (100 mg/mL), and 24.4 mL of ddH$_2$O for a total of 80 mL. Filter through the 0.22-μ Sterile Filter System and warm in a 45°C water bath for 45 min.
6. Mix the top agarose with the medium very well. Keep the bottle in a 45°C water bath.
7. Harvest the cells from 90% confluent monolayer culture. Resuspend the cells in culture medium at a concentration of 10^5 cells/mL of medium.
8. Aliquot 8 mL of top agarose medium. Incubate in a 37°C water bath for 3–10 min.
9. Mix 100 μL of cell suspension with 1.9 mL of the top agarose medium. Pour the mixture on hardened bottom agarose medium in a 60-mm dish. Plate at least three dishes for each cell line.
10. Leave the dishes at 4°C for 30 min.
11. Place the dishes in a 37°C incubator with 5% CO_2. Count the colonies after 3 to 4 wk of culture.

4. Notes

The cDNA microarrays provide an unprecedented high throughput technology for detection of genomewide gene expression. Microarray, array hybridization, scanning image, and data analysis are essential components of this technology. The number of cDNA clones (or unigenes) has been increasing greatly owing to the advancement of the Human Genome Project. The easy access to cDNA clones, array robots, and image scanners has made this technology available widely. The techniques for robotic microarrays, array hybridization, and scanning image have become mature. In addition, many kits are available to facilitate microarray-related expression studies. There has been a dramatic increase in the use of cDNA microarrays.

We wish to address a few areas related to the microarrays. First, analysis of genomewide gene expression is a daunting task, especially on a large sample. How one can extract a nature law out of expression patterns is extremely challenging. Expertise combining biology, computer science, and statistics would be quite helpful in analyzing expression data. Second, microarrays frequently reveal hundreds of genes with the differential expression. To determine which genes play an important role in determining a given phenotypic feature remains to be solved. It is extremely important to design an experiment to ask and answer a precise question. We demonstrated that the comparison of expression profiles between multiple genetically close-linked and phenotypically distinguishable cell lines led to the identification of tumor suppressor genes *(6)*. This rationale can be generalized because it allows the recognition of a small number of genes critical to the determination of phenotype. Third, if the aim of experiments is to find an unknown gene, that gene may not be included in a particular microarray. The methods such as cDNA subtraction *(19)*, differential display *(20)*, and representational difference analysis *(21)* may be considered to complement this limitation. Fourth, it is desirable to be able to compare expression profiles of the same cells between experiments, even if they are carried out under different experimental designs. The cross-comparison would expand our knowledge of expression changes of the same genes under the different conditions and decrease experimental costs. However, because of the lack of a "common" reference, gene expression levels of the same cells derived from different experiments or from different laboratories cannot be cross-compared currently. Finally, microarrays allow the detection of RNA levels. If RNA levels are different, the protein level may be different too. If RNA levels are the same, the protein levels may or may not be the same. The microarray detects only one of layers of gene expression. One should use other experiments to confirm or verify microarray data.

Acknowledgments

We thank Lian Tao and Jun Yang for their assistance. This work was supported in part by Lombardi Cancer Center Research Grant GX4395687, Latham Charitable Trust Foundation, and The Coloney Family.

References

1. Su, Y. A. and Trent, J. M. (1995) Genetics of cutaneous malignant melanoma. *Cancer Control* **2,** 392–397.
2. Trent, J. M., Stanbridge, E. J., McBride, H. L., Meese, E. U., Casey, G., Araujo, D. E., Witkowski, C. M., and Nagle, R. B. (1990) Tumorigenicity in human melanoma cell lines controlled by introduction of human chromosome 6. *Science* **247,** 568–571.
3. Welch, D. R., Chen, P., Miele, M. E., McGary, C. T., Bower, J. M., and Stanbridge, E. J. (1994) Microcell-mediated transfer of chromosome 6 into metastatic human C8161 melanoma cells suppresses metastasis but does not inhibit tumorigenicity. *Oncogene* **9,** 255–262.
4. Miele, M. E., Robertson, G., Lee, J. H., Coleman, A., McGary, C. T., Fisher, P. B., Lugo, T. G., and Welch, D. R. (1996) Metastasis suppressed, but tumorigenicity and local invasiveness unaffected, in the human melanoma cell line MelJuSo after introduction of human chromosome 1 or 6. *Mol. Carcinog.* **16,** 284–299.
5. Su, Y. A., Ray, M. E., Lin, T., Seidel, N. E., Bodine, D. M., Meltzer, P. S., and Trent, J. M. (1996) Reversion of monochromosome-mediated suppression of tumorigenicity in malignant melanoma by retroviral transduction. *Cancer Res.* **56,** 3186–3191.
6. Su, Y. A., Bittner, M. L., Chen, Y., Tao, L., Jiang, Y., Zhang, Y., Stephan, D., and Trent, J. M. (2000) Identification of tumor suppressor genes in human melanoma cell lines UACC903, UACC903(+6), and SRS3 by analysis of expression profiles. *Mol. Carcinog.* **28,** 1–9.
7. Schena, M., Shalon, D., Davis, R. W., and Brown, P. O. (1995) Quantitative monitoring of gene expression patterns with a complementary DNA microarray. *Science* **270,** 467–470.
8. DeRisi, J., Penland, L., Brown, P. O., Bittner, M. L., Meltzer, P. S., Ray, M., Chen, Y., Su, Y. A., and Trent, J. M. (1996) Use of a cDNA microarray to analyze gene expression patterns in human cancer. *Nat. Genet.* **14,** 457–460.
9. Welford, S. M., Gregg, J., Chen, E., Garrison, D., Sorensen, P. H., Denny, C. T., and Nelson, S. F. (1998) Detection of differentially expressed genes in primary tumor tissues using representational differences analysis coupled to microarray hybridization. *Nucleic Acids Res.* **26,** 3059–3065.
10. Khan, J., Simon, R., Bittner, M., Chen, Y., Leighton, S. B., Pohida, T., Smith, P. D., Jiang, Y., Gooden, G. C., Trent, J. M., and Meltzer, P. S. (1998) Gene expression profiling of alveolar rhabdomyosarcoma with cDNA microarrays. *Cancer Res.* **58,** 5009–5013.
11. Yang, G. P., Ross, D. T., Kuang, W. W., Brown, P. O., and Weigel, R. J. (1999) Combining SSH and cDNA microarrays for rapid identification of differentially expressed genes. *Nucleic Acids Res.* **27,** 1517–1523.
12. Wang, K., Gan, L., Jeffery, E., Gayle, M., Gown, A. M., Skelly, M., Nelson, P. S., Ng, W. V., Schummer, M., Hood, L., and Mulligan, J. (1999) Monitoring gene expression profile changes in ovarian carcinomas using cDNA microarray. *Gene* **229,** 101–108.

13. Pollack, J. R., Perou, C. M., Alizadeh, A. A., Eisen, M. B., Pergamenschikov, A., Williams, C. F., Jeffrey, S. S., Botstein, D., and Brown, P. O. (1999) Genome-wide analysis of DNA copy-number changes using cDNA microarrays. *Nat. Genet.* **23,** 41–46.

14. Bubendorf, L., Kolmer, M., Kononen, J., et al. (1999) Hormone therapy failure in human prostate cancer: analysis by complementary DNA and tissue microarrays. *J. Natl. Cancer Inst.* **91,** 1758–1764.

15. Sgroi, D. C., Teng, S., Robinson, G., LeVangie, R., Hudson, J. R. Jr., and Elkahloun, A. G. (1999) In vivo gene expression profile analysis of human breast cancer progression. *Cancer Res.* **59,** 5656–5661.

16. Xu, J., Stolk, J. A., Zhang, X., Silva, S. J., Houghton, R. L., Matsumura, M., Vedvick, T. S., Leslie, K. B., Badaro, R., and Reed, S. G. (2000) Identification of differentially expressed genes in human prostate cancer using subtraction and microarray. *Cancer Res.* **60,** 1677–1682.

17. Carlisle, A. J., Prabhu, V. V., Elkahloun, A., Hudson, J., Trent, J. M., Linehan, W. M., Williams, E. D., Emmert-Buck, M. R., Liotta, L. A., Munson, P. J., and Krizman, D. B. (2000) Development of a prostate cDNA microarray and statistical gene expression analysis package. *Mol. Carcinog.* **28,** 12–22.

18. Sambrook, J., Fritsch, E. F., and Maniatis, T. (1989) *Molecular Cloning.* Cold Spring Harbor Laboratory Press, Cold Spring Harbor, NY.

19. Wang, Z. and Brown, D. D. (1991) A gene expression screen. *Proc. Natl. Acad. Sci. USA* **88,** 11,505–11,509.

20. Liang, P. and Pardee, A. B. (1992) Differential display of eukaryotic messenger RNA by means of the polymerase chain reaction. *Science* **257,** 967–971.

21. Lisitsyn, N., Lisitsyn, N., and Wigler, M. (1993) Cloning the differences between two complex genomes. *Science* **259,** 946–951.

3

Molecular Characterization
of Melanoma-Derived Antigens

Marten Visser, Markwin P. Velders, Michael P. Rudolf,
and W. Martin Kast

1. Introduction

In the last decade, many antigens expressed by tumors and recognized by
the immune system have been identified. Melanoma was among the first tumors
found to express such tumor-associated antigens, and, therefore, melanoma is
currently one of the best and extensively studied tumors for which new techniques have been introduced to optimize the characterization of tumor antigens. In this chapter, we discuss the techniques used for identification of
melanoma-expressed antigens recognized by cytotoxic T-lymphocytes (CTLs).
In more detail, we describe in **Subheading 3.** the reverse immunology method.

1.1. Antigenicity of Tumors

The first indication that antigens, which could induce tumor rejection,
existed was described in 1943 *(1)*. That study showed that sarcomas induced
with the chemical carcinogen methylcholanthrene (MCA) activated the
immune system when they were transplanted in syngeneic mice. A few years
later, it was proved that the rejection of transplanted MCA-induced sarcomas
was tumor specific and that transplanted normal tissue of the same inbred animal was not rejected after immunization with the tumor cells *(2,3)*. In subsequent years, it was demonstrated that the induction of tumor-specific
transplantation resistance was not only restricted to tumors induced by MCA.
Also, tumors induced with other chemicals or ultraviolet light and even spontaneous tumors could induce resistance against the tumors after vaccination
with tumor cells. However, it turned out that the tumor rejection antigens were
not shared by different independently induced tumors but were rather unique

From: *Methods in Molecular Medicine, Vol. 61: Melanoma: Methods and Protocols*
Edited by: B. J. Nickoloff © Humana Press Inc., Totowa, NJ

antigens, as demonstrated by cross-protection experiments *(4)*. Therefore, for broad use in cancer therapy, efforts were made to discover shared tumor antigens, expressed by a series of different tumors or within one tumor type.

An example of shared tumor-specific antigens can be found in virus-induced tumors, in which viral proteins serve as tumor rejection antigens. The rejection of these tumors was found to be primarily T-lymphocyte mediated *(5,6)*. In the late 1970s, the technology of cloning functional human T-cell subsets in vitro became a powerful tool in studies of the cellular immune response against tumor antigens. Thus, also human tumors could be tested for expression of rejection antigens, which was impossible with the transplantation models. In the following years, CD8+ T-cell responses against human melanoma were described *(7,8)*, showing that melanoma expressed antigens against which CTLs could be generated. It was also possible to isolate tumor-specific CTLs out of peripheral blood lymphocytes (PBLs) from patients with a history of melanoma *(9)* and out of the tumor (tumor-infiltrating lymphocytes [TILs]) *(10)*. In vitro, these CTLs specifically lysed the autologous tumor cells, and when adoptively transferred into the autologous patient in combination with interleukin-2 (IL-2), occasional remissions of the remaining tumor cells were reported *(11,12)*. Based on identification and generation of different CTL lines, it was postulated that melanomas express multiple antigenic peptides, which can be recognized by CD8+ T-cells *(13)*. Since then, a series of antigens and antigenic peptides has been identified for melanoma and also for other tumor types, using different techniques, discussed later in this chapter.

1.2. Melanoma Antigens

Almost all the antigens identified in melanoma, except HER2/*neu*, are tumor-expressed self-antigens, which means that in addition to being found in tumor tissue antigens can be found in normal, nonmalignant tissues (reviewed in **ref. 14**). **Table 1** lists melanoma-derived antigens discovered so far.

1.2.1. Oncospermatogonal Antigens

The first human tumor-derived antigen to be described was melanoma antigen-A1 (MAGE-A1) *(15)*. This antigen turned out to be the first member of a family of shared tumor antigens with great homology, which are expressed in various human tumors of different histologic types (e.g., melanomas; bladder, mammary, head, and neck squamous cell and renal carcinomas). The genes are located on the long arm of the X chromosome, and expression in normal tissues can be found only in the testis and, in some cases, the placenta. Therefore, antigens in this category are called oncospermatogonal antigens. When these antigens are used as targets in cancer therapy, the risk of inducing an eventual autoimmune response is minimized by the lack of major histocompatibility

Table 1
Melanoma-Expressed Antigens Recognized by Both CD8[+]
and CD4[+] T-Cells

Antigen	HLA restriction[a]	Epitope	Sequence[g]	Reference
Oncospermatogonal antigens				
MAGE-A1	A*01	161–169	EADPTGHSY	*105*
	A*03	96–104	SLFRAVITK	*140*
	A*24	147–155	NYKHCFPEI	*113*
	A*28	222–231	EVYDGREHSA	*140*
	B*3701	127–136	REPVTKAEML	*108*
	B*53	258–266	DPARYEFLW	*140*
	Cw*0201	62–70	SAFPTTINF	*140*
	Cw*0301	230–238	SAYGEPRKL	*140*
	Cw*1601	230–238	SAYGEPRKL	*90*
MAGE-A2	A*0201	112–120	KMVELVHFL	*60*
	A*0201	157–166	YLQVFGIEV	*60*
	B*3701	127–136	REPVTKAEML	*109*
MAGE-A3	A*01	168–176	EVDPIGHLY	*89*
	A*02	112–120	KVAELVHFL	*140*
	A*02	276–284	FLWGPRAYA	*121*
	A*2402	195–203	IMPKAGLLI	*114*
	A*2402	97–105	TFPDLESEFF	*116*
	B*3701	127–136	REPVTKAEML	*109*
	B*44	167–176	MEVDPIGHLY	*119*
	Drβ1*1301/2	114–127	AELVHFLLKYRAR	*38*
	Drβ1*1301/2	121–134	LLKYRAREPVTKAE	*38*
	DR11	286–300	TSYVKVLHHMVKISG	*17*
MAGE-4a	A*0201	254–263	GLYDGREHTV	*17*
MAGE-A6	A*3402	290–298	MVKISGGPR	*123*
	B*3701	127–136	REPVTKAEML	*109*
MAGE-A10	A*0201	254–262	GLYDGMEHL	*110*
MAGE-A12	A*0201	276–284	FLWGPRALV	*121*
MAGE-B1	A*0201	276–284	FLWGPRAYA	*121*
MAGE-B2	A*0201	276–284	FLWGPRAYA	*121*
BAGE	Cw*1601	2–10	AARAVFLAL	*124*
GAGE-1	Cw*6	9–16	YRPRPRRY	*125*
LAGE-1 (CAMEL)	A*0201	ORF2 1–11[b]	MLMMAQEALALFL	*126*
PRAME	A*24	301–309	LYVDSLFFL	*127*
NY-ESO-1	A*02	157–165	SLLMWITQC	*104*
	A*02	157–167	SLLMWITQCFL	*104*
	A*02	155–163	QLSLLMWIT	*104*
	A*31	ORF2	LAAQERRVPR	*94*
	A*31	ORF1	ASCPGGGAPR	*94*
DAM-6	A*02	271–279	FLWGPRAYA	*128*

(continued)

Table 1 *(continued)*

Antigen	HLA restriction[a]	Epitope	Sequence[g]	Reference
Melanocytic differentiation antigens				
Tyrosinase	A*01	243–251	KCDICTDEY	*113*
	A*01	146–156	SSDYVIPIGTY	*129*
	A*0201	1–9	MLLAVLYCL	*107*
	A*0201	369–377	YMNGTMSQV	*96,107*
	A*0201	369–377	YMDGTMSQV	*107*
	A*0201			*130*
	A*2402	206–214	AFLPWHRLF	*108*
	B*44	192–205	SEIWRDIDF	*131*
	DRβ1*0401	56–70	QNILLSNAPLGPQFP	*36*
	DRβ1*0401	448–462	DYSYKQDSDPDSFQD	*36*
	DRβ1*1501	386–406		*132*
MART-1/Melan-A	A*0201	27–35	AAGIGILTV	*112*
	A*0201	26–35	EAAGIGILTV	*70*
	A*0201	32–40	ILTVILGVL	*99*
	A*02	27–35	LAGIGILTV	*133*
	B*4501	24–33	AEEAAGIGIL	*130*
gp100	A*0201	154–162	KTWGQYWQV	*120*
	A*0201	209–217	ITDQVPFSV	*28*
	A*0201	280–288	YLEPGPVTA	*28*
	A*0201	457–466	LLDGTATLRL	*108*
	A*0201	476–485	VLYRYGSFSV	*28*
	A*0201	619–627	RLMKQDFSV	*129*
	A*0201	639–647	RLPRIFCSC	*129*
	A*03	17–25	ALLAVGATK	*118*
	A*03	614–622	LIYRRRLMK	*129*
	A*0301	87–96	ALNFPGSQK	*117*
	A*0301	86–96	IALNFPGSQK	*117*
	A*1101	87–96	ALNFPGSQK	*117*
	A*2402	INT-4 170-178[c]	VYFFLPDHL	*21*
	C*0802	71–78	SNDGPTLI	*134*
	DRβ1*0401	44–59	WNRQLYPEWTEAQRLD	*37*
TRP-1/gp75	A*31	1–9	MSLQRQFLR	*25*
TRP-2	A*31	197–205	LLPGGRPYR	*93,135*
	A*33	197–205	LLPGGRPYR	*134*
	A*0201	180–188	SVYDFFVWL	*136*
	C*0802	387–395	ANDPIFVVL	*134*
	A*68011	INT-2	EVISCKLIKR	*20*
MC1R	A*0201	244–252	TILLGIFFL	*137*
	A*0201	283–291	FLALIICNA	*137*
	A*0201	291–300	AIIDPLIYA	*137*

Table 1 *(continued)*

Antigen	HLA restriction[a]	Epitope	Sequence[g]	Reference
Other melanoma-expressed (mutated) antigens				
MUM-1	B*44	nt782–808[d]	EEKLIVVLF	*32*
CDK4	A*02	22–32	ACDPHSGHFV	*34*
β-Catenin	A*24	29–37	SYLDSGIHF	*33*
p15	A*24	NA[e]	AYGLDFYIL	*138*
GnT-V	A*02	INT	VLPDVFIRC(V)	*31*
TPI	DRβ1*0101	23–37	GELIGILNAAKVPAD	*40*
Annexin II	DRβ1*0401	208–223	DVPKWISIMTERSVPH	*37*
LDLR-FUT fused genes	DRβ1*01	Antisense[f]	WRRAPAPGAK	*41*
CDC27 (mutated)	DRβ1*0401	758–772	FSWAMDLDPKGA	*42*
Oncogene-derived antigens				
HER2/*neu*	A*0201	369–377	KIFGSLAFL	*139*
	A*0201	435–443	ILHNGAYSL	*139*
	A*0201	665–673	VVLGVVFGI	*139*
	A*0201	689–697	RLLQETELV	*139*
	A*0201	952–961	YMIMVKCWMI	*139*

[a]HLA-DR-restricted epitopes are recognized by CD4+ T-cells, others by CD8+ T-cells.
[b]ORF, epitope derived from an alternative ORF from the same gene.
[c]INT, epitope is encoded by an intronic region of the gene.
[d]Location is given in nucleotide sequence.
[e]NA, not available.
[f]Epitope is derived from an antisense product of the fused genes.
[g]Bold amino acids are point mutated.

complex-I (MHC-I) expression in the testis *(16)*. After MAGE-A1, a series of other antigens of this family recognized by CTLs were identified (*see* **Table 1**).

There are four MAGE subfamilies: MAGE-A, MAGE-B, MAGE-C, and MAGE-D *(17)*. Many melanoma-reactive CTLs have been identified directed against MAGE-A and MAGE-B gene-derived peptides, but not yet against peptides from MAGE-C and MAGE-D. The MAGE-A subfamily consists of 12 closely related genes *(18)*, from which MAGE-A1, MAGE-A2, MAGE-A3, MAGE-A4a, MAGE-A6, MAGE-A10 and MAGE-A12 were shown to contain CTL epitopes. The MAGE genes are expressed in a large percentage of melanoma tumor samples (MAGE-A1 in 40%, MAGE-A2 in 70% of metastatic melanomas, MAGE-A3 in 65% of melanoma samples, and MAGE-A10 in 21% of primary melanoma lesions and in 47% of metastatic melanoma tissues) and are therefore promising targets for immunotherapy.

At present it is not clear why these testis-specific genes are activated in certain malignancies and what their normal function is. A possible mechanism of activation is demethylation (an event that occurs in many tumors) of the promoter region. It was shown for MAGE-A1 that a demethylating agent could activate the gene in MAGE-A1-negative cells *(18,19)*. Because expression is observed only in placental or testis tissue, it is thought that the onco-spermatogonal antigens play a role in embryogenesis.

1.2.2. Melanocytic Differentiation Antigens

Melanocytic differentiation antigens are not only expressed in melanomas but also in normal melanocytes and in the retina. These proteins are specific for the melanocytic lineage and are often involved in melanin metabolism (tyrosinase, gp100, and tyrosinase-related protein-1 [TRP-1] and TRP-2). They are located in cytoplasmic organelles called melanosomes. The antigenic epitopes of these differentiation antigens are derived from normally processed nonmutated proteins, or sometimes from intronic regions in the gene (TRP-2 *[20]* and gp100 *[21]*). Tyrosinase-specific CTLs can be induced from healthy donor blood, which means that these autoreactive CTLs are not clonally deleted in most individuals, as is usually the case with self-proteins *(22)*. It is possible that in a normal situation, these CTLs are not activated, but when antigen levels increase, the T-cells can be stimulated. The first differentiation antigen described is tyrosinase *(23)*. This enzyme is expressed in virtually all melanoma samples and converts tyrosine into dihydroxyphenylalanine, a process that is involved in melanin production *(24)*. Two other differentiation antigens, TRP-1 and TRP-2, are closely related to tyrosinase (40% homology). Their biologic function is not completely known, but they are probably also involved in the melanin pathway. Until now only one CTL epitope was determined for TRP-1 from an alternative open reading frame (ORF) *(25)*. TRP-2 is one of the most highly expressed glycoproteins in human pigmented melanocytic cells and melanoma. Multiple epitopes recognized by CTLs are described for TRP-2, including one derived from an intronic region of the TRP-2 gene *(20)*. MART-1/ Melan A is a small membrane protein with an unknown function that was simultaneously discovered by two research groups *(26,27)*. Finally, the differentiation antigen gp100 was originally identified as a melanocytic lineage-specific antigen recognized by antibodies. However, in recent years a series of CTL peptides from the gp100 protein were identified for different human leukocyte antigen (HLA) alleles. Moreover, a significant correlation between T-cell recognition in vitro and tumor regression in patients receiving T-cell therapy has been demonstrated for gp100 *(28)*. Melanocyte destruction has occurred in several melanoma patients responding to immunotherapies but only in the skin as vitiligo and not in the eye or other organs *(29)*. Also, after vaccination with a recombinant Vaccinia virus encoding for mouse TRP-1, it was observed that besides tumor rejection, the mice also developed autoimmune vitiligo *(30)*. This suggests that melanocytic differentiation antigens can be recognized by the immune system.

1.2.3. Other Melanoma-Expressed (Mutated) Antigens

The third group of tumor-expressed antigens is proteins, which are mutated or alternatively expressed or processed. Mutations or differences in expression levels can give rise to CTLs specific for such endogenously expressed antigen. For example, an encrypted promoter of an intronic region of the *N*-acetylglucosaminyltransferase-V gene intronic region encodes a CTL epitope presented by HLA-A*0201, which is expressed in a large number of melanoma (approx 50%), brain, and sarcoma samples, but not in normal tissues *(31)*. The normally transcribed enzyme is expressed in the Golgi apparatus of cells from many nonmalignant tissues.

It is believed that mutated self-proteins can give rise to antigens that can be recognized by T-cells. The problem with mutations is that they often occur randomly, differing by individual. In melanoma, the first mutated protein shown to be antigenic was the melanoma ubiquitous mutated-1 (MUM-1) antigen *(32)*. The epitope contains a point mutation and is partly a transcription of an intron. The MUM-1 antigen was observed in only one patient. Other CTL epitopes derived from a mutated gene were found for the proteins β-catenin *(33)* and CDK4 *(34)*. Both normal genes are widely expressed.

1.2.4. Antigens Recognized by CD4⁺ T-Cells

In recent years, research on T-cell immunity against human tumors has focused mainly on identification of CD8$^+$ HLA class I–restricted CTL responses. Now a series of antigenic peptides presented by HLA class II molecules (only HLA-DR), which are recognized by another subset of T-cells (CD4$^+$ T-cells), also have been identified. CD4$^+$ T-cells have a supportive role in the cellular antitumor immune response *(35)*. In general, the strategies used for the identification of peptides recognized by CD4$^+$ T-cells are the same as the ones described for the identification of peptides recognized by CTLs later in this chapter.

The first antigenic peptides expressed by melanomas, for which it was shown that they were recognized by CD4$^+$ T-cells, were the nonmutated tyrosinase$_{56-70}$ and tyrosinase$_{448-462}$ peptides *(36)*. In addition to epitopes from known CTL-recognized antigens such as gp100 *(37)* and MAGE-3 *(38,39)*, new antigens are described for CD4$^+$ T-cells, such as annexin II *(37)*, triosephosphate *(40)*, low-density lipid receptor-2-α-ʟ-fucosyltransferase fused genes *(41)*, and CDC27 *(42)*.

1.3. Presentation of Antigens to CTLs

In melanoma, as in virus-induced tumors, the major immune response is mediated by CTLs. To define tumor-derived antigens that are recognized by CTLs, it is important to understand the process involved in the presentation of the antigen to T-cells.

In the case of viral infections or a malignancy, intracellular abnormalities have to be recognized by the immune system. Presentation of small peptide fragments of cellular proteins on the cell surface by MHC-I visualizes the interior cell content to the exterior *(43,44)*. Peptide fragments of mostly cytosolic proteins are generated by a cytoplasmic proteolytic complex called proteasome *(45)*. These small peptide fragments, usually 9–11 amino acids long, are transported to the endoplasmic reticulum (ER), where the empty MHC-I molecules are located. The transportation over the ER membrane is mediated by specialized adenosine triphosphate–dependent molecules called transporters associated with antigen presentation *(46,47)*. In the ER, the peptides bind the empty MHC-I molecules. This binding stabilizes the MHC-I and initiates transport of the MHC-I/peptide complex to the cell surface.

That CTL recognition of peptides was MHC-I restricted was first described in 1974 *(48)*. X-ray crystallography elucidated that MHC-I is a membrane-bound molecule, consisting of two noncovalently associated components: a 45-kDa heavy chain, with three extracellular domains (α1, α2, and α3); and a 12-kDa β_2-microglobulin molecule. The α1 and α2 domains fold together and form a groove wherein peptides are embedded and bound by hydrogen bonds and salt bridge interactions. The shape of the binding groove and the peptide sequence determine binding of a peptide to an MHC-I molecule. The groove is different for each MHC-I allele or haplotype, and therefore each haplotype will bind to other peptides. The majority of peptides bound to MHC-I molecules has a restricted size of about nine amino acids corresponding to the size of the binding groove and requires free N- and C-terminal ends *(49–51)*. The binding groove contains conserved residues that are indispensable for peptide binding. These locations are called pockets, and their configuration determines which peptides can bind a particular MHC-I molecule. Peptides that bind to a given MHC-I haplotype share similar amino acids, which bind the pocket in the MHC binding groove *(50,52)*. These amino acids do not need to be identical, but they must be related to each other and are mostly hydrophobic or aromatic. In addition, it is not necessary for the anchor residues to be located at the same place in the peptide sequence, because the peptide can bend when it is in the binding groove. Except for the anchor residues, amino acids in peptides are highly polymorphic, as reviewed in **ref. 53**. In this way a wide range of peptides with similar residues at the anchor sides can bind to the same MHC-I haplotype. The two main anchor residues alone are not sufficient for high-affinity binding. It was shown for HLA-A*0201 molecules that secondary anchor residues at positions 1, 3, and 7 also play a role in peptide binding to MHC-I *(54)*. All these factors determine the binding of a peptide to an MHC-I molecule, and therefore whether a peptide can be antigenic.

When a peptide is presented on the outside of the cell by MHC-I, CTLs can recognize the complex through their T-cell receptor (TCR) *(55)*. The TCR is a membrane-bound heterodimer, consisting of an α- and β-chain connected through disulfide bonds. Each chain contains a constant and a variable region. The specific recognition of the MHC-peptide complex is mediated through the TCR variable domains. On recognition, the CTL is triggered to produce different cytokines (e.g., IL-2, tumor necrosis factor-α [TNF-α], granulocyte macrophage colony-stimulating factor, and interferon-γ [IFN-γ]) and enzymes that can mediate lysis of the target cell. Identification of new tumor antigens in most of the methods described later in this chapter is dependent first on the possibility of a peptide to bind to an HLA molecule and second on the availability of a CTL clone, which recognizes such peptides presented by a specific MHC-I molecule.

1.4. Improvement of Immunotherapy Targeting Melanoma-Expressed Antigens

The peptides listed in **Table 1** can be recognized by CTLs in vitro and may be used in the treatment of cancer patients in the future. After the initial identification, different methods are employed to test the immunogenicity of the peptide in vivo (reviewed in **ref. 56**). This can be done in either patients (clinical trials) or mouse models.

It was first shown for two naturally processed virus-derived immunogenic peptides that they could be used for in vivo vaccination in mice *(57,58)*. This opened the possibility of studying the immunogenicity of peptides in vivo. HLA transgenic mice are now available and can be used to study the immune response against human antigens, because these mice express, in addition to their own murine MHC molecule, human HLA molecules on their cells, which can present peptides derived from human antigens (reviewed in **ref. 59**).

The HLA-A*0201 transgenic mouse is the most extensively studied HLA transgenic mouse model in melanoma antigen research. There are several examples of melanoma antigen studies in HLA-transgenic mice. For instance, three HLA-A*0201 binding motif and affinity-selected peptides from MAGE-

A2 were able to induce CTL responses in HLA-A*0201/K^b transgenic mice *(60)*. A method using the HLA-A*0201 model is described in detail subsequently.

To find an optimal protocol for the use of peptides as targets of immuno-therapy, different ways of introducing the antigen or specific CTLs to the immune system are also being tested in clinical trials *(61)*. Several studies have been conducted using either naked peptides or peptides admixed with adjuvants and different routes of administration *(62)*. Recently, e.g., it was reported that vaccination of 25 patients with the HLA-A1-restricted MAGE-A3$_{168-176}$ led to tumor regression in 7 patients, from which 2 remained disease free, without a detectable CTL response directed against the peptide *(63)*. Instead of vaccination with peptides, it is also possible to inject the patient with in vitro-generated and -expanded tumor-specific CTLs (adoptive transfer). It has been shown that occasional regression of the tumor occurs in melanoma patients after treatment with TILs and IL-2 *(64,65)*.

Most peptides derived from melanoma antigens are weakly immunogenic in comparison with peptides derived from viral antigens. Their low immunogenicity is possibly owing to poor or intermediate MHC-I binding *(66)*, the instability of the MHC-peptide complex *(67)*, or the fact that they are self-antigens. To improve their immunogenicity, peptides are being modified to enhance their affinity for MHC-I. The MART-1/Melan-A$_{26-35}$ epitope, e.g., has anchor residues that are not optimal for binding to HLA-A*0201. A dominant anchor amino acid residue (leucine or methionine) is lacking at position 2 and a negatively charged amino acid is found at position 1. Therefore, amino acid substitutes are made at these positions to enhance affinity and stability, but without interfering with the portion of the peptide that is recognized by the specific CTLs. Recently, MART-1/Melan-A$_{27-35}$ peptide analogs were tested in HLA-A*0201/K^b transgenic mice in comparison with normal peptide analogs. It was found that the analogs were potent immunogens for in vivo CTL priming, in contrast to their natural counterparts *(68)*. A similar study was done with gp100 peptide analogs, in which it was shown that three analogs generated stronger immune responses, and that these analogs could generate CTLs from human PBLs that recognized the unmodified peptide *(69)*. In general, it was shown that modified peptides bound with a higher affinity to the MHC-I molecule, that they could induce more easily specific T-cells, and that recognition by TILs was more efficient *(70,71)*. Also, for the gp100$_{209-217}$ HLA-A*0201 restricted epitope, modifications at the anchor residue positions were made that were shown to increase the affinity of the peptide for MHC-I and to improve the induction of melanoma-reactive CTLs *(72)*. This modified peptide has now been used in a clinical trial, in which a significant increase in CTL precursor frequency was observed. Unfortunately, despite the increase in CTL precursors in all patients, 10 of 11 patients did not show tumor responses. When evaluated in vitro, peripheral blood mononuclear cell–derived T-cells from the vaccinated patients recognized the peptides, but only few recognized melanoma cell lines, indicating that immunization with the modified peptide affected the T-cell repertoire with different fine specificity *(73,74)*.

Although many antigens recognized by T-cells have been identified, more work is being done to find new antigenic peptides. Synthetic peptides are simple to produce in large amounts and are easy to handle, which makes them suitable for broad use as vaccines. However, there are several disadvantages to the use of peptides for immunotherapy. For each HLA allele, new peptides that can bind the MHC-I molecule have to be identified, because the anchor residues, which fit in the pockets of the binding groove, are different. Most peptides identified to date are HLA-A*0201 restricted, the HLA allele found most widespread in the Caucasian population. Now more and more peptides, deriving from known antigens such as gp100 or tyrosinase, also are being identified for other HLA haplotypes. Frequently occurring problems in the peptide-based immunotherapy of cancer are the loss of either antigen or MHC-I haplotype expression of tumor cells under pressure of the treatment (reviewed in **ref. 75**). It was shown that heterogeneous expression of melanoma antigens and HLA-A*0201 in metastatic melanoma tissues could be detected *(76,77)*. Another study describes two melanoma cell lines derived from metastases removed from a patient several years apart. The patient developed a very strong CTL response against the initial tumor. But the second tumor resisted lysis by these CTLs because it lost expression of most MHC-I molecules under the selective pressure of an in vivo antitumor CTL response *(78,79)*. These findings underline the need for multiple targets in the immunotherapy of melanoma patients, and, therefore, it is necessary to find new peptides that can be recognized by tumor-specific CTLs, when presented on an MHC-I molecule, to increase the possibilities for treatment.

Much effort has to be put into the development of tumor antigen–directed vaccines before they can be used as immunotherapy in the treatment of cancer *(80)*. It was shown that synthetic peptides are able to both induce and tolerize T-cells, as was reported for a peptide derived from an H-2D^b-restricted lymphocytic choriomeningitis virus *(81)* and for a tumor model based on a human adenovirus type 5 E1A-region (Ad5E1A$_{234-243}$) *(82,83)*. In the Ad5E1A model, it was demonstrated that tumor outgrowth was enhanced after peptide vaccination. Therefore, besides peptide-based immunotherapy, other vaccinations, e.g., with protein DNA, RNA, or (in case of virus-induced cancers) virus-like particles, are being tested. These methods have the advantage of HLA independency because the entire antigen is used for vaccination and may not lead to tolerization of CTLs. However, it still remains important to identify new tumor-expressed antigens and antigenic peptides to open new possibilities for active immunization against cancer.

2. Methods Used for Identification of Melanoma-Derived Antigens

There are several strategies to identify and characterize new melanoma-derived antigens depending on the starting points. Different strategies are applied to identify a new antigenic peptide (e.g., for a different HLA haplotype) from a known antigen, or to identify an antigen without prior knowledge of the source protein. Also, the availability of tumor-specific CTLs is a factor that influences the method of choice. The most commonly used approaches are discussed next.

2.1. Generation of T-Cells

Several methods for the identification of new antigens start with the generation of CTLs that recognize the tumor from which the antigen will be identified. Only for the reverse immunology method discussed in **Subheadings 2.3.2. and 3.**, a CTL clone is not necessary at the start. In this section, the strategies to obtain melanoma-specific CTLs are described briefly.

The basis of generating CTLs is the mixed lymphocyte tumor cell culture (MLTC). CTL clones against an autologous melanoma were generated in an MLTC by cocultivation of peripheral blood mononuclear leukocytes with irradiated autologous tumor cells and IL-2. To get CTL clones, the MLTC responder lymphocytes were cloned by limiting dilution and restimulating each week with irradiated tumor cells and Epstein-Barr virus (EBV)-transformed feeder B-cells *(9,84)*. Another group used instead of peripheral blood–derived lymphocytes, lymphocytes isolated from the tumor (TILs) as a source for lymphocytes. These TILs were prepared from metastatic melanomas as reported in **ref. 85**. TILs were initially expanded with IL-2 and IL-4, followed by cocultivation with irradiated autologous tumor cells *(86)*. Later it was also shown that tumor-specific T-cells could be generated from healthy donor blood instead of blood derived from melanoma patients *(87)*. Also, tumor-specific CTLs could be induced by stimulation with antigenic peptides pulsed on antigen-presenting cells *(88)*. This finding was useful for the method described in **Subheading 3.**

When a CTL clone is available, it has to be tested for specificity and HLA restriction before it can be used for the identification of the peptide recognized by this clone. The strategy described is used by most of the groups that have identified melanoma antigens. Usually, tumor specificity is tested by measuring cytotoxicity in a standard 51-chromium release assay of the CTL clone with a panel of cells as targets, including nonmelanoma (e.g., autologous EBV-B-cells and other tumors) and the autologous melanoma, which is used for the generation of T-cells. Preferably, the CTLs should recognize only the autologous melanoma, which will be used for the identification of the antigen. To test MHC-independent cytotoxicity, usually the natural killer (NK) cell–sensitive cell line K562 is used as the target. HLA restriction can be determined by blocking monoclonal antibodies (MAbs) against the HLA haplotypes expressed by the patient from which the tumor was removed. Blocking MAbs are not available for every HLA allele, which makes it difficult to identify peptides presented by some HLA molecules.

2.2. Identification of an Antigenic Peptide Without Prior Knowledge of the Source Protein

One requirement for identifying antigens when the protein is unknown is the availability of a tumor-specific CTL clone (*see* **Subheading 2.1.**). To find new antigens, a few different approaches have been developed that are used by several groups. One method generates genomic or cDNA libraries from tumor cells recognized by the CTL, but express the same HLA haplotype as the original tumor, followed by transfection of progressively smaller subsets of these molecular clones into cells that lack the antigen. These libraries are then screened for recognition by tumor-specific CTLs. A second method is the elution of naturally presented peptides from the MHC molecules of the tumor cell, which are then fractionated and tested for recognition by tumor-specific CTLs. A third method is based on the existence of antibodies in serum from melanoma patients, which are directed against a tumor antigen. This tumor antigen is subsequently tested for recognition by CTLs. All these techniques are discussed next.

2.2.1. Screening of cDNA Expression Libraries

This method is the most commonly used approach for identification of new tumor antigens. There are differences in the several transfection models, but the strategies are essentially the same. Most researchers start with the generation of CTLs for their specific tumor model. First, tumor specificity HLA-restriction and eventual MHC-unrestricted cytotoxicity (by testing an NK cell–sensitive cell line) of CTLs is tested. The tumor cells that are specifically lysed by the CTLs are used to generate a cDNA expression library by transfecting into cells that are not recognized by the specific T-cells but express the appropriate HLA haplotype. In this library, theoretically, the genes that are activated, and therefore transcribed into messenger RNA (mRNA), are available, including genes encoding for the antigen recognized by the CTL clone.

2.2.1.1. CREATING cDNA CONSTRUCTS OF MELANOMA CELLS

Polyadenylated mRNA is obtained from the melanoma cells of interest by using a standard commercially available poly (A)$^+$ mRNA isolation kit (e.g., see **refs. *31* and *33***). The isolated mRNA is converted into cDNA by a reverse transcriptase polymerase chain reaction (RT-PCR) using a poly-T tail primer (oligo dT) or random hexamer primers that bind on different random places of the mRNA fragments. Usually, the research groups that made a cDNA library for identifying melanoma antigens used commercial kits, which contain all the reaction ingredients and both primer solutions. Restriction sites are connected to the ends of the PCR fragments, making the cDNA suitable for cloning into an expression vector with a eukaryotic promoter. This can be done by using blunt end adapters or a dT primer connected to a restriction site.

2.2.1.2. TRANSFECTION OF cDNA CONSTRUCTS INTO AN EXPRESSION SYSTEM

The pools of plasmids containing different fragments are transformed into bacteria, to amplify the cDNA. Pools of approx 100 bacteria clones containing the cDNA are used to isolate the plasmid DNA, which is used for transfection into cells that can process and express the protein derived from the inserted cDNA. Originally, recombinant genomic or cDNA libraries were introduced into antigen lacking MHC-matched tumor cells. For example, the cDNA library, which led to the discovery of the MAGE-1 gene, was transfected into a melanoma cell line of the original patient who had lost the antigen recognized by the CTLs *(15)*. However, tumor cells are much more difficult to transfect, and expression levels of the newly introduced DNA are relatively low. This was improved by using systems such as the highly transfectable COS-7 cells *(89,90)*, which is currently the most commonly used transfection system for tumor antigen identification. COS-7 cells require the Simian Virus-40 (SV40) replication, which results in a high expression level of plasmids with the SV40 long terminal repeat. Because the purpose is to screen the library with CTLs, it is necessary to cotransfect a plasmid with an HLA gene together with the cDNA construct.

HLA restriction is determined by blocking antibodies, as discussed in **Subheading 2.1**. Usually, HLA genes are obtained by isolating the HLA encoding mRNA from the autologous tumor cells and cloning the cDNA into an expression vector. This was done for the HLA-Cw*1601-restricted MAGE-A1$_{230-238}$ peptide by isolation from the cDNA library with a standard hybridization using an HLA- and an HLA-Cw-specific probe *(90)*. In many cases, however, blocking antibodies are not available for particular HLA alleles, making it difficult to identify the restriction element. To circumvent this problem, retrovirus-based melanoma-derived cDNA constructs are made that can be transfected into autologous EBV-transformed B-cells *(91)*.

2.2.1.3. SCREENING THE LIBRARY

Screening the library is done with the tumor-specific CTLs, which are reactive against the tumor or tumor cell line from which the cDNA library is derived. The readout systems are the common assays for testing recognition by CTLs, although 51-chromium release assays are not frequently used for screening the libraries. To identify cDNA pools containing an insert for a tumor antigen, the supernatants of the T-cell and transfectant cocultures are tested for cytokines, such as IFN-γ, TNF-α, and GM-CSF, which are released by activated CTLs. These cytokines can be measured in standard assays, such as the cellular WEHI assay for TNF-α release and sandwich enzyme-linked immunosorbent assays for IFN-γ and GM-CSF *(92,93)*. WEHI cells, which are sensitive to TNF-α, are cultured in the presence of supernatant. Dead cells can be visualized by adding MTT to the cells, which turns blue inside living cells. After lysis of the WEHI cells, absorbance at 595 nm can be measured as an indication of TNF-α produced by the T-cells.

For the sandwich ELISA, supernatants of the T-cell and transfectant cocultures are transferred into 96-well plates coated with MAbs against IFN-γ or GM-CSF, to which the soluble cytokines bind. A second cytokine-specific antibody, labeled with a marker, is used to detect the binding cytokines in two steps.

Positive pools are subcloned, so that each pool of bacteria represents one single cDNA fragment. These clones are tested in the same way as described in the preceding paragraph, to identify the bacteria with the plasmid containing the insert encoding for the antigen. The sequence of the insert is determined and compared with known sequences. This can be done by a Basic Local Alignment Search Tool search in a database such as GenBank on the Internet (www.ncbi.nlm.nih.gov). Antigenic peptides derived from proteins such as CDK4 *(34)*, tyrosinase *(23)*, and β-catenin *(33)* were matched to sequences previously added to the GenBank database. Other antigens, including most oncospermatogonal, were completely new proteins. Therefore, expression of these genes in normal and malignant tissues had to be explored *(17)*.

The insert is usually a fragment of a few thousand base pairs. To narrow the localization of the part that encodes for the peptide recognized by the CTLs, smaller parts can be made of the insert. There are several options to accomplish this. First, there is the exonuclease III method, which is used for the determination of many melanoma CTL epitopes *(90,93,94)*. Exonuclease III is an enzyme that digests a certain amount of double-stranded DNA from the 3′ end per time point. By digesting the DNA with exonuclease III for different periods and at different temperatures, truncations of variable sizes of the inserted DNA sequence are made. Plasmid DNA is amplified and isolated the same way as described and used for transfection in, e.g., COS-7 cells. Then, these cells can be screened with CTLs for recognition. Shorter fragments also can be made by

PCR amplification of different fragments or digestion with restriction enzymes, as was done for the intron encoded TRP-2 epitope *(20)*.

Another way to identify the recognized peptides is to synthesize all the possible peptides from the inserted sequence that can be presented by MHC-I and screen them for CTL activity. However, this is a laborious method. Therefore, similar but faster approaches are used. When the antigen is presented by an MHC-I haplotype such as HLA-A*0201, from which multiple binding peptides and anchor residues are known, possible binding peptides of the tumor antigen can be synthesized and tested. This strategy can be used only when the protein sequence is known; it is discussed in detail in **Subheadings 2.3.2.** and **3.**

2.2.2. Acid Elution of MHC-I Binding Peptides

Another approach is largely biochemistry based. In this method, peptides presented by MHC-I molecules are eluted, fractionated, and tested for their possibility to reconstitute recognition by melanoma-specific CTLs of peptide-pulsed target cells expressing the appropriate MHC molecule. In this way, only naturally processed and presented peptides are evaluated. In addition to identification of new epitopes such as $gp100_{280-288}$ *(95)*, using this assay it was also discovered that a tyrosinase-derived epitope (369-377) was posttranslationally modified *(96)*. However, owing to the technical difficulties and complexities associated with fractionation and sequencing of the eluted peptides, very few research groups have been able to isolate antigenic peptides recognized by CTLs in this manner.

Similar to the cDNA expression libraries, melanoma tumor samples or melanoma cell lines recognized by established CTLs must be available in order to use this method. The cells recognized by the CTLs are then used for the elution of MHC-I-presented peptides. The elution is done in an acid environment using citrate phosphate (pH 3.3) *(97)*, or acetic acid (pH 2.1) *(98)* to break the bonds between the peptide and the MHC molecule. It is optional to isolate specific HLA molecules, by solubilizing the cells and pouring the supernatant on protein A-Sepharose columns containing MAbs for the appropriate HLA molecule *(98)*. The small MHC-bound peptides are separated from other proteins by using a spin column or a filter that discriminates among peptides of a certain molecular weight (e.g., masses <5 kDa).

The isolated peptides are fractionated by reverse phase high-performance liquid chromatography (RP-HPLC), the best technique for peptide isolation and purification. The RP-HPLC fractions can subsequently be used to pulse cells lacking the antigen recognized by the CTLs, but expressing the correct HLA molecule *(95,98)*. The fractions are tested for reconstituting lysis by the melanoma-specific T-cells in the previously mentioned assays. The recognized peptide epitope within a reconstituting peptide fraction can be identified and sequenced by tandem mass spectrometry *(93,96,99)*. This is done by scanning the fragment ions resulting from collision with argon, which results in a spectrum corresponding to the peptide amino acid sequence *(99)*. Gaps in the sequence can be solved by coelution of different synthetic peptides with the naturally processed peptide and comparison of the spectra *(95,99)*.

Another difficulty of using this method is the uncertainty from which protein the identified peptide is derived. Screening a database only gives a list of possible sources. The most plausible variant is chosen and can be used for testing, e.g., when the sequence can be found in a previously discovered tumor antigen, as was the case for the MART-1/Melan-A$_{32-40}$ peptide and gp100$_{280-288}$ *(95,99)*.

2.2.3. A Serologic-Based Approach

A relatively new method is a combination of a serologic and a cellular strategy, based on the finding that multiple specific immune responses can be elicited against tumors *(100,101)*. This method is called serologic identification of antigens by recombinant expression screening with autologous sera (SEREX) and it provides another route for defining immunogenic human tumor antigens. It was shown that elevated melanoma CTL antigen- (e.g., MAGE-1 and tyrosinase) directed IgG antibody titers could be detected in serum of melanoma patients *(100,102)*. Based on this observation, the antibody screening of cDNA libraries prepared from human tumors was used to identify new antigens recognized by CTLs. The oncospermatogonal antigen NY-ESO-1 *(102)* was among the first tumor antigens discovered with the SEREX method. Later, NY-ESO-1 also was shown to contain epitopes that were recognized by CTLs.

SEREX requires the construction of a cDNA expression library from total tumor RNA. Poly(A)$^+$ RNA is isolated from this pool and reverse transcribed into cDNA. The cDNA is digested into smaller fragments that are cloned in a bacteriophage vector (e.g., λZAPII) and packaged into phage particles. The phage library is screened with patient serum *(100,103)*. The reactive cDNA clones are subcloned and sequenced and compared in a database with existing sequences. The antigen identified is an antigen recognized by antibodies. In addition, the tumor antigen must be tested for recognition by T-cells. There fore, a cell expressing the antigen and a tumor-reactive CTL line must be established. The procedures followed to identify NY-ESO-1 as a CTL-recognized antigen *(104)* are basically the same as those used to identify new antigenic peptides deriving from a known protein (*see* **Subheadings 2.3.** and **3.**).

2.3. Identification of an Antigenic Peptide with Prior Knowledge of the Source Protein

After the first discoveries of tumor antigens, the genes encoding these proteins were identified. With this knowledge, new peptides encoded by these genes for other HLA haplotypes can be easily identified. The first one described here is based on the strategy also used for screening a cDNA library (*see* **Subheading 2.2.1.**). The second synthetic peptides used were selected for their MHC-I binding motif and were then tested for their ability to induce tumor-specific cytotoxicity.

2.3.1. Cloning the Gene Encoding for the Antigen

This approach overlaps mainly with the cDNA screening strategy, except that the entire gene for a known antigen, placed in an expression vector, is used. This construct is transfected in an autologous cell line or in highly transfectable cells such as COS-7. The screening with CTLs and identification of the antigenic peptides can be done in the same way as described previously (*see* **Subheading 2.2.1.**). The original plasmid cloned from the tumor cDNA library is frequently used. The peptide encoded by the MAGE-A1 gene, presented by HLA-A*01, was identified using a plasmid from the cDNA library *(105)* that led to the discovery of MAGE-A1 *(15)*.

Transfection of cells with a plasmid containing the gene for a known antigen is useful when a new epitope, binding to the same or another MHC-I molecule, has to be identified. It starts mostly with a CTL clone, which is restricted to a certain HLA type, depending on the different haplotypes present in the patient from whom the CTL clone is derived. It is also useful when recognition of different cell lines by CTLs strongly correlates with expression of a known antigen, e.g., gp100 for an HLA-A*0201-restricted CTL *(106)*. To determine whether this was in fact the antigen recognized by the CTL, a construct was made containing the gene for gp100 and transfected into gp100 negative HLA-A*0201-expressing cells. To identify the antigenic peptide, the same methods are used as described in **Subheading 2.2.2.** *(107,108)*.

It is also possible to test a CTL clone on a panel of cells expressing different known antigens (e.g., all the members of the MAGE-A family) and the appropriate HLA molecule. Screening a panel of cells recently led to the identification of a peptide encoded by multiple members of the MAGE family *(109)*. Additionally, using this method a MAGE-A10-derived peptide was identified as a melanoma antigen *(110)*.

2.3.2. Prediction of MHC-I Binding Peptides

The prediction of MHC-I binding is based on the knowledge of the protein sequence and the residues necessary for binding to a particular HLA allele.

Because the structure of the MHC-I molecule was elucidated, the importance of anchor residues in peptides for binding to MHC-I was acknowledged (*see* **Subheading 1.3.**). It was proposed that a binding peptide could be predicted from the protein sequence in order to identify new antigenic epitopes encoded by a known antigen. In studies with the human papillomavirus type 16 E6 and E7 proteins, the role of binding motifs to different HLA alleles in predicting affinity underlined the usefulness of these motifs for identification of new CTL epitopes *(111)*. The first melanoma-derived peptide identified based on the HLA-binding motif and recognized by CTLs was MART-1/Melan-A$_{27-35}$, which is presented by HLA-A*0201. This epitope was recognized by multiple CTLs *(112)*. Most described antigenic peptides predicted by their HLA-binding motif bind HLA-A*02, which is the most frequently expressed allele in the Caucasian population (about 50% of individuals) and for which the best experimental models are available. With the increasing number of antigenic peptides, binding motifs for other HLA haplotypes also are available and used in the characterization of new melanoma CTL epitopes (such as HLA-A*01 *[113]*, HLA-A*24 *[114–116]*, HLA-A*03 *[117,118]*, and HLA B*44 *[119]*). A protocol for identification of HLA-A*0201 binding peptides by reversed immunology is described later in this chapter.

There are two different ways to use the HLA-binding motif in the identification of new epitopes. The first is based on an existent CTL clone and is a combination of the cDNA expression library method (*see* **Subheadings 2.2.1.** and **2.3.1.**) and the production of binding motif–based synthetic peptides from the sequence of the plasmid in the clones recognized by CTLs *(28,112, 113,118,120)*. This is an alternative for synthesizing all possible 8–11 amino acid peptides from the sequence or the exonuclease III and PCR method to narrow down the location of the antigenic epitope. The synthetic peptides are tested in the same way as described for the second method, except that the CTLs are already available.

The second method is called reverse immunology and does not require an established CTL clone recognizing a melanoma cell line to start with, in contrast to all the other described methods. The sequences of proteins that previously have been shown to be antigenic are screened for peptides containing the anchor residues necessary for binding to a specific HLA molecule. This is done by comparing the peptide sequence to the chemistry of previously identified peptides expressed by that particular HLA allele, which are available in the literature. MAGE-A3$_{271-279}$ was the first melanoma-expressed peptide found with the reverse immunology method. That leucine in position 2 or valine in position 9 or 10 was present in many peptides that bound to HLA-A*02 enabled the selection of 10 peptides from the MAGE-A3 sequence containing that binding motif *(121)*. A computer program has been developed to screen sequences for HLA-A*0201-binding motifs *(122)*. Now, databases are also available on the Internet to screen proteins for peptides with HLA binding motifs (*see* **Subheading 3.2.**). Peptides with the appropriate anchor residues are synthesized and tested in vitro for MHC-I binding in a peptide-binding competition assay in which the half-maximal binding of a control peptide is measured (for details see **Subheadings 3.1.** and **3.2.**). From the synthetic peptides, moderate to good binders are selected for further testing. The methods of generating specific CTLs against the selected peptides in vitro when pulsed on IL-4 and GM-CSF stimulated peripheral blood monocytes and cloning of these CTLs are basically the same as described previously. When a CTL clone is generated against a synthetic peptide, it has to be tested for recognition of naturally processed peptides. This can be done either by transfection of cells with the appropriate HLA-type with a plasmid containing the antigen or by using autologous cells that are known to express the antigen. These cells are tested in standard T-cell recognition assays as previously described in this chapter. Peptides that can induce specific CTLs in vitro that also recognize naturally processed peptide can be used for vaccination studies in HLA-transgenic mice. Immunogenicity can be tested by determination of the specific T-cell precursor frequency, or in a later phase by challenging the vaccinated mice with a tumor expressing the antigen harboring the peptide. For the identification of the MAGE-A2$_{112-120}$ and MAGE-A2$_{157-166}$ peptides, splenocytes derived from vaccinated HLA-A*0201/K^b mice were restimulated with peptide-loaded lymphoblasts for 1 wk. Then these cells were tested for cytotoxicity in a ^{51}Cr-release assay *(60)*. The tumor model is much more difficult to establish and is not yet available for human melanoma. Therefore, studies in HLA-transgenic mice have determined only in vivo induction of a CTL response.

3. Protocol for Reverse Immunology to Identify New Melanoma Antigens

3.1. Materials

3.1.1. Selecting the Peptides

1. Protein sequence

3.1.2. Peptide Binding Assay on T2-Cells

1. IMDM (BioWhittaker, Walkersville, MD) with 10% fetal calf serum (FCS) (HyClone, Logan, UT), L-glutamin, kanamycin, and 2-mercaptoethanol.
2. IMDM as described in **item 1**, but without FCS.
3. 174CEM.T2 (T2) cells (ATCCno. CRL-1992).
4. 96-Well flat- or U-bottomed cell culture plates.
5. Synthetic melanoma antigen–derived peptides, selected by HLA-binding motif (2 mg/mL).

6. β_2-Microglobulin (Biodesign, Kennebunk, ME).
7. Phosphate-buffered saline (PBS) with 0.5% bovine serum albumin (BSA). Store at 4°C.
8. Antibodies: BB7.2 (anti-HLA-A*02) and goat-anti-Mouse fluorescein isothiocyanate-γ [FITC-γ] (Roche, Indianapolis, IN). Store stocks at –80°C.
9. Ice.
10. Propidium iodide (200 μg/mL).
11. FACstar.

3.1.3. In Vitro Immunization Assay

1. RPMI-1640 (BioWhittaker) containing 5% human AB-serum (HS) (Sigma, St. Louis, MO), Dulbecco's modified Eagle medium, (Life Technologies, Grand Island, NY), nonessential amino acids (1 : 100), 10 mM pyruvic acid, L-glutamin, and kanamycin.
2. PBS (1% HS) and PBS (1% BSA).
3. Cell culture: 75-cm^2 flasks, 6- and 48-well plates.
4. Cytokines: rhIL-2, rhIL-4, rhIL-7, hIL-10, and GM-CSF.
5. Filters (0.25 and 0.45 μm).
6. SACS: Pansorbin cells (Calbiochem, San Diego, CA) (minimal binding capacity: 2 mg/mL, 10% solution).
7. PBLs from a healthy HLA-A*0201$^+$ donor collected by leukapheresis.
8. M-450 CD8 Dynabeads (Dynal, Oslo, Norway).
9. Detachabead antibody for dynabeads M-450 CD4 and CD8 (Dynal).
10. Magnetic particle concentrator-1 (MCP-1) (Dynal).
11. Titer plate shaker.
12. β_2-Microglobulin (Biodesign).
13. Synthetic melanoma-derived peptides, which were positive in the MHC-binding assay.
14. Cell irradiation equipment.

3.1.4. Cytotoxicity Assays

1. Medium as described in **Subheading 3.2.3.**
2. JY cells (HLA-A*0201$^+$).
3. K562 cells (NK sensitive; ATCC no. CCL-243).
4. Cells expressing autologous antigen.
5. Synthetic peptides that were used for the in vitro generation of CTLs.
6. ^{51}Cr radionuclide (NEN, Boston, MA).
7. Triton X-100 (Sigma), 1% solution in medium.
8. 96-Well U-bottomed plate.
9. Microscint scintillation liquid (Packard, Meriden, CT).
10. 96-Well OptiPlate scintillation filter (Packard).
11. TopCount microplate scintillation and luminescence counter (Packard).

3.1.5. In Vivo Immunogenicity of Selected Peptides in HLA-A*0201/K^b Transgenic Mice

1. HLA-A*0201/K^b transgenic mice.
2. Hank's balanced salt solution (HBSS) (Sigma).
3. HBV-core antigen-derived T-helper peptide (amino acids 127–140, sequence TPPAYRPPNAPIL), synthetic melanoma-derived peptides recognized in vitro by CTLs.
4. Syringes (1 mL) with 25-gage needles.
5. Incomplete Freund's adjuvant (IFA, Difco).
6. Lipopolysaccharide (LPS).
7. Cell culture flasks (25 and 75 cm^2).
8. Medium A: RPMI-1640 + L-glutamine; add 10% FCS, 0.2 μM 2-mercaptoethanol, 5 mM L-glutamine, and 100 IU/mL penicillin.
9. Medium B: RPMI-1640 + HEPES and L-glutamine; add 2% FCS.
10. Medium C: RPMI-1640 + HEPES and L-glutamine; add 10% FCS.
11. JY cells.
12. Equipment for ^{51}Cr-release assays (*see* **Subheading 3.2.4.**).

3.2. Methods

3.2.1. Selecting Peptides

To select peptides that bind HLA-A*0201, the protein sequence must be screened for 8–10 amino acid long peptides containing the binding motif for HLA-A*0201. Databases are available on the Internet, containing information on several MHC-binding motifs, where this can be done. We use the following Web sites: For BioInformatics & Molecular Analysis Section HLA Peptide Binding Predictions <http://bimas.dcrt.nih.gov/cgi-bin/molbio/ken_parker_comboform> or SYFPEITHI: Epitope prediction <http://134.2.96.221/scripts/hlaserver.dll/EpPredict.htm>.

All the peptides predicted by the database or a selection are synthesized (*see* **Note 1**) and used in an HLA-A*0201 peptide binding assay (*see* **Subheading 3.2.2.**).

3.2.2. Peptide Binding Assay on T2-Cells (see **Note 2**)

1. Grow the T2-cells in IMDM (10% FCS).
2. Wash the cells with serum-free IMDM (centrifuge at 400g for 4 min). Count the cells and adjust to 2 × 10^6 cells/mL in serum-free IMDM.
3. Add β$_2$-microglobulin from the stock solution at a concentration of 10 μg/mL to the cell suspension.
4. Transfer 80 μL of the cell suspension to a well of a 96-well culture plate (flat- or U-bottomed).

5. Add peptide solution to each well, with a final concentration of 100 μg/mL. Use as a positive control a known HLA-A*0201-binding peptide and as a negative control an irrelevant nonbinding peptide.
6. Incubate the plate with T2-cells and peptides for 16 h at 37°C.
7. Centrifuge at 1500 rpm for 4 min, remove the supernatant, and wash each well twice with 100 μL PBS (0.5% BSA). Centrifuge between steps at 350g for 1 min.
8. To detect BB7.2 binding, add per well 50 μL of MAb BB7.2 (anti-HLA-A*02) and incubate for 30 min on ice.
9. Wash twice with 100 μL of PBS (0.5% BSA).
10. Add per well 50 μL of FITC-γ labeled goat-anti-Mouse antibody and incubate for 30 min on ice.
11. Wash the cells twice with 100 μL of PBS (0.5% BSA).
12. Dissolve the cells in 100 μL of PBS (0.5% BSA), add 5 μL of propidium iodide (200 μg/mL), and analyze immediately by flow cytometry for HLA-A*0201 on the surface of the cells.

3.2.3. In Vitro Immunization Assay (see **Note 3**)

3.2.3.1. GENERATION OF DENDRITIC CELLS

1. Thaw PBLs in 10 mL of RPMI (5% HS).
2. Transfer the cell suspension (1×10^7 cells/3 mL of RPMI [5% HS]) to a 6 well-plate (3 mL/well) or in a 75-cm^2 culture flask (15 mL/flask) and incubate for 2 h at 37°C. Shake gently (*see* **Note 4**).
3. Remove the supernatant and refreeze nonadherent cells for CD8$^+$ T-cell purification (*see* **Subheading 3.2.3.3.**).
4. Wash adherent cells twice with RPMI (5% HS) and check under the microscope whether nonadherent cells are still remaining. In this case repeat washing steps.
5. Incubate with 3 mL/well (for the 6-well plate) or 15 mL (for the flask) of RPMI (5% HS) plus 1000 U/mL of IL-4 and 800 U/mL of GM-CSF at 37°C.
6. Every other day centrifuge for 5 min at 350g, take off half the supernatant from the culture, and resuspend the cell pellet in fresh medium containing 1000 U/mL of IL-4 and 1600 U/mL of GM-CSF.
7. On d 7, replace the medium with fresh medium containing 500 U/mL of IL-4, 800 U/mL of GM-CSF, and 25% conditioned medium (*see* **Subheading 3.2.3.2.**).
8. On d 10, the cells can be used for the in vitro immunization procedure (*see* **Note 5**).

3.2.3.2. CONDITIONED MEDIUM FOR GENERATION OF DENDRITIC CELLS

1. Thaw PBLs and incubate 10×10^7 cells in 15 mL of medium (RPMI-1640 + 5% HS) in a 75-cm^2 flask for 1 h at 37°C.
2. Remove the supernatant and wash away the nonadherent cells.
3. Add fresh medium containing SACS at a dilution of 1 : 10,000.
4. Incubate for 24 h at 37°C.
5. Remove the supernatant and centrifuge for 15 min at 2500g.

6. Sterilize the supernatant through a 0.45-μm filter and subsequently through a 0.2-μm filter. Store 1-mL aliquots at –20°C.

3.2.3.3. PURIFICATION OF CD8$^+$ T-CELLS FROM PBLS (*see* **Note 6**)

1. Thaw PBLs in 10 mL of RPMI (5% HS).
2. Transfer the cells (1×10^7 cells/3 mL of medium) to a 6-well plate (3 mL/well) or to a 75-cm^2 culture flask (15 mL), and incubate for 2 h at 37°C.
3. Shake gently, remove the supernatant, and centrifuge at 400g for 4 min.
4. Resuspend nonadherent cells at 2×10^7 cells/mL in PBS (1% HS).
5. Wash dynabeads (anti-CD8) three times with 10 mL of PBS (1% HS) on ice.
6. Add 140-μL beads/mL of cells in a 15-mL tube and incubate on ice for 1 h, periodically mixing (not too much or the bead-cell interactions will be disrupted).
7. Select the beads on a magnet in the MCP-1.
8. Wash the beads three times with 10 mL of PBS (1% HS).
9. Centrifuge and dissolve the pellet in 10×10^7 cells/mL in PBS (1% HS) according to the original cell number from **step 2**.
10. Add 100 μL/mL of detachabead reagent and incubate at room temperature for 1 h with continuous mixing.
11. Select the beads on the magnet and save the supernatant (which contains the CD8$^+$ cells).
12. Centrifuge the cells down at 400g for 4 min.
13. Count the cells.

3.2.3.4. IN VITRO IMMUNIZATION ASSAY

1. Collect dendritic cells (DCs) from **Subheading 3.2.3.1.**, wash with PBS (1% HS), and centrifuge at 350g for 4 min.
2. Resuspend at 1 to 2×10^6 cells/mL in PBS (1% BSA).
3. Incubate with peptides at 40 μg/mL in the presence of 3 μg/mL of β$_2$-microglobulin for 4 h at room temperature.
4. Irradiate with 50 gy.
5. Wash, centrifuge at 1200 rpm for 4 min, count, and distribute into 48-well plates at 2.5×10^4 cells/well in 200 μL of medium. Use one 48-well plate for each different peptide.
6. Add 5×10^5 CD8$^+$ T-cells per well in 200 μL of medium.
7. Incubate at 37°C.
8. After 24 h add IL-10 to a final concentration of 10 ng/mL and incubate for 6 d at 37°C.

3.2.3.4.1. Restimulation of Cultures at d 7

1. Thaw PBLs from the same donor and irradiate with 50 gy.
2. Plate 300 μL of medium with 2×10^6 PBLs/mL per well in a 48-well plate and incubate at 37°C for 2 h.
3. Wash the wells three times with 200 μL of medium (slightly tapping each time, resuspending medium in the wells) to remove nonadherent cells. Check under the microscope.

4. Incubate adherent cells with 100 µL/well of medium without serum containing 10 µg/mL of peptide and 3 µg/mL of β_2-microglobulin for 2 h at room temperature.
5. Remove the peptide solution and wash once with PBS (1% HS).
6. Remove 150 µL of the supernatant from the wells of the primary culture (*see* **Subheading 3.2.3.4., step 8**).
7. Add new medium and transfer the cells from every well to a new well with peptide-loaded autologous adherent cells (*see* **steps 1–5**), without pooling cells from different wells.
8. Add medium to an approximate total volume of 300–400 µL.
9. After incubating for 24 h at 37°C, add IL-10 to a final concentration of 10 ng/mL.
10. Incubate for another 24 h at 37°C and add IL-2 to a final concentration of 50 U/mL.
11. Incubate for 48 h at 37°C and add IL-2 to a final concentration of 50 U/mL.
12. Incubate for another 48 h at 37°C.
13. Repeat this restimulation on d 14.

3.2.3.4.2. Restimulation of Cultures at d 21

1. Remove the supernatant on d 21 (150–175 µL) so that approx 225 µL of medium is left per well. Transfer directly 75 µL from each well two times (*see* **Note 6**) to a 96-well plate for the cytotoxicity assay described in **Subheading 3.2.4.** (75 µL for wells with peptide-pulsed targets and 75 µL for wells with nonpulsed targets). Seventy-five microliters remains in the culture for expansion.
2. To the remaining cells, add medium containing 20 U/mL of IL-2. Proceed with restimulation and expansion within 48 h.

3.2.4. Cytotoxicity Assays

3.2.4.1. CYTOTOXICITY OF CTLs AGAINST SYNTHETIC PEPTIDE-PULSED TARGET

1. Spin down the JY cells, take off the supernatant, and resuspend 0.5 to 1.0×10^6 cells in a 1.5-mL Eppendorf tube containing a 100-µCi ^{51}Cr solution and incubate for 1 h at 37°C.
2. Wash three times with medium and centrifuge for 1 min at 400g in a tabletop centrifuge.
3. Pulse ^{51}Cr-labeled JY cells in medium with 10 µg/mL of synthetic peptide for 30 min at room temperature and wash the cells (*see* **step 2**).
4. Add to each well of the 96-well plate from the in vitro immunization (*see* **Subheading 3.2.3.4.2., step 1**) 2×10^3 labeled target cells and 2×10^5 unlabeled K562 cells (for labeling eventual NK activity, *see* **Note 7**) in 75 µL. The total volume is now 150 µL.
5. Use for maximum release ^{51}Cr-labeled JY cells in medium with 1% Triton X-100 and for spontaneous release ^{51}Cr-labeled JY cells in medium.
6. Spin the plate down for 3 min at 300g.
7. Incubate at 37°C for 4 h.
8. Harvest 50 µL of supernatant and transfer to a scintillation filter.

9. Count chromium release with a gamma counter.
10. Specific lysis can be determined by the following equation:

$$[(\text{cpm sample} - \text{cpm spontaneous release})/ \\ (\text{cpm maximum release} - \text{cpm spontaneous release})] \times 100\%$$

11. CTLs that show a specific lysis >10% are supposed to be peptide specific and can be used for the next step.

3.2.4.2. CYTOTOXICITY OF CTLS AGAINST TARGETS EXPRESSING THE ENDOGENOUS ANTIGEN

Here we follow the same protocol as described in **Subheading 3.2.4.**, but as targets autologous cells that express the antigen endogenously are used, e.g., a melanoma cell line or a cell line transfected with a plasmid containing the gene coding for the antigen.

3.2.5. In Vivo Immunogenicity of Selected Peptides in HLA-A*0201/K^b Transgenic Mice (see **Note 9**)

1. Mix and emulsify for 10 min on ice with a homogenizer (highest speed) 100 µg of synthetic peptide and 140 µg of HBV-core peptide in 100 µL of HBSS at a ratio of 1:1 with IFA.
2. Inject 200 µL of the peptide emulsion subcutaneously in the direction of the base of the tail of groups of at least two HLA-A*0201/K^b transgenic mice. IFA samples should be prepared at two times the amount needed for the injection, because considerable amounts are lost during emulsification and syringe loading. Mice are immunized at d 0 and boosted at d 14 with a fresh emulsion.
3. Prepare LPS blasts as follows. Isolate splenocytes of A*0201/K^b transgenic mice 72 h prior to use as stimulator cells. Pool the cells of several mice and resuspend in medium A containing LPS at 25 µg/mL and dextran sulfate at 7 µg/mL. Splenocytes from one spleen serve as stimulator cells for CTL cultures of two mice. Prepare cultures with 1.5×10^6 blast splenocytes/mL in a total volume of 30 mL of medium and incubate for 72 h at 37°C in vertical, standing 75-cm^2 flasks.
4. After 72 h, collect the blasts and centrifuge (400g for 4 min).
5. Resuspend the cells in medium B, select viable cells by a 100% Ficoll-gradient, adjust to 5×10^6 cells/mL, and irradiate with 25 gy. Wash the irradiated cells with medium C and adjust to 4×10^7 cells/mL in medium B.
6. Incubate 1-mL aliquots of the LPS blasts in medium B with 100 µg/mL of synthetic peptide for 1 h at 37°C on a shaker.
7. Wash the cells once and resuspend at 1×10^7 in medium A.
8. After in vivo priming for 28 d, sacrifice the mice and isolate the splenocytes. Incubate the splenocytes (30×10^6 cells/9 mL in 25-cm^2 flasks) in the presence of syngeneic peptide–loaded LPS blasts (*see* **step 6**) functioning as stimulator cells.

9. Add 1 mL of the LPS blast suspension to the 9-mL responder splenocyte suspension at an effector:stimulator ratio of 3:1.
10. Incubate for 6 d at 37°C.
11. For cytotoxicity assay, 1 d prior to the assay split the culture of the target cells to ensure an exponential growth phase for ^{51}Cr labeling. Use HLA-A*0201-expressing cells as targets.
12. Harvest the splenocytes from the restimulation culture and transfer them to 15-mL tubes. Centrifuge at 400g for 4 min. Resuspend the pellet in 1 mL of medium C and count the cells. Test these bulk cultures at effector:target ratios of 100, 50, 25, and 12.5. Add 100 μL of the splenocytes to each well of a U-bottomed 96-well plate.
13. Label JY cells with ^{51}Cr and load with peptide as described previously (*see* **Subheading 3.2.4.**). Add 100 μL of the target cells to the 96-well plate with the restimulated splenocytes. Controls are the same as described in **Subheading 3.2.4.**
14. Spin the plates for 3 min at 350g.
15. Incubate for 6 h at 37°C, 5% CO_2.
16. Harvest 100 μL of supernatant from each well and count the ^{51}Cr release with a gamma counter. Calculate specific lysis as described in **Subheading 3.2.4.**

4. Notes

1. How many peptides should be synthesized depends on how much you wish to invest in the identification of new antigenic peptides. Usually, when several binding peptides are found by the database search, a limitation is made in the number of peptides. A selection of only the peptides with the highest affinity from the search results does not necessarily include all the peptides that are immunogenic. Therefore, peptides with less affinity also can be chosen. Another method of selecting peptides is to choose peptides derived from a region in the protein that is important for the protein function or for transformation of the cell, which are less likely to mutate.
2. T2 (HLA-A*0201$^+$)-cells have a deficiency in the TAP genes and are therefore unable to transport peptides from the cytoplasm to the ER. The mostly empty MHC-I molecules are normally transported to the cell surface but are unstable. A peptide is considered a binding peptide when the fluorescence index is ≥0.5. The fluorescence index is calculated as the mean fluorescence of each peptide subtracted and divided by the mean fluorescence of a nonbinding peptide as background control. The T2 binding assay only can be used for HLA-A*0201 binding peptides. For other HLA haplotypes, methods such as the quantitative peptide-MHC-binding assay for HLA molecules using purified class I molecules *(54)* or competition with a known fluorescent labeled binding peptide for the particular HLA haplotype must be used *(111)*.
3. Use PBLs from the same donor for generating DCs and CD8$^+$ T-cells. It is necessary to collect leukocytes by leukapheresis, because large numbers of cells must

be used in this assay. Usually 6 to 10×10^7 PBLs can be obtained from one donor. Only peptides that showed moderate to high binding affinity in the binding assay are tested for in vitro generation of CTLs. Again, how many peptides will be tested depends on how much effort and money you wish to put in the identification.

4. Do this carefully, because the DCs are slightly adherent and will come loose when shaken too hard.
5. It is important that mature DCs be used for the in vitro immunization.
6. PBLs from the same donor or the nonadherent cells mentioned in **Subheading 3.2.3.1.** should be used for the purification of CD8$^+$ T-cells.
7. Just transfer 75 µL without taking the effector:target ratio into account.
8. Instead of K562, also YAC-1 cells (ATCC no. TIB-160) can be used for testing NK activity.
9. There are two different ways to test the in vivo immunogenicity of peptides. One is the induction of an in vivo immune response by injection of peptide and restimulation of splenocytes of immunized mice in vitro test the precursor frequency of specific T-cells. This method is described here. Another, but more difficult method, is the use of a tumor model. Establishing a tumor model for a specific antigen is difficult, and it takes much testing before an antigen-expressing tumor with the appropriate growth features in the HLA-transgenic mice is available. Once a tumor model is established, it can be used for testing in vivo immunogenicity of a peptide by challenging the mice with tumor cells 2 wk after immunization with the peptide and by subsequent monitoring of tumor development.

Acknowledgments

Research in this review was supported in part by grants from Illinois Department of Public Health and National Institutes of Health grant R01-CA74397.

References

1. Gross, L. (1943) Intradermal immunization of C3H mice against a sarcoma that originated in an animal of the same line. *Cancer Res.* **3,** 326–333.
2. Foley, E. J. (1953) Antigenic properties of methylcholanthrene-induced tumors in mice of the strain of origin. *Cancer Res.* **13,** 835–837.
3. Prehn, R. T. and Main, J. M. (1957) Immunity to methylcholanthrene-induced sarcomas. *J. Natl. Cancer. Inst.* **18,** 769–778.
4. Basombrio, M. A. (1970) Search for common antigenicities among twenty-five sarcomas induced by methylcholanthrene. *Cancer Res.* **30,** 2458–2462.
5. Leclerc, J. C., Gomard, E., and Levy, J. P. (1972) Cell-mediated reaction against tumors induced by oncornaviruses. I. Kinetics and specificity of the immune response in murine sarcoma virus (MSV)-induced tumors and transplanted lymphomas. *Int. J. Cancer* **10,** 589–601.
6. Tevethia, S. S., Blasecki, J. W., Vaneck, G., and Goldstein, A. L. (1974) Requirement of thymus-derived theta-positive lymphocytes for rejection of DNA virus (SV 40) tumors in mice. *J. Immunol.* **113,** 1417–1423.

7. Mukherji, B. and MacAlister, T. J. (1983) Clonal analysis of cytotoxic T cell response against human melanoma. *J. Exp. Med.* **158,** 240–245.

8. de Vries, J. E. and Spits, H. (1984) Cloned human cytotoxic T lymphocyte (CTL) lines reactive with autologous melanoma cells. I. In vitro generation, isolation, and analysis to phenotype and specificity. *J. Immunol.* **132,** 510–519.

9. Herin, M., Lemoine, C., Weynants, P., Vessiere, F., Van Pel, A., Knuth, A., Devos, R., and Boon, T. (1987) Production of stable cytolytic T-cell clones directed against autologous human melanoma. *Int. J. Cancer* **39,** 390–396.

10. Topalian, S. L., Solomon, D., and Rosenberg, S. A. (1989) Tumor-specific cytolysis by lymphocytes infiltrating human melanomas. *J. Immunol.* **142,** 3714–3725.

11. Rosenberg, S. A., Spiess, P., and Lafreniere, R. (1986) A new approach to the adoptive immunotherapy of cancer with tumor-infiltrating lymphocytes. *Science* **233,** 1318–1321.

12. Rosenberg, S. A. (1988) Immunotherapy of cancer using interleukin 2: current status and future prospects. *Immunol. Today* **9,** 58–62.

13. Van den Eynde, B., Hainaut, P., Herin, M., Knuth, A., Lemoine, C., Weynants, P., Van der Bruggen, P., Fauchet, R., and Boon, T. (1989) Presence on a human melanoma of multiple antigens recognized by autologous CTL. *Int. J. Cancer* **44,** 634–640.

14. Kirkin, A. F., Dzhandzhugazyan, K., and Zeuthen, J. (1998) Melanoma-associated antigens recognized by cytotoxic T lymphocytes. *APMIS* **106,** 665–679.

15. Van der Bruggen, P., Traversari, C., Chomez, P., Lurquin, C., De Plaen, E., Van den, Eynde, B., Knuth, A., and Boon, T. (1991) A gene encoding an antigen recognized by cytolytic T lymphocytes on a human melanoma. *Science* **254,** 1643–1647.

16. Tomita, Y., Kimura, M., Tanikawa, T., Nishiyama, T., Morishita, H., Takeda, M., Fujiwara, M., and Sato, S. (1993) Immunohistochemical detection of intercellular adhesion molecule-1 (ICAM-1) and major histocompatibility complex class I antigens in seminoma. *J. Urol.* **149,** 659–663.

17. Lucas, S., Brasseur, F., and Boon, T. (1999) A new *MAGE* gene with ubiquitous expression does not code for known MAGE antigens recognized by T cells. *Cancer Res.* **49,** 4100–4103.

18. De Plaen, E., Arden, K., Traversari, C., et al. (1994) Structure, chromosomal localization, and expression of 12 genes of the MAGE family. *Immunogenetics* **40,** 360–369.

19. Weber, J., Salgaller, M., Samid, D., Johnson, B., Herlyn, M., Lassam, N., Treisman, J., and Rosenberg, S. A. (1994) Expression of the MAGE-1 tumor antigen is up-regulated by the demethylating agent 5-aza-2′-deoxycytidine. *Cancer Res.* **54,** 1766–1771.

20. Lupetti, R., Pisarra, P., Verrecchia, A., Farina, C., Nicolini, G, Anichini, A., Bordignon, C., Sensi, M., Parmiani, G., and Traversari, C. (1998) Translation of a retained intron in tyrosinase-related protein (TRP) 2 mRNA generates a new cytotoxic T lymphocyte (CTL)-defined and shared human melanoma antigen not expressed in normal cells of the melanocytic lineage. *J. Exp. Med.* **188,** 1005–1016.

21. Robbins, P. F., El-Gamil, M., Li, Y. F., Fitzgerald, E. B., Kawakami, Y., and Rosenberg, S. A. (1997) The intronic region of an incompletely spliced gp100 gene transcript encodes an epitope recognized by melanoma-reactive tumor-infiltrating lymphocytes. *J. Immunol.* **159**, 303–308.
22. Visseren, M. J., Van Elsas, A., van der Voort, E. I., Ressing, M. E., Kast, W. M., Schrier, P. I., and Melief, C. J. M. (1995) CTL specific for the tyrosinase autoantigen can be induced from healthy donor blood to lyse melanoma cells. *J. Immunol.* **154**, 3991–3998.
23. Brichard, V., Van Pel, A., Wolfel, T., Wolfel, C., De Plaen, E., Lethe, B., Coulie, P., and Boon, T. (1993) The tyrosinase gene codes for an antigen recognized by autologous cytolytic T lymphocytes on HLA-A2 melanomas. *J. Exp. Med.* **178**, 489–495.
24. Bouchard, B., Fuller, B. B., Vijayasaradhi, S., and Houghton, A. N. (1989) Induction of pigmentation in mouse fibroblasts by expression of human tyrosinase cDNA. *J. Exp. Med.* **169**, 2029–2042.
25. Wang, R. F., Parkhurst, M. R., Kawakami, Y., Robbins, P. F., and Rosenberg, S. A. (1996) Utilization of an alternative open reading frame of a normal gene in generating a novel human cancer antigen. *J. Exp. Med.* **183**, 1131–1140.
26. Coulie, P. G., Brichard, V., Van Pel, A., et al. (1994) A new gene coding for a differentiation antigen recognized by autologous cytolytic T lymphocytes on HLA-A2 melanomas. *J. Exp. Med.* **180**, 35–42.
27. Kawakami, Y., Eliyahu, S., Delgado, C. H., Robbins, P. F., Rivoltini, L., Topalian, S. L., Miki, T., and Rosenberg, S. A. (1994) Cloning of the gene coding for a shared human melanoma antigen recognized by autologous T cells infiltrating into tumor. *Proc. Natl. Acad. Sci. USA* **91**, 3515–3519.
28. Kawakami, Y., Eliyahu, S., Jennings, C., Sakaguchi, K., Kang, X., Southwood, S., Robbins, P. F., Sette, A., Appella, E., and Rosenberg, S. A. (1995) Recognition of multiple epitopes in the human melanoma antigen gp100 by tumor-infiltrating T lymphocytes associated with in vivo tumor regression. *J. Immunol.* **154**, 3961–3968.
29. Rosenberg, S. A. and White, D. E. (1996) Melanoma, Vitiligo, Immunotherapy, Antigens, and melanocyte-differentiation. Vitiligo in patients with melanoma—normal tissue antigens can be targets for cancer immunotherapy. *J. Immunother.* **19**, 81–84.
30. Overwijk, W. W., Lee, D. S., Surman, D. R., Irvine, K. R., Touloukian, C. E., Chan, C. C., Carroll, M. W., Moss, B., Rosenberg, S. A., and Restifo, N. P. (1999) Vaccination with a recombinant vaccinia virus encoding a "self" antigen induces autoimmune vitiligo and tumor cell destruction in mice: requirement for CD4(+) T lymphocytes. *Proc. Natl. Acad. Sci. USA* **96**, 2982–2987.
31. Guilloux, Y., Lucas, S., Brichard, V. G., Van Pel, A., Viret, C., De Plaen, E., Brasseur, F., Lethe, B., Jotereau, F., and Boon, T. (1996) A peptide recognized by human cytolytic T lymphocytes on HLA-A2 melanomas is encoded by an intron sequence of the N-acetylglucosaminyltransferase V gene. *J. Exp. Med.* **183**, 1173–1183.

32. Coulie, P. G., Lehmann, F., Lethe, B., Herman, J., Lurquin, C., Andrawiss, M., and Boon, T. (1995) A mutated intron sequence codes for an antigenic peptide recognized by cytolytic T lymphocytes on a human melanoma. *Proc. Natl. Acad. Sci. USA* **92,** 7976–7980.

33. Robbins, P. F., El-Gamil, M., Li, Y. F., Kawakami, Y., Loftus, D., Appella, E., and Rosenberg, S. A. (1996) A mutated beta-catenin gene encodes a melanoma-specific antigen recognized by tumor infiltrating lymphocytes. *J. Exp. Med.* **183,** 1185–1192.

34. Wolfel, T., Hauer, M., Schneider, J., Serrano, M., Wolfel, C., Klehmann-Hieb, E., De Plaen, E., Hankeln, T., Meyer, zum Buschenfelde, K. H., and Beach, D. (1995) A p16INK4a-insensitive CDK4 mutant targeted by cytolytic T lymphocytes in a human melanoma. *Science* **269,** 1281–1284.

35. Toes, R. E. M., Ossendorp, F., Offringa, R., and Melief, C. J. M. (1999) Commentary: CD4 T cells and their role in antitumor immune responses. *J. Exp. Med.* **189,** 753–756.

36. Topalian, S. L., Gonzales, M. I., Parkhurst, M., Li, Y. F., Southwood, S., Sette, A., Rosenberg, S. A., and Robbins, P. F. (1996) Melanoma-specific CD4+ T cells recognize nonmutated HLA-DR-restricted tyrosinase epitopes. *J. Exp. Med.* **183,** 1965–1971.

37. Li, K., Adibzadeh, M., Halder, T., Kalbacher, H., Heinzel, S., Mueller, C., Zeuthen, J., and Pawelec, G. (1998) Tumour-specific MHC-class-II-restricted responses after in vitro sensitization to synthetic peptides corresponding to gp100 and annexin II eluted from melanoma cells. *Cancer Immunol. Immunother.* **47,** 32–38.

38. Chaux, P., Vantomme, V., Stroobant, V., Thielemans, K., Corthals, J., Luiten, R., Eggermont, A. M. M., Boon, T., and Van der Bruggen, P. (1999) Identification of MAGE-3 epitopes presented by HLA-DR molecules to CD4+ T lymphocytes. *J. Exp. Med.* **189,** 767–777.

39. Manici, S., Sturniolo, T., Imro, M. A., Hammer, J., Sinigaglia, F., Noppen, C., Spagnoli, G., Mazzi, B., Bellone, M., Dellabona, P., and Protti, M. P. (1999) Melanoma cells present a MAGE-3 epitope to CD4+ cytotoxic T cells in association with histocompatibility leukocyte antigen DR11. *J. Exp. Med.* **189,** 871–876.

40. Pieper, R., Christian, R. E., Gonzales, M. I., Nishimura, M. I., Gupta, G., Settlage, R. E., Shabanowitz, J., Rosenberg, S. A., Hunt, D. F., and Topalian, S. L. (1999) Biochemical identification of a mutated human melanoma antigen recognized by CD4+ T cells. *J. Exp. Med.* **189,** 757–765.

41. Wang, R. F., Wang, X., and Rosenberg, S. A. (1999) Identification of a novel major histocompatibility complex class-II restricted tumor antigen resulting form a chromosomal rearrangement recognized by CD4+ T cells. *J. Exp. Med.* **189,** 1659–1667.

42. Wang, R. F., Wang, X., Atwood, A. C., Topalian, S. L., and Rosenberg, S. A. (1999) Cloning genes encoding MHC class II-restricted antigens: mutated CDC27 as a tumor antigen. *Science* **284,** 1351–1354.

43. Townsend, A. R., Bastin, J., Gould, K., and Brownlee, G. G. (1986) Cytotoxic T lymphocytes recognize influenza haemagglutinin that lacks a signal sequence. *Nature* **324,** 575–577.
44. Buus, S., Sette, A., Colon, S. M., Miles, C., and Grey, H. M. (1987) The relation between major histocompatibility complex (MHC) restriction and the capacity of Ia to bind immunogenic peptides. *Science* **235,** 1353–1358.
45. Goldberg, A. L. and Rock, K. L. (1992) Proteolysis, proteasomes and antigen presentation. *Nature* **357,** 375–379.
46. Kelly, A., Powis, S. H., Kerr, L. A., Mockridge, I., Elliott, T., Bastin, J., Uchanska-Ziegler, B., Ziegler, A., Trowsdale, J., and Townsend, A. (1992) Assembly and function of the two ABC transporter proteins encoded in the human major histocompatibility complex. *Nature* **355,** 641–644.
47. Spies, T. and DeMars, R. (1991) Restored expression of major histocompatibility class I molecules by gene transfer of a putative peptide transporter see comments. *Nature* **351,** 323–324.
48. Zinkernagel, R. M. and Doherty, P. C. (1974) Restriction of in vitro T cell-mediated cytotoxicity in lymphocytic choriomeningitis within a syngeneic or semiallogeneic system. *Nature* **248,** 701–702.
49. Rotzschke, O., Falk, K., Deres, K., Schild, H., Norda, M., Metzger, J., Jung, G., and Rammensee, H. G. (1990) Isolation and analysis of naturally processed viral peptides as recognized by cytotoxic T cells. *Nature* **348,** 252–254 (see comments).
50. Falk, K., Rotzschke, O., Stevanovic, S., Jung, G., and Rammensee, H. G. (1991) Allele-specific motifs revealed by sequencing of self-peptides eluted from MHC molecules. *Nature* **351,** 290–296.
51. Schumacher, T. N., De Bruijn, M. L., Vernie, L. N., Kast, W. M., Melief, C. J. M., Neefjes, J. J., and Ploegh, H. L. (1991) Peptide selection by MHC class I molecules. *Nature* **350,** 703–706.
52. Rotzschke, O., Falk, K., Stevanovic, S., Jung, G., Walden, P., and Rammensee, H. G. (1991) Exact prediction of a natural T cell epitope. *Eur. J. Immunol.* **21,** 2891–2894.
53. Rammensee, H. G. (1995) Chemistry of peptides associated with MHC class I and class II molecules. *Curr. Opin. Immunol.* **7,** 85–96.
54. Ruppert, J., Sidney, J., Celis, E., Kubo, R. T., Grey, H. M., and Sette, A. (1993) Prominent role of secondary anchor residues in peptide binding to HLA-A2.1 molecules. *Cell* **74,** 929–937.
55. Bjorkman, P. J., Saper, M. A., Samraoui, B., Bennett, W. S., Strominger, J. L., and Wiley, D. C. (1987) The foreign antigen binding site and T cell recognition regions of class I histocompatibility antigens. *Nature* **329,** 512–518.
56. Velders, M. P., Nieland, J. D., Rudolf, M. P., Loviscek, K., Weijzen, S., de Visser, K. E., Macedo, M. F., Carbone, M., and Kast, W. M. (1998) Identification of peptides for immunotherapy of cancer: it is still worth the effort. *Crit. Rev. Immunol.* **18,** 7–27.
57. Kast, W. M., Roux, L., Curren, J., Blom, H. J., Voordouw, A. C., Meloen, R. H., Kolakofsky, D., and Melief, C. J. M. (1991) Protection against lethal Sendai virus

infection by in vivo priming of virus-specific cytotoxic T lymphocytes with a free synthetic peptide. *Proc. Natl. Acad. Sci. USA* **88,** 2283–2287.

58. Schulz, M., Zinkernagel, R. M., and Hengartner, H. (1991) Peptide-induced antiviral protection by cytotoxic T cells. *Proc. Natl. Acad. Sci. USA* **88,** 991–993.

59. Faulkner, L., Borysiewicz, L. K., and Man, S. (1998) The use of human leucocyte antigen class I transgenic mice to investigate human immune function. *J. Immunol. Methods* **221,** 1–16.

60. Visseren, M. J. W., van der Burg, S. H., van der Voort, E. I. H., Brandt, R. M. P., Schrier, P. I., Van der Bruggen, P., Boon, T., Melief, C. J. M., and Kast, W. M. (1997) Identification of HLA-A*0201-restricted CTL epitopes encoded by the tumor-specific MAGE-2 gene product. *Int. J. Cancer* **73,** 326–333.

61. Restifo, N. P. and Rosenberg, S. A. (1999) Developing recombinant and synthetic vaccines for the treatment of melanoma. *Curr. Opin. Oncol.* **11,** 50–57.

62. Melief, C. J. M., Offringa, R., Toes, R. E. M., and Kast, W. M. (1996) Peptide based cancer vaccines. *Curr. Opin. Immunol.* **8,** 651–657.

63. Marchand, M., Van Baren, N., Weynants, P., et al. (1999) Tumor regressions observed in patients with metastatic melanoma treated with an antigenic peptide encoded by gene MAGE-3 and presented by HLA-A1. *Int. J. Cancer* **80,** 219–230.

64. Rosenberg, S. A., Packard, B. S., Aebersold, P. M., et al. (1988) Use of tumor-infiltrating lymphocytes and interleukin-2 in the immunotherapy of patients with metastatic melanoma. *N. Engl. J. Med.* **319,** 1676–1680.

65. Rosenberg, S. A., Yannelli, J. R., Yang, J. C., Topalian, S. L., Schwartzentruber, D. J., Weber, J. S., Parkinson, D. R., Seipp, C. A., Einhorn, J. H., and White, D. E. (1994) Treatment of patients with metastatic melanoma with autologous tumor-infiltrating lymphocytes and interleukin 2. *J. Nat. Cancer Inst.* **86,** 1159–1166.

66. Sette, A., Vitiello, A., Reherman, B., et al. (1994) The relationship between class I binding affinity and immunogenicity of potential cytotoxic T cell epitopes. *J. Immunol.* **153,** 5586–5592.

67. van der Burg, S. H., Visseren, M. J., Brandt, R. M. P., Kast, W. M., and Melief, C. J. M. (1996) Immunogenicity of peptides bound to MHC class I molecules depends on the MHC-peptide complex stability. *J. Immunol.* **156,** 3308–3314.

68. Men, Y., Miconnet, I., Valmori, D., Rimoldi, D., Cerottini, J. C., and Romero, P. (1999) Assessment of immunogenicity of human melan-A peptide analogues in HLA-A*0201/Kb transgenic mice. *J. Immunol.* **162,** 3566–3573.

69. Bakker, A. B., van der Burg, S. H., Huijbens, R. J., Drijfhout, J. W., Melief, C. J., Adema, G. J., and Figdor, C. G. (1997) Analogues of CTL epitopes with improved MHC class-I binding capacity elicit anti-melanoma CTL recognizing the wild-type epitope. *Int. J. Cancer* **70,** 302–309.

70. Romero, P., Gervois, N., Schneider, J., Escobar, P., Valmori, D., Pannetier, C., Steinle, A., Wolfel, T., Lienard, D., Brichard, V., Van Pel, A., Jotereau, F., and Cerottini, J. C. (1997) Cytolytic T lymphocyte recognition of the immunodominant HLA-A*0201-restricted Melan-A/MART-1 antigenic peptide in melanoma. *J. Immunol.* **159,** 2366–2374.

71. Valmori, D., Fonteneau, J. F., Lizana, C. M., Gervois, N., Lienard, D., Rimoldi, D., Jongeneel, V., Jotereau, F., Cerottini, J. C., and Romero, P. (1998) Enhanced generation of specific tumor-reactive CTL in vitro by selected Melan-A/MART-1 immunodominant peptide analogues. *J. Immunol.* **160,** 1750–1758.
72. Parkhurst, M. R., Salgaller, M. L., Southwood, S., Robbins, P. F., Sette, A., Rosenberg, S. A., and Kawakami, Y. (1996) Improved induction of melanoma-reactive CTL with peptides from the melanoma antigen gp100 modified at HLA-A*0201-binding residues. *J. Immunol.* **157,** 2539–2548.
73. Rosenberg, S. A., Yang, J. C., Schwartzentruber, D. J., et al. (1998) Immunologic and therapeutic evaluation of a synthetic peptide vaccine for the treatment of patients with metastatic melanoma. *Nat. Med.* **4,** 321–327.
74. Clay, T. M., Custer, M. C., McKee, M. D., Parkhurst, M., Robbins, P. F., Kerstann, K., Wunderlich, J., Rosenberg, S. A., and Nishimura, M. I. (1999) Changes in the fine specificity of gp100(209-217)-reactive T cells in patients following vaccination with a peptide modified at an HLA-A2.1 anchor residue. *J. Immunol.* **162,** 1749–1755.
75. Fleuren, G. J., Gorter, A., Kuppen, P. J. K., Litvinov, S. V., and Warnaar, S. O. (1995) Tumor heterogeneity and immunotherapy of cancer. *Immunol. Rev.* **145,** 91–122.
76. Cormier, J. N., Panelli, M. C., Hackett, J. A., Bettinotti, M. P., Mixon, A., Wunderlich, J., Parker, L. L., Restifo, N. P., Ferrone, S., and Marincola, F. M. (1999) Natural variation of the expression of HLA and endogenous antigen modulates CTL recognition in an in vitro melanoma model. *Int. J. Cancer* **80,** 781–790.
77. Cormier, J. N., Hijazi, Y. M., Abati, A., Fetsch, P., Bettinotti, M., Steinberg, S. M., Rosenberg, S. A., and Marincola, F. M. (1998) Heterogeneous expression of melanoma-associated antigens and HLA-A2 in metastatic melanoma in vivo. *Int. J. Cancer* **75,** 517–524.
78. Lehmann, F., Marchand, M., Hainaut, P., Pouillart, P., Sastre, X., Ikeda, H., Boon, T., and Coulie, P. G. (1995) Differences in the antigens recognized by cytolytic T cells on two successive metastases of a melanoma patient are consistent with immune selection. *Eur. J. Immunol.* **25,** 340–347.
79. Coulie, P. G., Ikeda, H., Baurain, J. F., and Chiari, R. (1999) Antitumor immunity at work in a melanoma patient. *Adv. Cancer Res.* **76,** 213–242.
80. Velders, M. P., Schreiber, H., and Kast, W. M. (1998) Active immunization against cancer cells: impediments and advances. *Semin. Oncol.* **25,** 1–10.
81. Aichele, P., Brduscha-Riem, K., Zinkernagel, R. M., Hengartner, H., and Pircher, H. (1995) T cell priming versus T cell tolerance induced by synthetic peptides. *J. Exp. Med.* **182,** 261–266.
82. Toes, R. E. M., Blom, R. J. J., Offringa, R., Kast, W. M., and Melief, C. J. M. (1996) Enhanced tumor outgrowth after peptide vaccination. Functional deletion of tumor-specific CTL induced by peptide vaccination can lead to the inability to reject tumors. *J. Immunol.* **156,** 3911–3918.
83. Toes, R. E. M., Offringa, R., Blom, R. J. J., Melief, C. J. M., and Kast, W. M. (1996) Peptide vaccination can lead to enhance tumor growth through specific T-cell tolerance induction. *Proc. Natl. Acad. Sci. USA* **93,** 7855–7860.

84. Knuth, A., Wolfel, T., Klehmann, E., Boon, T., Meyer zum Buschenfelde, K. H. (1989) Cytolytic T-cell clones against an autologous human melanoma: specificity study and definition of three antigens by immunoselection. *Proc. Natl. Acad. Sci. USA* **86**, 2804–2808.

85. Lotze, M. T., Grimm, E. A., Mazumder, A., et al. (1981) In vitro growth of cytotoxic human lymphocytes. IV: lysis of fresh and cultured autologous tumors by lymphocytes cultured in T cell growth factor (TCGF). *Cancer Res.* **41**, 4420–4425.

86. Kawakami, Y., Rosenberg, S. A., and Lotze, M. T. (1988) Interleukin 4 promotes the growth of tumor-infiltrating lymphocytes cytotoxic for human autologous melanoma. *J. Exp. Med.* **168**, 2183–2191.

87. Houssaint, E. and Flajnik, M. (1990) The role of thymic epithelium in the acquisition of tolerance. *Immunol. Today* **11**, 357–360.

88. Celis, E., Tsai, V., Crimi, C., DeMars, R., Wentworth, P. A., Chesnut, R. W., Grey, H. M., Sette, A., and Serra, H. M. (1994) Induction of anti-tumor cytotoxic T lymphocytes in normal humans using primary cultures and synthetic peptide epitopes. *Proc. Natl. Acad. Sci. USA* **91**, 2105–2109.

89. Gaugler, B., Van den Eynde, B., Van der Bruggen, P., Romero, P., Gaforio, J. J., De Plaen, E., Lethe, B., Brasseur, F., and Boon, T. (1994) Human gene MAGE-3 codes for an antigen recognized on a melanoma by autologous cytolytic T lymphocytes. *J. Exp. Med.* **179**, 921–930.

90. Van der Bruggen, P., Szikora, J. P., Boel, P., Wildmann, C., Somville, M., Sensi, M., and Boon, T. (1994) Autologous cytolytic T lymphocytes recognize a MAGE-1 nonapeptide on melanomas expressing HLA-Cw*1601. *Eur. J. Immunol.* **24**, 2134–2140.

91. Wang, R. F., Wang, X., Johnston, S. L., Zeng, G., Robbins, P. F., and Rosenberg, S. A. (1998) Development of a retrovirus-based complementary DNA expression system for the cloning of tumor antigens. *Cancer Res.* **58**, 3519–3525.

92. Wang, R. F., Robbins, P. F., Kawakami, Y., Kang, X. Q., and Rosenberg, S. A. (1995) Identification of a gene encoding a melanoma tumor antigen recognized by HLA-A31-restricted tumor-infiltrating lymphocytes. *J. Exp. Med.* **181**, 799–804 (published erratum appeared in *J. Exp. Med.* 1995;181[3]:1261).

93. Wang, R. F., Appella, E., Kawakami, Y., Kang, X., and Rosenberg, S. A. (1996) Identification of TRP-2 as a human tumor antigen recognized by cytotoxic T lymphocytes. *J. Exp. Med.* **184**, 2207–2216.

94. Wang, R. F., Johnston, S. L., Zeng, G., Topalian, S. L., Schwartzentruber, D. J., and Rosenberg, S. A. (1998) A breast and melanoma-shared tumor antigen: T cell responses to antigenic peptides translated from different open reading frames. *J. Immunol.* **161**, 3598–3606.

95. Cox, A. L., Skipper, J., Chen, Y., Henderson, R. A., Darrow, T. L., Shabanowitz, J., Engelhard, V. H., Hunt, D. F., and Slingluff, C. L. Jr. (1994) Identification of a peptide recognized by five melanoma-specific human cytotoxic T cell lines. *Science* **264**, 716–719.

96. Skipper, J. C., Hendrickson, R. C., Gulden, P. H., Brichard, V., Van Pel, A., Chen, Y., Shabanowitz, J., Wolfel, T., Slingluff, C. L., Jr., Boon, T., Hunt, D. F.,

and Engelhard, V. H. (1996) An HLA-A2-restricted tyrosinase antigen on melanoma cells results from posttranslational modification and suggests a novel pathway for processing of membrane proteins. *J. Exp. Med.* **183,** 527–534.

97. Storkus, W. J., Zeh, H. J. III, Maeurer, M. J., Salter, R. D., and Lotze, M. T.
    (1993) Identification of human melanoma peptides recognized by class I
    restricted tumor infiltrating T lymphocytes. *J. Immunol.* **151,** 3719–3727.

98. Slingluff, C. L. Jr., Cox, A. L., Henderson, R. A., Hunt, D. F., and Engelhard, V. H.
    (1993) Recognition of human melanoma cells by HLA-A2.1-restricted cytotoxic
    T lymphocytes is mediated by at least six shared peptide epitopes. *J. Immunol.*
    150, 2955–2963.

99. Castelli, C., Storkus, W. J., Maeurer, M. J., Martin, D. M., Huang, E. C.,
    Pramanik, B. N., Nagabhushan, T. L., Parmiani, G., and Lotze, M. T. (1995)
    Mass spectrometric identification of a naturally processed melanoma peptide
    recognized by CD8+ cytotoxic T lymphocytes. *J. Exp. Med.* **181,** 363–368.

100. Sahin, U., Tureci, O., Schmitt, H., Cochlovius, B., Johannes, T., Schmits, R.,
     Stenner, F., Luo, G., Schobert, I., and Pfreundschuh, M. (1995) Human neo-
     plasms elicit multiple specific immune responses in the autologous host. *Proc.
     Natl. Acad. Sci. USA* **92,** 11,810–11,813.

101. Old, L. J. and Chen, Y. T. (1998) New paths in human cancer serology. *J. Exp.
     Med.* **187,** 1163–1167.

102. Chen, Y.-T., Stockert, E., Chen, Y., Garin-Chesa, P., Rettig, W. J., Van der
     Bruggen, P., Boon, T., and Old, L. J. (1994) Identification of the *MAGE-1* gene
     product by monoclonal and polyclonal antibodies. *Proc. Natl. Acad. Sci. USA*
     91, 1004–1008.

103. Tureci, O., Sahin, U., Schobert, I., Koslowski, M., Scmitt, H., Schild, H. J.,
     Stenner, F., Seitz, G., Rammensee, H. G., and Pfreundschuh, M. (1996) The
     SSX-2 gene, which is involved in the t(X;18) translocation of synovial sarcomas,
     codes for the human tumor antigen HOM-MEL-40. *Cancer Res.* **56,** 4766–4772.

104. Jager, E., Chen, Y. T., Drijfhout, J. W., Karbach, J., Ringhoffer, M., Jager, D.,
     Arand, M., Wada, H., Noguchi, Y., Stockert, E., Old, L. J., and Knuth, A. (1998)
     Simultaneous humoral and cellular immune response against cancer-testis anti-
     gen NY-ESO-1—definition of human histocompatibility leukocyte antigen
     (HLA)-A2-binding peptide epitopes. *J. Exp. Med.* **187,** 265–270.

105. Traversari, C., Van der Bruggen, P., Luescher, I. F., Lurquin, C., Chomez, P.,
     Van Pel, A., De Plaen, E., Amar-Costesec, A., and Boon, T. (1992) A
     nonapeptide encoded by human gene MAGE-1 is recognized on HLA-A1 by
     cytolytic T lymphocytes directed against tumor antigen MZ2-E. *J. Exp. Med.*
     176, 1453–1457.

106. Bakker, A. B., Schreurs, M. W., de Boer, A. J., Kawakami, Y., Rosenberg, S. A.,
     Adema, G. J., and Figdor, C. G. (1994) Melanocyte lineage-specific antigen
     gp100 is recognized by melanoma-derived tumor-infiltrating lymphocytes.
     J. Exp. Med. **179,** 1005–1009.

107. Wolfel, T., Van Pel, A., Brichard, V., Schneider, J., Seliger, B., Meyer zum
     Buschenfelde, K. H., and Boon, T. (1994) Two tyrosinase nonapeptides recog-

nized on HLA-A2 melanomas by autologous cytolytic T lymphocytes. *Eur. J. Immunol.* **24,** 759–764.

108. Kang, X., Kawakami, Y., El-Gamil, M., Wang, R., Sakaguchi, K., Yannelli, J. R., Appella, E., Rosenberg, S. A., and Robbins, P. F. (1995) Identification of a tyrosinase epitope recognized by HLA-A24-restricted, tumor-infiltrating lymphocytes. *J. Immunol.* **155,** 1343–1348.

109. Tranzarella, S., Russo, V., Lionello, B., Dalerba, P., Bordignon, C., and Traversari, C. (1999) Identification of a promiscuous T-cell epitope encoded by multiple members of the MAGE family. *Cancer Res.* **59,** 2668–2674.

110. Huang, L.-Q., Brasseur, F., Serrano, A., De Plaen, E., Van der Bruggen, P., Boon, T., and Van Pel, A. (1999) Cytolytic T lymphocytes recognize an antigen encoded by MAGE-A10 on a human melanoma. *J. Immunol.* **162,** 6849–6854.

111. Kast, W. M., Brandt, R. M. P., Sidney, J., Drijfhout, J. W., Kubo, R. T., Grey, H. M., Melief, C. J. M., and Sette, A. (1994) Role of HLA-A motifs in identification of potential CTL epitopes in human papillomavirus type 16 E6 and E7 proteins. *J. Immunol.* **152,** 3904–3912.

112. Kawakami, Y., Eliyahu, S., Sakaguchi, K., Robbins, P. F., Rivoltini, L., Yannelli, J. R., Appella, E., and Rosenberg, S. A. (1994) Identification of the immunodominant peptides of the MART-1 human melanoma antigen recognized by the majority of HLA-A2-restricted tumor infiltrating lymphocytes. *J. Exp. Med.* **180,** 347–352.

113. Kittlesen, D. J., Thompson, L. W., Gulden, P. H., Skipper, J. C., Colella, T. A., Shabanowitz, J. A., Hunt, D. F., Engelhard, V. H., and Slingluff, C. L. Jr. (1998) Human melanoma patients recognize an HLA-A1-restricted CTL epitope from tyrosinase containing two cysteine residues: implications for tumor vaccine development. *J. Immunol.* **160,** 2099–2106.

114. Tanaka, F., Fujie, T., Tahara, K., Mori, M., Takesako, K., Sette, A., Celis, E., and Akiyoshi, T. (1997) Induction of antitumor cytotoxic T lymphocytes with a MAGE-3-encoded synthetic peptide presented by human leukocytes antigen-A24. *Cancer Res.* **57,** 4465–4468.

115. Fujie, T., Tahara, K., Tanaka, F., Mori, M., Takesako, K., and Akiyoshi, T. A. (1999) MAGE-1-encoded HLA-A24-binding synthetic peptide induces specific anti-tumor cytotoxic T lymphocytes. *Int. J. Cancer* **80,** 169–172.

116. Oiso, M., Eura, M., Katsura, F., Takiguchi, M., Sobao, Y., Masuyama, K., Nakashima, M., Itoh, K., and Ishikawa, T. (1999) A newly identified MAGE-3-derived epitope recognized by HLA-A24-restricted cytotoxic T lymphocytes. *Int. J. Cancer* **81,** 387–394.

117. Kawashima, I., Tsai, V., Southwood, S., Takesako, K., Celis, E., and Sette, A. (1998) Identification of gp100-derived, melanoma-specific cytotoxic T-lymphocyte epitopes restricted by HLA-A3 supertype molecules by primary in vitro immunization with peptide-pulsed dendritic cells. *Int. J. Cancer* **78,** 518–524.

118. Skipper, J. C., Kittlesen, D. J., Hendrickson, R. C., Deacon, D. D., Harthun, N. L., Wagner, S. N., Hunt, D. F., Engelhard, V. H., and Slingluff, C. L. Jr. (1996) Shared epitopes for HLA-A3-restricted melanoma-reactive human CTL

include a naturally processed epitope from Pmel-17/gp100. *J. Immunol.* **157,** 5027–5033.

119. Herman, J., Van der Bruggen, P., Luescher, I. F., Mandruzzato, S., Romero, P., Thonnard, J., Fleischhauer, K., Boon, T., and Coulie, P. G. (1996) A peptide encoded by the human MAGE3 gene and presented by HLA-B44 induces cytolytic T lymphocytes that recognize tumor cells expressing MAGE3. *Immunogenetics* **43,** 377–383.

120. Bakker, A. B., Schreurs, M. W., Tafazzul, G., de Boer, A. J., Kawakami, Y., Adema, G. J., and Figdor, C. G. (1995) Identification of a novel peptide derived from the melanocyte-specific gp100 antigen as the dominant epitope recognized by an HLA-A2.1-restricted anti-melanoma CTL line. *Int. J. Cancer* **62,** 97–102.

121. Van der Bruggen, P., Bastin, J., Gajewski, T., Coulie, P. G., Boel, P., De Sme, C., Traversari, C., Townsend, A., and Boon, T. (1994) A peptide encoded by human gene MAGE-3 and presented by HLA-A2 induces cytolytic T lymphocytes that recognize tumor cells expressing MAGE-3. *Eur. J. Immunol.* **24,** 3038–3043.

122. D'Amaro, J., Houbiers, J. G., Drijfhout, J. W., Brandt, R. M. P., Schipper, R., Bavinck, J. N., Melief, C. J. M., and Kast, W. M. (1995) A computer program for predicting possible cytotoxic T lymphocyte epitopes based on HLA class I peptide-binding motifs. *Hum. Immunol.* **43,** 13–18.

123. Zorn, E. and Hercend, T. (1999) A MAGE-6-encoded peptide is recognized by expanded lymphocytes infiltrating a spontaneously regressing human primary melanoma lesion. *Eur. J. Immunol.* **29,** 602–607.

124. Boel, P., Wildmann, C., Sensi, M. L., Brasseur, R., Renauld, J. C., Coulie, P., Boon, T., and Van der Bruggen, P. (1995) BAGE: a new gene encoding an antigen recognized on human melanomas by cytolytic T lymphocytes. *Immunity* **2,** 167–175.

125. Van den Eynde, B., Peeters, O., De Backer, O., Gaugler, B., Lucas, S., and Boon, T. (1995) A new family of genes coding for an antigen recognized by autologous cytolytic T lymphocytes on a human melanoma. *J. Exp. Med.* **182,** 689–698.

126. Aarnoudse, C. A., Van den Doel, P. B., Heemskerk, B., and Schrier, P. I. (1999) Interleukin-2-induced, melanoma-specific T cells recognize CAMEL, an unexpected translation product of LAGE-1. *Int. J. Cancer* **82,** 442–448.

127. Ikeda, H., Lethe, B., Lehmann, F., Van Baren, N., Baurain, J. F., De Smet, C., Chambost, H., Vitale, M., Moretta, A., Boon, T., and Coulie, P. G. (1997) Characterization of an antigen that is recognized on a melanoma showing partial HLA loss by CTL expressing an NK inhibitory receptor. *Immunity* **6,** 199–208.

128. Fleischhauer, K., Gattinoni, L., Dalerba, P., Lauvau, G., Zanaria, E., Dabovic, B., van Endert, P. M., Bordignon, C., and Traversari, C. (1998) The DAM gene family encodes a new group of tumor-specific antigens recognized by human leukocyte antigen A2-restricted cytotoxic T lymphocytes. *Cancer Res.* **58,** 2969–2972.

129. Kawakami, Y., Robbins, P. F., Wang, X., Tupesis, J. P., Parkhurst, M. R., Kang, X., Sakaguchi, K., Appella, E., and Rosenberg, S. A. (1998) Identification of new melanoma epitopes on melanosomal proteins recognized by tumor infiltrating T lymphocytes restricted by HLA-A1, -A2, and -A3 alleles. *J. Immunol.* **161,** 6985–6992.

130. Schneider, J., Brichard, V., Boon, T., Meyer zum Buschenfelde, K. H., and Wolfel, T. (1998) Overlapping peptides of melanocyte differentiation antigen Melan-A/MART-1 recognized by autologous cytolytic T lymphocytes in association with HLA-B45.1 and HLA-A2.1. *Int. J. Cancer* **75,** 451–458.

131. Brichard, V. G., Herman, J., VanPel, A., Wildmann, C., Gaugler, B., Wolfel, T., Boon, T., and Lethe, B. (1996) A tyrosinase nonapeptide presented by HLA-B44 is recognized on a human melanoma by autologous cytolytic T lymphocytes. *Eur. J. Immunol.* **26,** 224–230.

132. Kobayashi, H., Kokubo, T., Sato, K., Kimura, S., Asano, K., Takahashi, H., Iizuka, H., Miyokawa, N., and Katagiri, M. (1998) CD4+ T cells from peripheral blood of a melanoma patient recognize peptides derived from nonmutated tyrosinase. *Cancer Res.* **58,** 296–301.

133. Rivoltini, L., Squarcina, P., Loftus, D. J., Castelli, C., Tarsini, P., Mazzocchi, A., Rini, F., Viggiano, V., Belli, F., and Parmiani, G. (1999) A superagonist variant of peptide MART1/Melan A27-35 elicits anti-melanoma CD8+ T cells with enhanced functional characteristics: implication for more effective immunotherapy. *Cancer Res.* **59,** 301–306.

134. Castelli, C., Tarsini, P., Mazzocchi, A., Rini, F., Rivoltini, L., Ravagnani, F., Gallino, F., Belli, F., and Parmiani, G. (1999) Novel HLA-Cw8-restricted T cell epitopes derived from tyrosinase-related protein-2 and gp100 melanoma antigens. *J. Immunol.* **162,** 1739–1748.

135. Wang, R. F., Johnston, S. L., Southwood, S., Sette, A., and Rosenberg, S. A. (1998) Recognition of an antigenic peptide derived from tyrosinase-related protein-2 by CTL in the context of HLA-A31 and -A33. *J. Immunol.* **160,** 890–897.

136. Parkhurst, M. R., Fitzgerald, E. B., Southwood, S., Sette, A., Rosenberg, S. A., and Kawakami, Y. (1998) Identification of a shared HLA-A*0201-restricted T-cell epitope from the melanoma antigen tyrosinase-related protein 2 (TRP2). *Cancer Res.* **58,** 4895–4901.

137. Salazaronfray, F., Nakazawa, T., Chhajlani, V., Petersson, M., Karre, K., Masucci, G., Celis, E., Sette, A., Southwood, S., Appella, E., and Kiessling, R. (1997) Synthetic peptides derived from the melanocyte-stimulating hormone receptor MC1R can stimulate HLA-A2-restricted cytotoxic T lymphocytes that recognize naturally processed peptides on human melanoma cells. *Cancer Res.* **57,** 4348–4355.

138. Robbins, P. F., El-Gamil, M., Kawakami, Y., and Rosenberg, S. A. (1994) Recognition of tyrosinase by tumor-infiltrating lymphocytes from a patient responding to immunotherapy. *Cancer Res.* **54,** 3124–3126.

139. Rongcun, Y., Salazar-Onfray, F., Charo, J., Malmberg, K. J., Evrin, K., Maes, H., Kono, K., Hising, C., Petersson, M., Larsson, O., Lan, L., Appella, E., Sette, A., Celis, E., and Kiessling, R. (1999) Identification of new Her2/neu-derived peptide epitopes that can elicit specific CTL against autologous and allogeneic carcinomas and melanomas. *J. Immunol.* **163,** 1037–1044.
140. Chaux, P., Luiten, R., Demotte, N., Vantomme, V., Stroobant, V., Traversari, C., Russo, V., Schultz, E., Cornelis, G. R., Boon, T., and Van der Bruggen, P. (1999) Identification of five MAGE-A1 epitopes recognized by cytolytic T lymphocytes obtained by in vitro stimulation with dendritic cells transduced with *MAGE-A1*. *J. Immunol.* **163,** 2928–2936.

4

Experimental Induction of Human Atypical Melanocytic Lesions and Melanoma in Ultraviolet-Irradiated Human Skin Grafted to Immunodeficient Mice

Carola Berking and Meenhard Herlyn

1. Introduction

The development of melanoma and its precursor lesions has been associated with intense intermittent sun exposure and the deleterious effects of ultraviolet (UV) light *(1)*. This is supported by epidemiologic data as well as several animal models in which melanoma could be induced or promoted by UV irradiation (**Table 1**). It remains to be elucidated what changes UV light induces in the human pigment cells at the molecular level that trigger malignant transformation. Experimental animal models established to date have helped us to understand the etiology and pathobiology of melanoma, but they do not necessarily mirror the biology of human melanoma development. The skin morphology in animals differs substantially from that in humans, and melanocytes show a different distribution pattern. In mice, melanocytes are mainly located in the hair follicles, whereas in humans, melanocytes are found epidermally at the basement membrane zone. The number of cell layers of the epidermis is, for the most part, markedly less in mice than in humans (**Fig. 1**).

Using immunodeficient laboratory animals, it has become possible to graft human skin without inducing a host-vs-graft response and to subsequently use this skin for experimental in vivo studies. The first grafts were done in the 1970s with athymic nude mice *(15,16)*. More recently, mouse strains with genetic immunodefects such as severe combined immunodeficiency (SCID) *(17,18)* and recombinase activating gene-1 (RAG-1) mutant mice *(19)* have been used for grafting human skin *(20–28)*. Their inability to produce functional T- and

From: *Methods in Molecular Medicine, Vol. 61: Melanoma: Methods and Protocols*
Edited by: B. J. Nickoloff © Humana Press Inc., Totowa, NJ

Table 1
Animal Models for Melanoma[a]

Species	Model	Induction	Reference
Mouse	Transgenic	Tyrosinase promoter fused to the simian virus 40 early region oncogenic sequences	2
Mouse	Transgenic	Metallothionein fused to transmembrane tyrosine kinase oncogene *ret*	3
Mouse	Transgenic	Metallothionein fused to hepatocyte growth factor/scatter factor	4
Mouse	Transgenic	Tyrosinase promoter for H-RAS on an INK4a-null background	5
Mouse	Transgenic	Active DNA clones (Clone B)	6
Fish genus *Xiphophorus*	Hybrid with a dominant oncogene	Spontaneous, UV light	7
South American opossum genus *Monodelphis domestica*	UV radiation-induced mutagenesis	UV light	8
Sinclair swine	Genetic inheritance	Spontaneous	9
Syrian hamster	Genetic inheritance	Spontaneous, DMBA	10
Mouse	Chemically induced	DMBA	11
Guinea pig	Chemically induced	DMBA	12
Human/mouse	Human melanoma xenograft	Transplantation of human melanomas to immunodeficient mice	13
Mouse	Murine melanoma allograft	Transplantation of murine melanoma cell lines (B16, Cloudman S91, Harding Passey, K-1735) to mice	
Human/mouse	Human skin xenograft	Transplantation of human skin to immunodeficient mice, topical DMBA application and UVB irradiation	14

[a]DMBA, 9,10-dimethyl-2,2-benzanthracene; UV, ultraviolet.

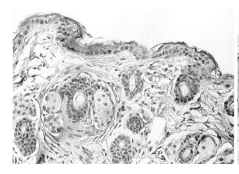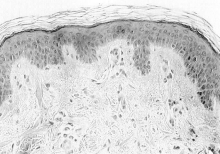

Fig. 1. Histologic section of normal mouse (**left**) and human (**right**) skin from the trunk (hematoxylin and eosin [H&E] stain, ×400). There are many hair follicles in the murine dermis, and the epidermis is composed of only two cell layers as opposed to the multilayered human epidermis.

B-cells leads to the absence of immunoglobulin production. However, macrophages and natural killer cell activities are unimpaired, enabling a nonspecific host defense. **Table 2** lists the characteristics of nude, SCID, and RAG-1 mice. The type of hair and pigmentation of the various background strains are important for UV irradiation studies, because mice of albino background or nude mice are less protected from the development of murine tumors and cataracts than mice with pigmentation and hair *(14,29,30)*.

The skin to be grafted can be derived from different sources. Foreskins are commonly available from circumcisions of newborns. Breast, abdominal, facial, and eyelid skin from adults can be obtained from plastic surgery. Skin adjacent to skin lesions can be derived from wide surgical excisions, and fetal skin is obtained from aborts. Human skin equivalents generated as three-dimensional, organotypic cultures in vitro also can be grafted to immunodeficient mice *(31,32)*. The advantage of skin substitutes is that they can be engineered in numerous copies with identical genetic and biologic features, which facilitates standardization of experiments and avoids the interindividual variability seen in human skin. On the other hand, skin substitutes only contain a portion of all the different cell types and extracellular matrix components that form the human skin.

The quality of the grafts is influenced by the donor's age; pigmentation type; medical, occupational, and recreational history; and body site from which they are taken. **Table 3** summarizes the main differences between neonatal foreskin and adult skin specimens. The high engraftment rates for foreskins is most likely owing to rich vascularization, the thin skin, and the donor's age. Typical features of foreskin grafts are a wrinkled skin surface (**Fig. 2**) and smooth muscle bundles in the dermis. Adult skin has been grafted as split-thickness

Table 2
Comparison of Immunodeficient Mice Used for Grafting Experiments

	Nude mouse	SCID mouse	RAG-1 mouse
First description	1966	1983	1992
Genetic defect	Homozygous for the nude mutation on chromosome 11	Homozygous for the SCID mutation on chromosome 16	Homozygous for a mutation in RAG-1
V(D)J recombination	Intact	Defect	Defect
T-lymphocytes	Deficient	Deficient	Deficient
B-lymphocytes	Abortive	Deficient, but frequent leakage	Deficient
Immunoglobulin production	Low IgM	None, but frequent leakage	None
Macrophages	Activity increased	Unimpaired	Unimpaired
Natural killer cells	Activity increased	Unimpaired	Unimpaired
Granulocytes	Unimpaired	Unimpaired	Unimpaired
Megakaryocytes	Unimpaired	Unimpaired	Unimpaired
Erythrocytes	Unimpaired	Unimpaired	Unimpaired
Thymus	Aplastic	Hypoplastic	Hypoplastic
DNA repair	No known defect	Double-strand break repair defect	No known defect
Availability	Inbred strains (Balb/c, C57BL/6) and hybrids (B6cBy, cByB6) between the two strains	Different congenic backgrounds including C3H, C57BL/6, NOD/L, Balb/c	Different congenic backgrounds including B6, C57BL/6
Pelage	Hairless	Normal	Normal

(26,27) or full-thickness skin *(22,24,28)*. Split-thickness skin can show higher take rates than full-thickness skin, because it is less prone to dry out during the first critical weeks of engraftment. However, fewer human dermal structures including hair follicles and sebaceous glands will survive in split-thickness skin.

Figure 3 shows an example of an abdominal skin graft. Histologically epidermis and upper dermis resemble the human morphology in vivo (**Fig. 4**).

For optimal engraftment results, the skin specimens are surgically trimmed before grafting to remove excess fat and fibrous tissue. A favorable anatomic site of the graft on the mouse was found to be just above and behind the shoulder, leaving the well-vascularized panniculus carnosus muscle intact.

In this chapter, we describe in detail the technique of grafting human neonatal foreskin and full-thickness adult skin to SCID mice. The surgical procedure

Table 3
Characteristics of Human Skin for Grafting

Parameter	Foreskin from newborns	Skin from adults
Availability	Local hospitals, private practice	Specialized centers
Specimen size	Small	Large
Exposure to sunlight	No	Yes
External irritation (chemicals, cosmetics, etc.)	No	Yes
Tanning ability	Unknown	Known
Medical history	Unknown	Known
Engraftment rates	90%	70–90%

for the well-vascularized and elastic foreskins from newborns differs slightly from that for normal adult skin, as described in **Subheading 3.2., step 9.**

For the induction of melanocytic lesions, skin from donors with fair skin, which easily sunburns and freckles (i.e., skin phototype I and II [Fitzpatrick]) and from high-risk melanoma patients is recommended. The induction is performed by a single topical application of 9,10-dimethyl-1,2-benzanthracene (DMBA) and subsequent UVB irradiations at regular intervals *(14)*.

2. Materials
2.1. Skin Preparation

All materials are sterile. Surgical instruments are made of stainless steel and autoclavable.

1. Human foreskins from newborns (1 to 2 cm^2) or human adult skin from trunk, extremities, scalp, or face (*see* **Notes 1** and **2**).
2. Transport and storage medium: Hank's balanced salt solution (HBSS) or RPMI-1640 (Gibco, Gaithersburg, MD) supplemented with 0.1 mg/mL of gentamycin (Mediatech, Herndon, VA) and 0.02 mg/mL of penicillin-streptomycin (Mediatech). Store refrigerated at 4°C; stable for 3 mo.
3. Petri dishes (100 × 15 mm) (Fisher, Pittsburgh, PA).
4. Tissue forceps (Roboz, Rockville, MD).
5. Straight operating scissors and curved microdissecting scissors (Roboz).
6. Scalpel handle (no. 4) (Martin, Germany).
7. Surgical blades (single use, no. 22) (Feather, Japan).
8. 70% Ethanol.
9. Phosphate-buffered saline (PBS).
10. Plastic tubes (50 mL) (Falcon, Fisher Scientific).

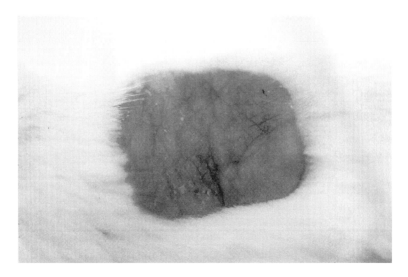

Fig. 2. Well-healed human foreskin from a newborn donor 4 wk after grafting to a SCID mouse. Note the typical wrinkled appearance.

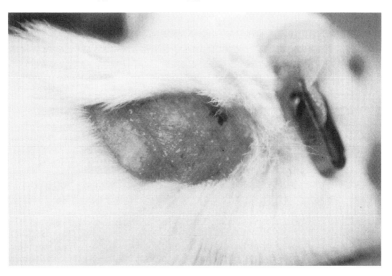

Fig. 3. Well-healed human abdominal skin from an adult donor 7 wk after grafting to a SCID mouse.

2.2. Animal Surgery

Mice are housed in groups in autoclavable filter-topped cages with sterile bedding, water bottles, and chow (*see* **Note 9**). All procedures with the animals are performed in a biologic laminar flow safety cabinet with a sterile drape.

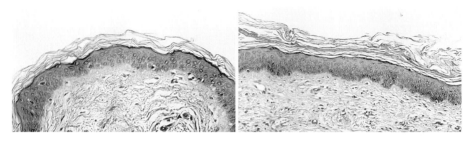

Fig. 4. Histologic section of human breast skin from an adult donor before (**left**) and 6 wk after (**right**) grafting to a SCID mouse (H&E, ×200).

1. C.B-17 SCID mice, both sexes, 6 wk of age or older (Jackson, Bar Harbor, ME) (*see* **Note 10**).
2. Anesthesia: 20 mg/mL of xylazine, injectable; and 100 mg/mL of ketamine (both Phoenix Pharmaceutical, St. Joseph, MI). Dilute 3.65 mL of ketamine and 0.54 mL of xylazine in 5.8 mL of sterile PBS. Store and inject at room temperature.
3. Insulin syringes (1 cc, single use, 28-g needle, 0.5 in.) (Becton Dickinson, Franklin Lakes, NJ).
4. Electric clipper (A5, blade size 40) (Oster, Milwaukee, WI).
5. 70% Isopropyl alcohol swabs (Becton Dickinson).
6. Sterile gloves (Baxter, CA).
7. Petri dish (100 × 15 mm) (Fisher).
8. Scissors (microdissecting, straight, sharp S-114, S-136) (Delasco, Council Bluffs, IA).
9. Microdissecting forceps (straight and slightly curved, tip width 0.5–0.8 mm) (Roboz).
10. Needle holder (Delasco).
11. Polyviolene nonabsorbable surgical suture (6/0, C-22 cutting) (Look, Boston, MA) (*see* **Note 6**).
12. Sponges (7.5 × 7.5 cm, sterile) (Versalon; Kendall, Cincinnati, OH).
13. Nonadhering dressing (7.6 × 7.6 cm, sterile) (Adaptic; Johnson&Johnson, Arlington, TX) (*see* **Note 7**).
14. Surgical tape (1.25 cm × 9.1 m) (Durapore; 3M Health Care, St. Paul, MN).
15. Bandage scissors (Roboz).

2.3. Chemicals

1. 9,10-Dimethyl-1,2-benzanthracene (DMBA) (approx. 95%, carcinogenic) (Sigma, St. Louis, MO).
2. Acetone (≥99.5%) (Fisher): Add 10 mL of acetone to 100 mg of DMBA into the manufacturer's bottle and store light-protected at –20°C until use. Dilute stock 1 : 10 in acetone for use.

2.4. UV Irradiation Equipment

1. UVB/UVA lamp: UVA-340 (300–400 nm, peak emission at 340 nm) (Q-Panel, Cleveland, OH).
2. UVB lamp: FS72T12 (280–370 nm, peak emission at 313 nm) (Westinghouse lamps, Ultraviolet Resources, Athens, Cleveland, OH).
3. Cellulose triacetate sheets (Kodacel TA407) (Eastman Kodak, Rochester, NY).
4. Radiometer with UVA and UVB detectors (PMA 2100) (Solar Light, Philadelphia, PA).

3. Methods
3.1. Skin Preparation

All procedures are performed aseptically and all materials are sterile. Dissecting instruments may be repeatedly sterilized by dipping in 70% ethanol and rinsed in sterile PBS. Alternatively, instruments may be dipped in 95% ethanol, burned in a gas flame, and cooled before contacting the tissue. Skin specimens are always kept humid.

1. Store skin specimens in medium (HBSS or RPMI supplemented with antibiotics) at 4°C and transport on ice. Neonatal foreskins can be used up to 3 d and adult skin up to 1.5 d after excision from the donor. Optimum performance is achieved by using the specimens as fresh as possible.
2. Place the specimen in a Petri dish and thoroughly trim off sc fat and excess fibrous tissue with scissors.
3. Rinse the specimen in PBS and cut with a scalpel into square grafts of 1 to 2 × 1 to 2 cm.
4. Transfer the grafts into tubes containing transport medium (antibiotic supplement can be omitted), and keep on ice until surgery.

3.2. Animal Surgery

All care and use of animals is approved by The Wistar Institutional Animal Care and Use Committee. All procedures are performed with aseptic techniques, and all materials are sterile.

1. Cover the inside of the biologic safety cabinet with a sterile drape. Place the surgical instruments and suture and bandage material on a sterile operating field.
2. Place the grafts in a Petri dish slightly covered with medium at room temperature.
3. Anesthetize a mouse by sc injection of 800–1200 µL of xylazine/ketamine mixture (*see* **Subheading 2.2., item 2**). Put the mouse back into the cage and close the top. After 1–3 min verify complete anesthesia by negative response to toe pinch.
4. Shave back and side hair close to the shoulders of the mouse with an electric clipper. Stretch the skin of the animal with hands to facilitate shaving without injury to the skin (*see* **Note 5**).

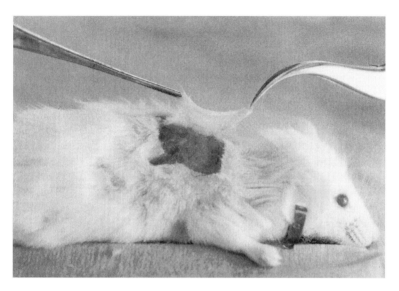

Fig. 5. Creation of a wound bed for the human skin graft above the shoulder of a SCID mouse. The mouse skin (lifted up with forceps in the Figure) is cut off, leaving the murine panniculus carnosus muscle intact.

5. Cleanse the shaved area with 70% isopropanol swabs and place the animal on an operating field with the right flank facing the surgeon.
6. Put on new sterile surgical gloves, grasp the graft with forceps, and trim it to a thickness of 1 to 2 mm with scissors by holding the graft in one hand.
7. Estimate the size of the graft and choose an appropriate area for the wound bed on the mouse. The ideal localization is just behind or above the shoulders (*see* **Note 3**).
8. For preparation of a wound bed, lift the skin with straight fine forceps parallel to the spine of the mouse and cut carefully along the lifted line. The incision into the dermis is performed as flat as possible to preserve the panniculus carnosus muscle. Parallel to the first incision at a distance of 0.5–2 cm depending on the graft's size, make another incision of the same length. Then connect the parallel ends of both incisions by two further incisions. Grasp with fine forceps one corner of the square formed by the incisions and carefully pull off the murine skin leaving the panniculus carnosus muscle intact by dissecting it from the dermis with the help of another pair of forceps (**Fig. 5**) (*see* **Note 4**).
9. Place the graft epidermis onto the wound and secure it with single-type sutures to the wound margins at four to eight points (**Fig. 6**). Stretching of the graft by the sutures supports an even contact of its dermal side with the wound bed. Sutures are omitted when foreskins or very thin and well-vascularized adult skin (e.g., eyelid) is grafted. Ideally, the graft size should exactly match the size of the wound bed.

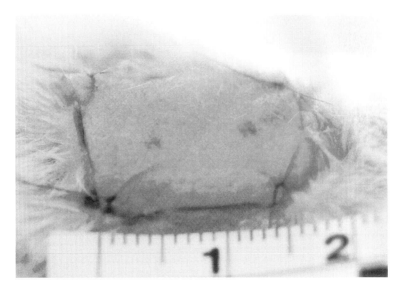

Fig. 6. Human skin graft is placed on the wound bed of a SCID mouse. The skin graft is secured to the murine wound margins with sutures at the corners.

3.3. Bandaging

1. Cut the nonadhering dressing into a square and cover the graft and the wound edges.
2. Cut the sponges into 2- to 2.5-cm-wide strips and cut the tape into 15- to 20-cm-long strips. Cover the graft with one end of a sponge and hold it in place by slightly pressing it against the animal with one hand. Then lift the mouse and wrap the other end of the sponge very tightly around the mouse. Hold the sponge in place by wrapping the tape several times very tightly around the mouse.
3. Check whether the mouse is breathing normally and put it back into the cage (*see* **Note 11**). After 30 min to 1 h, the mouse will recover from the anesthesia.

3.4. Dressing Control and Care

1. Check daily whether the bandage is on and is not causing discomfort to the animal. If it has come off or is too loose, replace it immediately (*see* **Note 8**); otherwise the graft will dry out and eventually be lost.
2. After 1.5–2 wk anesthetize the mouse with a sc injection of 200–600 µL of the xylazine/ketamine mixture and remove the bandage with bandage scissors.
3. Repeat the bandaging as described in **Subheading 3.3.**
4. Remove the bandage completely 4 wk after grafting.
5. Start experiments when the grafts look well healed. Foreskins are usually well healed after 4 wk, whereas adult skins require 5 to 6 wk.

3.5. Application of DMBA

Measure the graft and calculate the total volume for topical application. For example, if a concentration of 15 μg/cm^2 is intended, apply 15 μL of the DMBA/acetone solution per 1 × 1 cm graft. Apply the solution extremely cautiously with a standard pipet under sterile conditions and try not to contaminate the mouse skin. Protect yourself accordingly, avoiding any skin, eye, or other direct contact with DMBA.

3.6. UV Irradiation

1. Let the UV bulbs burn 10–20 min before use and check the lamp's UV output with the radiometer.
2. Place the mice in appropriate cages under the UV lamps at a distance between 20 and 100 cm. The irradiation field is more homogeneous when the distance is far. However, the farther the distance, the lower the light intensity of the lamp becomes, which requires a longer irradiation time to achieve the same UV dose as with a closer distance.
3. Monitor the UV output with the radiometer during irradiation and note the cumulative dose and time.

4. Notes

1. Split-thickness skin generally results in higher engraftment rates and shorter healing periods than full-thickness skin, particularly when thick and poorly vascularized skin, such as from the trunk, is used. Split-thickness skin can be obtained from the donor in vivo or ex vivo with the help of a dermatome. A dermatome is a surgical instrument with a blade that is pushed forward along the skin of the donor in order to harvest a graft of uniform thickness and size. Ex vivo the skin specimen can be stretched and held in place with needles on a sterile, covered styrofoam block. If preservation of human dermal structures such as appendages and vessels is intended, use full-thickness skin and trim off excess fat and fibrous tissue by hand.
2. Take rates are highest for foreskins from newborns, followed by eyelid skin or skin from the face, which is thin and very well vascularized. Adult skin from any other part of the body is more difficult to graft and needs thorough surgical preparation as described earlier.
3. It is possible to graft two different skin specimens to the same mouse, e.g., on the left and on the right side behind the shoulders. This can be done at one surgery session or at a later time.
4. Quality surgical instruments are essential for successful surgery. Only use sharp scissors and fine forceps. Operating scissors dull rapidly when used for cutting bandage material or paper. Scissors can be sharpened manually after each use with a scissors sharpener (Miltex™; Delasco, Council Bluffs, IA).

5. Instead of shaving the animal, hair can also be treated with a hair remover cream or lotion (Nair®, Carter, New York, NY). It is applied thickly onto the fur, and after 3–5 min, the hair and the cream can be wiped off with a wet cloth.
6. Dark blue or black sutures are difficult to see when used on darkly pigmented mice. Suture material of brighter colors can be purchased instead.
7. The use of self-adhesive transparent dressings, such as OpSite® or TegaDerm®, tends to create an air-impermeable sealing of the wound, which is not advantageous for successful engraftment.
8. When replacing the bandage, use only about one third of the quantity of the anesthetic used for the surgery to avoid overdose in the more sensitive and less tolerant animals.
9. Up to five mice of the same gender can be housed in one cage. Occasionally, males must be separated from each other to avoid serious injuries to themselves or damage to the grafts caused by fighting. Female mice are less fierce than their male counterparts and easier to handle. However, they are usually smaller, which limits the grafting area.
10. Some young adult SCID mice can generate a few clones of functional B- and T-lymphocytes, which can impair their tolerance of heterologous tissue. Hence, at age 6 wk, screening for high IgM titers (>3.0 µg/mL) by enzyme-linked immunosorbent assay before use is recommended.
11. Anesthetized mice are separated from nonanesthetized mice until recovery to avoid possible injuries from biting.

References

1. Gilchrest, B. A., Eller, M. S., Geller, A. C., and Yaar, M. (1999) The pathogenesis of melanoma induced by ultraviolet radiation. *N. Engl. J. Med.* **340,** 1341–1348.
2. Bradl, M., Klein-Szanto, A., Porter, S., and Mintz, B. (1991) Malignant melanoma in transgenic mice. *Proc. Natl. Acad. Sci. USA* **88,** 164–168.
3. Iwamoto, T., Takahashi, M., Ito, M., Hamatani, K., Ohbayashi, M., Wajjwalku, W., Isobe, K., and Nakashima, I. (1991) Aberrant melanogenesis and melanocytic tumour development in transgenic mice that carry a metallothionein/ret fusion gene. *EMBO J.* **10,** 3167–3175.
4. Takayama. H., LaRochelle, W. J., Sharp, R., Otsuka, T., Kriebel, P., Anver, M., Aaronson, S. A., and Merlino, G. (1997) Diverse tumorigenesis associated with aberrant development in mice overexpressing hepatocyte growth factor/scatter factor. *Proc. Natl. Acad. Sci. USA* **94,** 701–706.
5. Chin, L., Pomerantz, J., Polsky, D., Jacobson, M., Cohen, C., Cordon-Cardo, C., Horner, J. W. II, and DePinho, R. A. (1997) Cooperative effects of INK4a and ras in melanoma susceptibility in vivo. *Genes Dev.* **11,** 2822–2834.
6. Zhu, H., Reuhl, K., Zhang, X., Botha, R., Ryan, K., Wei, J., and Chen, S. (1998) Development of heritable melanoma in transgenic mice. *J. Invest. Dermatol.* **110,** 247–252.

7. Setlow, R. B., Woodhead, A. D., and Grist, E. (1989) Animal model for ultraviolet radiation-induced melanoma: platyfish-swordtail hybrid. *Proc. Natl. Acad. Sci. USA* **86,** 8922–8926.
8. Ley, R. D., Applegate, L. A., Padilla, R. S., and Stuart, T. D. (1989) Ultraviolet radiation-induced malignant melanoma in Monodelphis domestica. *Photochem. Photobiol.* **50,** 1–5.
9. Millikan, L. E., Hook, R. R., and Manning, P. J. (1973) Immunobiology of melanoma: gross and ultrastructural studies in a new melanoma model: the Sinclair swine. *Yale J. Biol. Med.* **46,** 631–645.
10. Chernozemski, I. and Raichev, R. (1966) Two transplantable lines from melanomas induced in Syrian hamsters with 9,10 dimethyl-1,2-benz(a)anthracene (DMBA). *Neoplasma* **13,** 577–582.
11. Epstein, J. H., Epstein, W. L., and Nakai, T. (1967) Production of melanomas from DMBA-induced "blue nevi" in hairless mice with ultraviolet light. *J. Natl. Cancer Inst.* **38,** 19–30.
12. Clark, W. H. Jr., Min, B. H., and Kligman, L. H. (1976) The developmental biology of induced malignant melanoma in guinea pigs and a comparison with other neoplastic systems. *Cancer Res.* **36,** 4079–4091.
13. Rofstad, E. K. and Lyng, H. (1996) Xenograft model systems for human melanoma. *Mol. Med. Today* **2,** 394–403.
14. Atillasoy, E. S., Seykora, J. T., Soballe, P. W., Elenitsas, R., Nesbit, M., Elder, D. E., Montone, K. T., Sauter, E., and Herlyn, M. (1998) UVB induces atypical melanocytic lesions and melanoma in human skin. *Am. J. Pathol.* **152,** 1179–1186.
15. Reed, N. D. and Manning, D. D. (1973) Long-term maintenance of normal human skin on congenitally athymic (nude) mice. *Proc. Soc. Exp. Biol. Med.* **143,** 350–353.
16. Sundberg, J. P. (1994) The nude (nu) and streaker (nu^{str}) mutations, chromosome 11, in *Handbook of Mouse Mutations with Skin and Hair Abnormalities: Animal Models and Biomedical Tools* (Sundberg, J. P., ed.), CRC Press, Boca Raton, FL, pp. 379–389.
17. Sundberg, J. P. and Shultz, L. D. (1994) The severe combined immunodeficiency (scid) mutation, chromosome 16, in *Handbook of Mouse Mutations with Skin and Hair Abnormalities: Animal Models and Biomedical Tools* (Sundberg, J. P., ed.), CRC Press, Boca Raton, FL, pp. 423–429.
18. Bosma, M. J. and Carroll, A. M. (1991) The SCID mouse mutant: definition, characterization, and potential uses. *Annu. Rev. Immunol.* **9,** 323–350.
19. Mombaerts, P., Iacomini, J., Johnson, R. S., Herrup, K., Tonegawa, S., and Papaioannou, V. E. (1992) RAG-1-deficient mice have no mature B and T lymphocytes. *Cell* **68,** 869–877.
20. Kim, Y. H., Woodley, D. T., Wynn, K. C., Giomi, W., and Bauer, E. A. (1992) Recessive dystrophic epidermolysis bullosa phenotype is preserved in xenografts using SCID mice: development of an experimental in vivo model. *J. Invest. Dermatol.* **98,** 191–197.

21. Kawamura, T., Niguma, T., Fechner, J. H. Jr., Wolber, R., Beeskau, M. A., Hullett, D. A., Sollinger, H. W., and Burlingham, W. J. (1992) Chronic human skin graft rejection in severe combined immunodeficient mice engrafted with human PBL from an HLA-presensitized donor. *Transplantation* **53,** 659–665.

22. Yan, H.-C., Juhasz, I., Pilewski, J., Murphy, G. F., Herlyn, M., and Albelda, S. M. (1993) Human/severe combined immunodeficient mouse chimeras: an experimental in vivo model system to study the regulation of human endothelial cell-leukocyte adhesion molecules. *J. Clin. Invest.* **91,** 986–996.

23. Juhasz, I., Albelda, S. M., Elder, D. E., Murphy, G. F., Adachi, K., Herlyn, D., Valyi-Nagy, I. T., and Herlyn, M. (1993) Growth and invasion of human melanomas in human skin grafted to immunodeficient mice. *Am. J. Pathol.* **143,** 528–537.

24. Nickoloff, B. J., Kunkel, S. L., Burdick, M., and Strieter, R. M. (1995) Severe combined immunodeficiency mouse and human psoriatic skin chimeras: validation of a new animal model. *Am. J. Pathol.* **146,** 580–588.

25. Atillasoy, E. S., Elenitsas, R., Sauter, E. R., Soballe, P. W., and Herlyn, M. (1997) UVB induction of epithelial tumors in human skin using a RAG-1 mouse xenograft model. *J. Invest. Dermatol.* **109,** 704–709.

26. Kaufmann, R., Mielke, V., Reimann, J., Klein, C. E., and Sterry, W. (1993) Cellular and molecular composition of human skin in long-term xenografts on SCID mice. *Exp. Dermatol.* **2,** 209–216.

27. Murray, A. G., Schechner, J. S., Epperson, D. E., Sultan, P., Hughes, C. C., Lorber, M. I., Askenase, P. W., and Pober, J. S. (1998) Dermal microvascular injury in the human peripheral blood lymphocyte reconstituted-severe combined immunodeficient (HuPBL-SCID) mouse/skin allograft model is T-cell mediated and inhibited by a combination of cyclosporine and rapamycin. *Am. J. Pathol.* **153,** 627–638.

28. Grichnik, J. M., Burch, J. A., Burchette, J., and Shea, C. R. (1998) The SCF/KIT pathway plays a critical role in the control of normal human melanocyte homeostasis. *J. Invest. Dermatol.* **111,** 233–238.

29. Soballe, P. W., Montone, K. T., Satyamoorthy, K., Nesbit, M., and Herlyn, M. (1996) Carcinogenesis in human skin grafted to SCID mice. *Cancer Res.* **56,** 757–764.

30. Nomura, T., Nakajima, H., Hongyo, T., et al. (1997) Induction of cancer, actinic keratosis, and specific p53 mutations by UVB light in human skin maintained in severe combined immunodeficient mice. *Cancer Res.* **57,** 2081–2084.

31. Hansbrough, J. F., Morgan, J. L., Greenleaf, G. E., and Bartel, R. (1993) Composite grafts of human keratinocytes grown on a polyglactin mesh-cultured fibroblast dermal substitute function as a bilayer skin replacement in full-thickness wounds on athymic mice. *Burn Care Rehabil.* **14,** 485–494.

32. Boyce, S. T. (1999) Methods for the serum-free culture of keratinocytes and transplantation of collagen-GAG-based skin substitutes, in *Methods in Molecular Medicine*, vol. 18 (Morgan, J. R. and Yarmush, M. L., eds.), Humana, Totowa, NJ, pp. 365–389.

5

Dissection of Immunosuppressive Effects of Ultraviolet Radiation

Stephen E. Ullrich and David A. Schmitt

1. Introduction

For nearly 100 yr physicians and scientists have appreciated the carcinogenic potential of the ultraviolet (UV) radiation present in sunlight (*1,2*). During the latter part of the twentieth century, immunologists and dermatologists realized that UV radiation suppressed the immune response (*3–5*). Moreover, the immune suppression induced by UV radiation is a major risk factor for the induction of nonmelanoma skin cancer (*6*). The association between nonmelanoma skin cancer induction and immune suppression has fueled the efforts of many to study the immunologic mechanism underlying UV-induced immune suppression. This chapter focuses on describing the methods used to dissect the suppressive effects of UV on the immune system, concentrating particularly on in vivo models of immunity.

Data indicating that UV exposure is immune suppressive was initially provided by Kripke (*4*). In those experiments nonmelanoma skin tumors were induced by a chronic course of UV exposure. Unlike most murine tumors, the UV-induced nonmelanoma skin tumors failed to grow progressively when transplanted into normal syngeneic hosts. Progressive growth only occurred if the UV-induced skin cancers were transplanted into immune-compromised animals. This observation indicated that the UV-induced skin tumors were recognized and rejected by the intact immune system of the normal syngeneic host and suggested that unlike most murine tumors, the skin cancers induced by UV radiation were highly antigenic. What was not readily apparent from these findings, however, was a mechanism to explain how the highly antigenic UV-induced skin tumors could escape immune rejection and develop in the

From: *Methods in Molecular Medicine, Vol. 61: Melanoma: Methods and Protocols*
Edited by: B. J. Nickoloff © Humana Press Inc., Totowa, NJ

UV-irradiated host. Subsequent studies demonstrated that subcarcinogenic exposure to UV radiation caused the activation of CD3$^+$, CD4$^+$, CD8$^-$ antigen-specific suppressor T-cells that suppressed the development of tumor immunity in the UV-irradiated autochthonous host *(5,7,8)*. These studies relied on transferring suppressor T-cells from the UV-irradiated mice into normal syngeneic recipients, where they presumably suppress the immune response of the recipient and permit the progressive growth of the antigenic tumors. Although quite informative, this approach is difficult owing to the large numbers of mice required; the chronic UV irradiation protocol needed to induce suppressor T cells; and the end point of tumor growth in the recipient mice, which requires a 6- to 8-wk follow-up. Because of these problems, most investigators have used a surrogate model system—UV-induced suppression of delayed-in-time hypersensitivity reactions (contact and/or delayed-type hypersensitivity [DTH] reactions)—to dissect the mechanisms involved in UV-induced immune suppression. The advantages of this model system include suppression following a single exposure to UV radiation; immunization with well-known, well-characterized antigens; and end points (ear and/or footpad swelling) that are easily quantified, amenable to standard statistical analysis, and measured 10–15 d after the initiation of the experiment.

In this chapter, we describe the protocol for measuring the effects of UV radiation on the induction of DTH and contact hypersensitivity. We pay particular attention to describing the methods and procedures that have been useful in dissecting the mechanisms through which UV exposure suppresses the immune response.

2. Materials

2.1. Mice

Specific pathogen-free mice are obtained from the National Cancer Institute Frederick Cancer Research Facility Animal Production Area (Frederick, MD). Female C3H/HeN, Balb/c, or C57BL/6 mice, between 10 and 12 wk of age (weighing approx 20 g) are used. The animals are maintained in facilities approved by the Association for Assessment and Accreditation of Laboratory Care International, in accordance with current regulations of the US Department of Health and Human Services. The animal procedures described herein were all reviewed and approved by the Institutional Animal Care and Use Committee. Within each experiment the mice are age and sex matched (*see* **Note 1**).

2.2. Source of UV Radiation

The mice are irradiated with a bank of six FS-40 sunlamps (National Biological, Twinsberg, OH). These lamps emit a continuous spectrum from 270 to

390 nm, with a peak emission at 313 nm. Approximately 60% of the energy emitted by the FS-40 is within the UVB region of the solar spectrum. The irradiance of the source is measured by an IL-1700 research radiometer using an SEE 240 UVB detector equipped with an A127 quartz diffuser (International Light, Newburyport, MA) (*see* **Notes 2** and **3**).

2.3. Antigens and Haptens

To immunize for DTH, allogeneic spleen cells are used. To sensitize for CHS, haptens such as 4-ethoxymethylene-2-phenyl-2-oxasolon-5-one or 1,4-dinitroflurobenzene are purchased from Sigma (St. Louis, MO) and diluted in acetone.

2.4. Antibodies and Biologic Reagents

Recombinant interleukin-10 (IL-20), IL-12, and interferon-γ, as well as the antibodies specific for these cytokines are purchased from PharMingen (San Diego, CA). On receipt the recombinant cytokines are aseptically dispensed into microcentrifuge tubes and held at –80°C. Once thawed, the tubes are held at 4°C until completely used. The antibodies are generally held at 4°C. Care is taken to avoid multiple freezing and thawing of any cytokine or antibody. Cocktails of cell surface antibodies used for negative and positive enrichment of cells by immunomagnetic selection are purchased from Stem Cell Technologies (Vancouver, BC) and stored at 4°C.

2.5. Miscellaneous Supplies

Electric clippers (Oster model no. 01-331) equipped with a size 40 blade set can be purchased from Fisher (Houston, TX). Engineer's micrometers are acquired from Mitutoyo (Tokyo, Japan). RPMI-1640 tissue culture medium is from Gibco (Grand Island, NY). Nembutal (sodium pentobarbital; 0.1 mL of a 5 mg/mL solution 10 g of body weight) or 0.1 mL/10 g of body weight of a ready-to-use ketamine hydrochloride/xylazine hydrochloride solution is used to immobilize the mice (Research Biochemicals, Natick, MA). Guinea pig complement is purchased from Pel-Freeze (Rodgers, AK). Immunomagnetic beads and magnets are acquired from Dynal (Great Neck, NY) or from Stem Cell Technologies.

3. Methods
3.1. Suppression of DTH by UV Radiation

Figure 1 illustrates the general scheme of the experimental protocol. The first step in the procedure is to shave the mice. Place the mouse on a cage top, hold the tail, and clip off the hair. Generally we shave from the midline of the

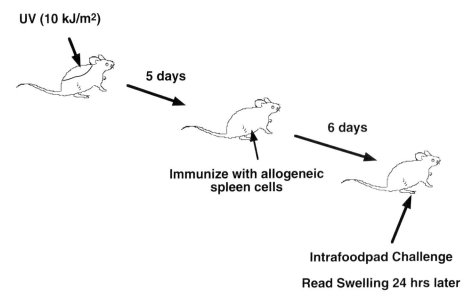

Fig. 1. General scheme for inducing immune suppression following UV exposure.

back to a point about halfway down the flank (**Fig. 2A**). Then place the mice are into standard-sized animal cages into which have been placed specially constructed Plexiglas dividers to prevent the animals from climbing on each other's backs and interfering with the irradiation (**Fig. 2B**). Place the cages under the FS-40 bulbs and expose to UV radiation. We strongly suggest that a series of different irradiation times be used in the initial experiments to construct a dose response curve.

Three to 5 d after exposure, immunize the mice with the antigen. To induce DTH, allogeneic spleen cells are used. For example, if the animals receiving the UV radiation are C3H/HeN, we prepare spleen cells from C57BL/6 or Balb/c mice. Kill the spleen cell donors, remove the spleens, and prepare single cell suspensions by gently pressing the spleens between two glass microscope slides. Collect the cells, resuspend in RPMI-1640 medium, wash, and count. Resuspend the cells at a concentration of 10^8/mL and inject 0.25 mL of this suspension (sc injection) into each flank.

Six days later challenge the mice with allogeneic spleen cells. The site of challenge is the footpad (**Fig. 2C**). Use Nembutal or ketamine/xylazine anesthesia to immobilize the mice. Measure the baseline footpad thickness with the engineer's micrometer and record the thickness. Prepare allogeneic spleen cells as described above. Resuspend the cells at a concentration of 2×10^8/mL and using a 1-cc insulin syringe, inject both hind footpads with 50 µL of this cell

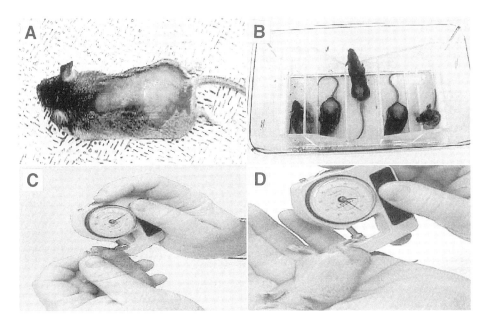

Fig. 2. Exposing mice to UV radiation and measuring ear and/or footpad swelling. **(A)** A mouse after removal of dorsal hair; **(B)** use of cage dividers to prevent cagemates from climbing on each other and interfering with UV exposure; **(C)** where ears are measured before and after challenge; **(D)** where footpads are measured before and after challenge.

suspension. The next day (18–24 h later) immobilize the mouse with anesthesia, and remeasure the hind footpads. Record this number. The footpad swelling, which is a measure of the DTH reaction and is comparable to the wheal and flare reaction seen in humans, is determined by subtracting the initial baseline thickness from the value obtained after challenge (*9*) (*see* **Notes 4** and **5**).

3.2. Suppression of CHS by UV Radiation

Alternatively, one may choose to use CHS as the immunologic end point. This requires two modifications of the procedure described in **Subheading 3.1.** First, because the site of challenge, the ears, will be exposed to UV radiation during the first step, they must be protected. To do this, place a piece of electrical tape over the ears. The use of anesthesia, such as Nembutal or ketamine/xylazine may facilitate application of the tape. Second, the hapten must be applied directly to the skin rather than sc injection as described in **Subheading 3.1.** To accomplish this, first remove the abdominal hair with electric clippers. Then remove any remaining hair by shaving with a razor blade. Care must be taken to avoid abrading the skin at this stage because it may interfere with proper sensitization. Then apply the hapten with a micropipet, using the tip of the pipet to distribute the solution evenly over the skin. Because the hapten is diluted in acetone or ethanol containing vehicles, we suggest that the animal be shaved 1 d prior to sensitization to minimize the discomfort that may result from applying the solution to freshly shaved skin.

Six days after sensitization, challenge the mice. Immobilize the animals with anesthesia, measure the ear thickness, and record the measurements (**Fig. 2D**). The next day (18–24 h later) immobilize the mouse with anesthesia, remeasure the ears, and record this number. The ear swelling, which is a measure of the CHS is determined by subtracting the initial baseline thickness from the value obtained after challenge *(9)* (*see* **Notes 4** and **5**).

3.3. Adoptive Transfer of Immune Suppression

The existence of suppressor cells is denoted based on function—the ability of these cells to suppress the induction of DTH/CHS when transferred into naïve mice. A two-part procedure is used (**Fig. 3**). The first part of the procedure is described above: induction of immune suppression by UV exposure. To determine whether suppressor cells were induced in the UV-irradiated animal, an adoptive transfer procedure is used. Immediately after reading the challenge site, kill the mice and remove their spleens. Make a single cell suspension and wash the cells and resuspend in RPMI-1640 medium. Count the cells and adjust to 2×10^8 cells/mL. Insert 0.5 mL of this cell suspension into the tail veins of normal syngeneic age- and sex-matched recipient mice. Then immediately immunize the recipients with antigen or paint with the contact allergen. Six days later, challenge the mice, and measure DTH/CHS 18–24 h later, as described above. Suppression of the induction of immunity in the recipient mice indicates the induction of suppressor cells in the irradiated donor mice *(10)*. Specificity of suppression can be ascertained by immunizing the recipient mice with an irrelevant antigen. For example, if the donor UV-irradiated C3H/HeN mice were immunized with Balb/c spleen cells, inject cells from these mice into two groups of syngeneic recipients. Immunize and challenge one group with the same antigen as the donor (Balb/c) and immunize and challenge the other group with C57BL/6 spleen cells. If the suppressor cells are specific then only the response in the recipient mice immunized with the Balb/c spleen cells will be suppressed *(11)* (*see* **Note 6**).

3.3.1. Depletion of Cell Subsets

The nature of the cells that transfer immune suppression can be elucidated by several methods. We have regularly employed two: depletion of function by antibody-mediated complement lysis, or depletion of function by removing a cell population with antibody-coated magnetic beads. Depletion with antibody

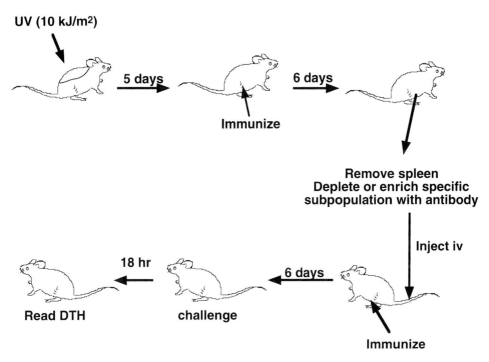

Fig. 3. Scheme for determining the induction of suppressor T-cells.

and complement is accomplished by the following procedure. First, lyse contaminating erythrocytes with ammonium chloride (0.83% in 0.001 M Tris-HCl, pH 7.2, 10 min at room temperature; wash the cells in RPMI-1640). Resuspend the cells at a concentration of 10^7/mL in RPMI-1640 medium supplemented with 5% bovine serum albumin (BSA) and 10 μg/mL of monoclonal anti-CD3, or anti-CD4, or anti-CD8, and so on. Hold the cells at 4°C for 30 min to 1 h, and then wash and resuspend in medium containing guinea pig complement (1:8 dilution) for 1 h at 37°C. Next, wash, count, and inject the cells into the recipient animals *(11)*.

Alternatively, one may remove or enrich a population of cells by using antibody-coated magnetic beads. Lyse the erythrocytes and treat the cells with antibody (i.e., anti-CD3) as described above. After washing resuspend the cells in medium containing 1% BSA at a concentration of 1 to 2×10^7/mL. Then add sheep antirat IgG-coated immunomagnetic beads to the cell suspension at a ratio of four beads per cell and incubate at 4°C for 30 min. CD3-positive cells attach to the beads and can be removed by passing the cells over a strong magnet; the cells of interest are held up by the magnet, and all others pass through. The negative population can then be injected into the recipient mice and the effect removing a specific population has on the transfer of immune suppression is noted. However, the real advantage of using this technique to isolate a cell population is the ability to enrich for the cells of interest. The CD3-positive cells can be detached mechanically by vigorous pipeting and washing, culturing overnight at 37°C, or using a new generation of beads (Dynal) in which the antibody is attached to the bead by a nucleic acid linker. Treating the cells with DNase digests the linker and liberates the cells from the magnetic bead *(12)* (*see* **Note 7**).

3.4. Determination of Tolerance Induction

The induction of long-term immunologic tolerance is measured by a modification of the procedures described above. The protocol for shaving the mice, exposing the mice to UV radiation, and immunization is the same. The difference is in the challenge step. In tolerance induction experiments, we want to expose the mice to UV radiation, determine whether this treatment induces immune suppression, and then wait a period of time (2–4 wk) and remeasure the ability of the animal to mount an immune response. Because we need to challenge the same animal twice, we need to avoid challenging both feet and both ears after the initial immunization. Thus, 6 d after immunization challenge only the right hind footpad (or right ear) (generally we double the numbers of mice in each group to ensure sufficient statistical power). Record the swelling and return the mice to the animal facility. Fourteen days later, immunize the mice a second time. The site of immunization is important; the hapten and/or antigen is always applied or injected at a site distant from the original site. Six days after the second immunization, inject the allogeneic spleen cells into the left hind footpad (or paint the hapten on the left ear). Failure to respond to the second immunization indicates tolerance induction. Specificity of tolerance induction can be determined by using an irrelevant antigen during the reimmunization step *(13)* (*see* **Note 8**).

3.5. Mechanisms of UV-Induced Immune Suppression

Up to this point, we have described the basic mechanisms for measuring UV-induced systemic immune suppression. These procedures have served as the foundation for determining the mechanisms through which UV radiation interferes with the induction of an immune response. Because a review of all the pertinent literature in this area is beyond the scope of this chapter (For a review, *see* **ref. 14**), we use a schematic representation to illustrate the approaches that have been used (**Fig. 4**). Generally, the approaches that have been successful include the following:

1. Blocking the immune suppression induced by UV with monoclonal antibodies to some of the mediators involved such as *cis*-urocanic acid, IL-4, and IL-10.

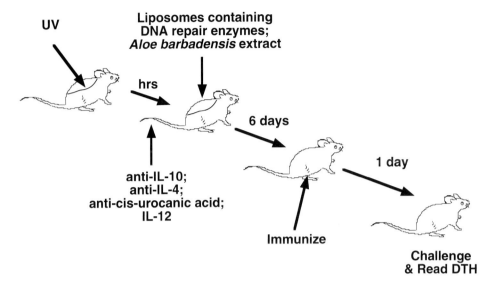

Fig. 4. Strategies used to interfere with UV-induced immune suppression, thereby determining mechanisms involved.

2. Blocking prostaglandin E_2 production with specific cyclooxygenase-2 inhibitors.
3. Mimicking the effects of UV radiation with purified *cis*-urocanic acid or recombinant IL-10.
4. Repairing DNA damage by using liposomes to deliver DNA repair enzymes directly to UV-irradiated skin.
5. Reversing UV-induced immune suppression with immune modulators such as IL-12.

4. Notes

1. Healthy animals, maintained in a state-of-the-art animal facility, are critical to the success of these experiments. The temperature, humidity, ambient lighting conditions, and microbial load of the mice must be rigorously controlled to ensure success. The age of the mice is also critical; generally, we find that mice between 8 and 12 wk of age perform best in the DTH and CHS experiments described. As they become older, the magnitude of the immune response generated subsides. For proper statistical analysis of the data, groups of 5–10 mice are required. Some investigators use hairless (Skh/Hr-1) mice in these types of experiments. The use of this strain of animals eliminates the requirement for shaving; however, if cell transfer experiments are conducted, inbred syngeneic mice are required and the availability of inbred hairless mice can sometimes present a problem.

2. For the bulk of the experiments done in our laboratory and in most other photobiology laboratories, the UV radiation is supplied by a bank of FS-40 or FS-20 sunlamps. The spectral output of an FS-20 is the same as that of an FS-40; the 20 and 40 refer to the overall size of the lamp. The advantage of the FS-40 is that it is an inexpensive fluorescent lightbulb that can be used in a standard lighting fixture to irradiate a large surface area. The bulb emits approx 0.5% of its energy in the UVC (200–280 nm) region of the solar spectrum, 60% of its energy in the UVB (280–320 nm), and 40% of its energy in the UVA (320–400 nm). The problem with the FS-40 is that it does not mimic the spectral output of sunlight. All the UVC in sunlight and the UVB radiation below 300 nm is removed by the atmospheric ozone layer. In addition, sunlight contains a much higher proportion of UVA radiation than that emitted by an FS-40 sunlamp. If you need to mimic the radiation emitted by the sun in your experiments (i.e., measuring the efficacy of sunscreens in preventing UV-induced immune suppression), a solar simulator is required. We use an Oriel 1000W Solar UV simulator equipped with an atmospheric attenuation filter (Schott WG-320; 1 mm thick), a visible/infrared bandpass blocking filter (Schott UG-11; 1 mm thick), and a dichroic mirror to further reduce visible and infrared energy (Oriel, Stratford, CT). No UVC is emitted by this light source, all UVB below 295 nm is filtered out, and a large proportion of the energy emitted by this light source is in the UVA region of the solar spectrum. The disadvantages of using a solar simulator is the purchase price (>$35,000), the relative small field of irradiation, and the time and costs associated with maintaining the machine.

3. Because of shielding by the metal cage lids (approx 50% of the energy is filtered out by the wire cage tops), we place the detector in an empty mouse cage, put the metal cage lid in place, put the cage under the FS-40 sunlamps, and proceed with the measurements. The intensity of irradiation along the FS-40 bulb varies; it is most intense at the center, and the intensity decreases as near the end of the bulb. For this reason, we take measurements at the center of the bulb and approximately one third of the length of the bulb from the end, and use the average of the three measurements when calculating the output of the bulb. Generally, the variation from the readings at the center to the end of the bulb is in the range of 5–7%. For this reason, we do not use the end of the bulb to irradiate mice.

4. The controls for these experiments are critical. The positive control consists of a group of normal nonirradiated mice that are immunized (or sensitized) and challenged. The negative control consists of a group of mice that are not immunized (or sensitized) but are challenged. The background response of the negative controls is then subtracted from the values obtained in the positive control group and the experimental groups to yield the specific swelling response. Some investigators inject the contralateral foot with phosphate-buffered saline (PBS) or paint the contralateral ear with the vehicle (i.e., acetone) and use this as the background value. We caution against this practice. In addition to being contact allergens, the haptens used here are also, to a degree, irritants. Similarly, injecting 10^7 cells into

a footpad will induce a degree of footpad swelling. Simply injecting 50 μL of PBS into a foot or painting the ears with acetone will not adequately mimic the irritant effect. It is better to control for this effect by challenging a group of mice that are not immunized.

5. There are several tricks in measuring ear and footpad thickness that will decrease error. First, one person should do both measurements (pre- and postchallenge). Second, the same spot on the foot and ear should be measured on both days (**Fig. 2C,D**). Third, the same micrometer should be used to do the pre- and postchallenge measurements. The micrometers are spring loaded; we take care to avoid allowing the piston of the micrometer to smash down on the ear or foot, because this will distort the reading. Usually one person does all the measurements and another records all the data. The added advantage of having two people do the measurements is that they can be done in a blinded fashion to minimize investigator bias.

6. Although it is a natural tendency of cell biologists to place a tubefull of cells into an ice bucket, this must be avoided during this procedure. Injecting 0.5–1 mL of cold media IV will induce acute hypothermia, and we have lost mice to cold shock. Another cause of fatality is induction of a pulmonary embolism owing to cell clumping. We filter out cell clumps by twice passing the cell suspension through sterile gauze. In every cell transfer experiment the following controls are run: the negative control (not immunized but challenged), the positive control (immunized and challenged), and a control in which 10^8 normal spleen cells are injected into normal mice that are then immunized and challenged. This last control documents that the simple procedure of transferring spleen cells is not affecting, either positively or negatively, the induction of immunity in the recipient mice.

7. Complement depletion of cells is sometimes hampered by nonspecific toxicity. Treating the target cells with an irrelevant antibody and complement to ensure that the results obtained are not owing to nonspecific killing is an essential control in these experiments. Although somewhat more expensive, the use of magnetic bead technology offers a number of distinct advantages. First and foremost, this procedures enables having two pools of cells at the end of the day, one enriched for the population in question and one depleted of that population. Second, it offers the capability of recovering large numbers of cells in a relatively short time, with a high degree of purity. Third, it is amenable to both positive and negative selection. This is an important consideration in studies in which cellular function is the readout. For example, if naïve splenic CD4-positive cells are desired, an antibody cocktail that will stain CD8 cells, B-cells, dendritic cells, erythrocytes, and macrophages can be purchased (Stem Cell Technologies). All the undesired cells bind to the beads and are retained by the magnet, leaving a relatively pure population of unstained, naïve CD4-positive cells behind. Because some of the antibodies used here, especially anti-CD3, will activate cells, this is an important consideration.

8. In addition to the negative and positive controls described in **Note 6**, one additional control must be run in tolerance induction experiments. During the second

immunization step it is necessary to include one group of naïve animals that are being immunized (sensitized) for the first time. A positive response in these mice means that the antigen or hapten that you are using is potent and capable of immunizing. Because tolerance is a failure to respond to a second exposure to antigen, if, for some reason, the antigen loses its potency over 14–21 d, the end result would functionally be similar and interfere with the proper interpretation of the data.

References

1. Urbach, F. (1978) Evidence and epidemiology of UV-induced carcinogenesis in man. *Natl. Cancer Inst. Monogr.* **50,** 5–10.
2. Urbach, F. (1997) Ultraviolet radiation and skin cancer of humans. *J. Photochem. Photobiol. B: Biol.* **40,** 3–7.
3. Fisher, M. S. and Kripke, M. L. (1977) Systemic alteration induced in mice by ultraviolet light irradiation and its relationship to ultraviolet carcinogenesis. *Proc. Natl. Acad. Sci. USA* **74,** 1688–1692.
4. Kripke, M. L. (1974) Antigenicity of murine skin tumors induced by UV light. *J. Natl. Cancer Inst.* **53,** 1333–1336.
5. Fisher, M. S. and Kripke, M. L. (1982) Suppressor T lymphocytes control the development of primary skin cancers in UV-irradiated mice. *Science* **216,** 1133–1134.
6. Yoshikawa, T., Rae, V., Bruins-Slot, W., Van den Berg, J. W., Taylor, J. R., and Streilein, J. W. (1990) Susceptibility to effects of UVB radiation on induction of contact hypersensitivity as a risk factor for skin cancer in humans. *J. Invest. Dermatol.* **95,** 530–536.
7. Fisher, M. S. and Kripke, M. L. (1978) Further studies on the tumor-specific suppressor cells induced by ultraviolet radiation. *J. Immunol.* **121,** 1139–1144.
8. Ullrich, S. E. and Kripke, M. L. (1984) Mechanisms in the suppression of tumor rejection produced in mice by repeated UV irradiation. *J. Immunol.* **133,** 2786–2790.
9. Kim, T.-K., Ullrich, S. E., Ananthaswamy, H. N., Zimmerman, S., and Kripke, M. L. (1998) Suppression of delayed and contact hypersensitivity responses in mice have different UV dose responses. *Photchem. Photobiol.* **68,** 738–744.
10. Schmitt, D. A., Owen-Schaub, L., and Ullrich, S. E. (1995) Effect of IL-12 on immune suppression and suppressor cell induction by ultraviolet radiation. *J. Immunol.* **154,** 5114–5420.
11. Magee, M. J., Kripke, M. L., and Ullrich, S. E. (1989) Suppression of the elicitation of the immune response to alloantigen by ultraviolet radiation. *Transplantation* **47,** 1008–1013.
12. Moodycliffe, A. M., Maiti, S., and Ullrich, S. E. (1999) Splenic NK1.1-negative, TCR intermediate CD4+ T cells exist in naive NK1.1 allelic positive and negative mice, with the capacity to rapidly secrete large amounts of IL-4 and IFN-γ upon primary TCR stimulation. *J. Immunol.* **162,** 5156–5163.

13. Niizeki, H. and Streilein, J. W. (1997) Hapten-specific tolerance induced by acute, low-dose ultraviolet B radiation of skin is mediated via interleukin-10. *J. Invest. Dermatol.* **109,** 25–30.
14. Ullrich, S. E. (2000) The effects of ultraviolet radiation on the immune response, in *Biochemical Modulation of Skin Reactions in Dermal and Transdermal Delivery of Drugs* (Kydonieus, A. F. and Wille, J. J., eds.), CRC Press, Boca Raton, FL, pp. 281–300.

6

Antisense Oligonucleotides as Research Tools

Jennifer K. Taylor, Scott R. Cooper, and Nicholas M. Dean

1. Introduction

The use of antisense oligonucleotides as both research tools and therapeutic molecules has emerged as a powerful alternative to small molecule inhibitors. Antisense oligonucleotides are short pieces of chemically modified DNA designed to hybridize to specific mRNA sequences present in the target gene. The oligonucleotide interaction with the targeted mRNA can lead to inhibition in the translation of the protein encoded by the targeted transcript through a variety of reasonably well-characterized mechanisms *(1–3)*.

Because antisense oligonucleotides hybridize to the mRNA in a sequence-specific manner, knowledge of the function, structure, and localization of the target protein is not required. The only information needed is the nucleic acid sequence of the target gene. Because of recent advances in large-scale genomic sequencing, there has been a rapid increase in the rate and amount of sequence information available. Antisense technology may be useful in determining the function of unknown proteins because it allows the direct use of DNA sequence information to identify inhibitors of gene expression.

Antisense oligonucleotides can serve as therapeutic molecules in their own right. To this end, oligonucleotides have demonstrated pharmacologic activity in a number of animal models of human disease. Several human clinical trials have been undertaken in autoimmune diseases (Crohn disease, inflammatory bowel disease, psoriasis, rheumatoid arthritis) *(4)*, and cancer *(5,6)*. Recently, the Food and Drug Administration issued approval for the antisense compound Vitravene™ as an inhibitor of cytomegalovirus retinitis.

Because antisense oligonucleotide inhibitors can be extremely specific and selective in reducing gene expression, several groups of investigators have used

From: *Methods in Molecular Medicine, Vol. 61: Melanoma: Methods and Protocols*
Edited by: B. J. Nickoloff © Humana Press Inc., Totowa, NJ

this approach to inhibit expression of genes that may be involved in melanoma. These gene targets include Bcl-2, c-*myc*, protein kinase Cα (PKCα), and myb. A recent study examined the role of the apoptosis inhibitor protein, Bcl-2, in chemoresistance of melanoma *(7)*. Using antisense oligonucleotide inhibitors of Bcl-2, this study demonstrated that the reduction in Bcl-2 resulted in chemosensitization of human melanoma in severe combined immuno-deficiences (SCID) mice. The combination of Bcl-2 antisense oligonucleotides and the chemotherapeutic agent dacarbazine resulted in complete ablation of the tumor in three of six animals. Thus, in this xenotransplantation model, it is apparent that Bcl-2 has a role in protecting melanoma cells from chemothera-peutic agents.

Another potential gene involved in melanoma is c-*myc*. It is five- to ninefold more highly expressed in melanoma cells relative to that observed in normal melanocytes *(8–10)*. Treatment of human melanoma cells in vitro and in human melanoma xenografts in CD-1 nude mice demonstrated that c-*myc* antisense oligonucleotide inhibitors were able to inhibit the growth of all tested melanoma cultures and that this growth inhibition was associated with the induction of apoptosis *(8)*. Furthermore, the combination of c-*myc* and cisplatinum treatment exerted a significantly greater antiproliferative effect than either agent used alone *(11,12)*.

Previous evidence suggested that PKCα expression levels increase with melanoma metastasis *(13)*. Recently, it was shown that when C8161 cells were treated with an antisense inhibitor of PKCα and injected intravenously into athymic mice, metastasis was suppressed by 75% *(14)*. These results suggest that PKCα expression may be important in the regulation of human melanoma metastasis.

There is also evidence that the altered myb expression may be involved in the pathogenesis of melanoma *(15,16)*. Growth of representative melanoma cell lines was inhibited in vitro in a concentration- and sequence-dependent manner by targeting the myb gene with an antisense oligonucleotide inhibitor *(17)*. In SCID mice containing human melanoma tumors, infusion of the myb inhibitor resulted in long-term growth suppression of transplanted tumor cells *(17)*. These results suggest that myb may play a role in the growth of some human melanomas.

In this chapter, we focus on various aspects of how to apply antisense oligo-nucleotide technology to research purposes in melanoma-derived cell lines. We focus on the steps of oligonucleotide sequence identification, oligonucle-otide uptake, and in vitro pharmacology of antisense oligonucleotides.

2. Materials

The reagents needed for antisense oligonucleotide technology are fairly stan-dard in most laboratories. However, because different types of oligonucleotides are available, we present some background on oligonucleotide chemistry. Unmodified phosphodiester oligonucleotides are rapidly degraded in most biologic systems, and, therefore, they are not practical to use as antisense inhibitors. Considerable effort has been made to develop chemical modifications to improve oligonucleotide pharmacology. This area has been covered by excellent reviews *(18,19)*. The most commonly used and commercially available chemically modified oligonucleotides are phosphorothioate (P=S) oligodeoxynucleotides. In this modification, the nonbridging oxygen atoms are replaced by sulfur in the DNA backbone of the molecule. This modification results in a 100- to 300-fold increase in nuclease resistance compared with a phosphodiester oligonucleotide *(20)*. When carefully designed and used, this class of oligonucleotide provides effective and specific inhibitors of gene expression.

3. Methods
3.1. Oligonucleotide Sequence Identification

The selection of effective oligonucleotide sequence targets on a given mRNA transcript is a key issue. Antisense oligonucleotides are proposed to function through three different mechanisms: translation arrest, splicing arrest, and RNase H degradation. For the P=S oligodeoxynucleotides, the best characterized mechanism of action is through target mRNA degradation by RNase H, a class of ubiquitous enzymes found within eukaryotic cells in the nucleus and cytoplasm that degrades the RNA strand of an RNA:DNA duplex.

Several strategies to predict effective mRNA target sequences have been investigated. For the researcher interested in finding an oligonucleotide inhibitor of a specific gene product, we suggest a simple approach, that we have successfully employed *(21–23)*. This method requires the synthesis of a series of oligonucleotide sequences designed to hybridize to multiple sites throughout the target mRNA. These oligonucleotides are then evaluated for their ability to reduce the expression of either the target mRNA or protein. The "hit rate" for identifying active sequences varies from sequence to sequence, but, in general, the hit rate for P=S oligodeoxynucleotides is between 10 and 20%. Therefore, it is usually sufficient to evaluate between 10 and 15 oligonucleotides for activity. Two simple guidelines for oligonucleotide design are avoiding multiple contiguous G residues, which can affect oligonucleotide secondary structure, and avoiding oligonucleotide self-complementation.

3.2. Oligonucleotide Uptake

The ability of antisense oligonucleotides to reduce target gene expression in tissue culture cells is greatly enhanced by the use of uptake enhancers, and the use of such compounds is strongly recommended. Various agents have been used including cationic lipids *(21,24)*, liposomes *(25)*, peptides *(26)*, dendrimers *(27)*, polycations *(28)*, conjugation with cholesterol *(29)*, aggregation with cell-surface ligands *(11)*, streptolysin O *(30)*, and electroporation *(31)*. Commercially available cationic lipid preparations work well to enhance oligonucleotide activity for many cells and are a good first choice.

Cationic lipids appear not just to increase oligonucleotide accumulation in treated cells, but also to change oligonucleotide intracellular distribution *(21)*. This is characterized by increased oligonucleotide accumulation in the nucleus *(21)*, which may be required for the oligonucleotide to reduce target mRNA expression.

3.3. Antisense In Vitro Pharmacology

The most common mechanism of action for P=S oligonucleotides transfected into tissue culture cells is through a reduction in target mRNA expression by RNase H. The pharmacology of inhibition of gene expression by such a mechanism is fairly typical and reproducible. If the target gene is constitutively expressed, then one should expect greater than an 80% reduction at P=S oligodeoxynucleotide concentrations of between 0.2 and 1 μM *(22)*. This inhibition lasts between 24 and 48 h, depending on the cell line used *(22,32)*.

The use of proper controls is extremely important, and a number of suggestions have been proposed *(33)*. Briefly, at the very least, one should demonstrate a reduction in targeted mRNA and/or protein, determine the effects of the active oligonucleotide on another gene product, and determine the effects of mismatched oligonucleotides on the targeted gene product. If these simple rules are followed, the chances of misinterpreting data should be minimized.

4. Notes

1. Two common problems encountered using antisense oligonucleotides are no reduction in targeted RNA and nonspecific reduction of target RNA. The most frequent reasons that targeted RNA is not reduced by antisense oligonucleotides are either that cells are not efficiently transfected with oligo or that the optimal oligonucleotide sequence has not been identified. It is also important to remember that some cells are easier to transfect than others. By altering the cationic lipid or trying electroporation, one may be able to improve the transfection efficiency. We have successfully transfected human melanoma C8161 and Mel Juso cells, as well as human epidermal melanocytes.

   To transfect these cells successfully, the following procedure can be used. Work from a 1 mM stock oligonucleotide solution diluted to a working 1 or 10 μM solution. The concentration of the stock solution can be determined by the following procedure. Dilute a small aliquot 1 : 1000 (e.g., 5 μL in 5 mL) in 0.9%

saline solution in duplicate. Read the absorbance on a spectrophotometer at 260 nm. (The optical density should be between 0.1 and 1.0. If it is significantly higher than 1, you should dilute the sample further.) To calculate the amount of actual oligo present, multiply the absorbance value obtained by 1000 (or the dilution factor you used) and divide by the extinction coefficient for the oligonucleotide (usually provided by the commercial supplier of the oligonucleotide). This will give the millimolar concentration. To treat the cells with oligonucleotide, start with cells that are approx 80–90% confluent, and then do the following:

a. Wash the cells to remove serum-containing media.
b. Prepare lipofectin solution. We routinely use this to greatly (up to 1000-fold) increase oligo potency in vitro. Use 1–5 µL of lipofectin/(mL·100 n*M* oligo) (e.g., 10 µL of lipofectin/mL of media for a 200 n*M* oligo concentration). This procedure maintains a constant ratio between the oligo and the lipid. Add the lipofectin to the media (without serum) and shake vigorously to disperse the lipofectin (extremely important). Do this in the absence of antibiotics. Add this to the cells (typically 4 to 5 mL to a T-75 flask). Add the oligo to a final concentration of 50–400 n*M* from 1 or 10 µ*M* stock for the first screen for activity. shake the flask well again to fully complex the oligo/lipofectin (extremely important). The oligo and lipofectin solution can alternatively be preformulated before addition to the cells.
c. Allow the cells to incubate for 4 h. Occasionally swirl the solution around the cells to prevent drying.
d. Remove lipofectin solution and replace with media.
e. Allow the cells to incubate overnight and measure the target mRNA or protein expression. We normally measure mRNA expression, not protein expression, initially because some proteins have a long half-life, which can make further characterization necessary.

The 4-h incubation of cells with oligo and lipofectin effectively "loads" the cells with oligo and should keep mRNA expression down for up to 72 h. It is important to do these studies before looking at "phenotypic" changes in the cells, to confirm that the oligo effects are specific for a given target.

It is also important to demonstrate the specificity of the antisense oligonucleotide on the targeted mRNA and protein. By introducing mismatched bases into the oligonucleotide sequence, one should observe that the mRNA level of the targeted gene is not affected. Occasionally, one will continue to see a reduction in mRNA in spite of mismatched bases. This could be because too high a concentration of oligonucleotide has been used. It is important to optimize the concentration of antisense oligonucleotides used by performing a dose response. Then, when examining the specificity of the oligonucleotide, one should use the lowest, most effective concentration of oligonucleotide to avoid nonspecific effects.

The length of the oligonucleotide sequence is important for maintaining adequate specificity and optimal efficacy. Based on an estimate of approx 3 to 4 billion bp in the human genome and assuming a random distribution of bases, several investigators have calculated the minimum size needed to recognize a single specific sequence in the genome at between 12 and 15 bases *(34)*.

References

1. Crooke, S. T. (1998) Basic principles of antisense therapeutics, in *Antisense Research and Application* (Crooke, S. T., ed.), Springer-Verlag, Berlin, pp 1–50.
2. Crooke, S. T. and Bennett, C. F. (1996) Progress in antisense oligonucleotide therapeutics. *Annu. Rev. Pharmacol. Toxicol.* **36,** 107–129.
3. Gewirtz, A. M. (1997) Developing oligonucleotide therapeutics for human leukemia. *Anticancer Drug Des.* **12,** 341–358.
4. Shanahan, W. R. (1998) Properties of ISIS 2302, an inhibitor of intercellular adhesion molecule-1, in humans, in *Antisense Research and Application* (Crooke, S. T., ed.), Springer-Verlag, Berlin, pp. 499–524.
5. Dorr, F. A. and Kisner, D. L. (1998) Antisense oligonucleotides to protein kinase C-α and C-raf kinase: rationale and clinical experience in patients with solid tumors, in *Antisense Research and Applications* (Crooke, S. T., ed.), Springer-Verlag, Berlin, pp. 461–476.
6. Gerwitz, A. M. (1998) Nucleic acid therapeutics for human leukemia: development and early clinical experience with oligodeoxynucleotides directed against c-myb, in *Antisense Research and Applications* (Crooke, S. T., ed.), Springer-Verlag, Berlin, pp. 477–497.
7. Jansen, B., Schlagbauer-Wadl, H., Brown, B. D., Bryan, R. N., Van Elsas, A., Muller, M., Wolff, K., Eichler, H.-G., and Pehamberger, H. (1998) Bcl-2 antisense therapy chemosensitizes human melanoma in SCID mice. *Nat. Med.* **4,** 232–234.
8. Leonetti, C., D'Agnano, I., Lozypone, F., Valentini, A., Geiser, T., Zon, G., Calabretta, B., Citro, G., and Zupi, G. (1996) Antitumor effect of c-myc antisense phosphorothioate oligodeoxynucleotides on human melanoma cells in vitro and in mice. *J. Natl. Cancer Inst.* **88,** 419–429.
9. Grover, R., Ross, D. A., Richman, P. I., Robinson, B., and Wilson, G. D. (1996) C-myc oncogene expression in human melanoma and its relationship with tumor antigenicity. *Eur. J. Surg. Oncol.* **22,** 342–-346.
10. Schlagbauer-Wadl, H., Griffioen, M., Van Elsas, A., Schrier, P. I., Pastelnik, T., Eichler, H.,G., Wolff, K., Pehamberger, H., and Jansen, B. (1999) Influence of increased c-myc expression on the growth characteristics of human melanoma. *J. Invest. Dermatol.* **112,** 332–336.
11. Citro, G., D'Agnano, I., Leonetti, C., Perini, R., Bucci, B., Zon, G., Calabretta, B., and Zupi, G. (1998) C-myc antisense oligodeoxynucleotides enhance the efficacy of cisplatin in melanoma chemotherapy in vitro and in nude mice. *Cancer Res.* **58,** 283–289.
12. Leonetti, C., Biroccio, A., Candiloro, A., Citro, G., Fornari, C., Mottolese, M., Del Bufalo, D., and Zupi, G. (1999) Increase of cisplatin sensitivity by c-myc antisense oligodeoxynucleotides in a human metastatic melanoma inherently resistant to cisplatin. *Clin. Cancer Res.* **5,** 2588–2595.

13. Blobe, G. C., Obeid, L. M., and Hannun, Y. A. (1994) Regulation of protein kinase C and role in cancer biology. *Cancer Metast. Rev.* **13,** 411–431.

14. Dennis, J. U., Dean, N. M., Bennett, C. F., Griffith, J. W., Lang, C. M., and Welch, D. R. (1998) Human melanoma metastasis is inhibited following ex vivo treatment with an antisense oligonucleotide to protein kinase C-α. *Cancer Lett.* **128,** 65–70.

15. Dasgupta, P., Linnenbach, P., Giaccia, A. J., Stamato, T. D., and Reddy, E. P. (1989) Molecular cloning of the breakpoint region on chromosome 6 in cutaneous malignant melanoma: evidence for deletion in the c-myb locus and translocation of a segment of chromosome 12. *Oncogene* **4,** 1201–1205.

16. Gewirtz, A. M. (1999) Myb targeted therapeutics for the treatment of human malignancies. *Oncogene* **18,** 3056–3062.

17. Hijiya, N., Zhang, J., Ratajczak, M. Z., Kant, J. A., DeRiel, K., Herlyn, M., Zon, G., and Gewirtz, A. M. (1994)Biologic and therapeutic significance of MYB expression in human melanoma. *Proc. Natl. Acad. Sci. USA* **91,** 4499–4503.

18. Cook, P. D. (1998) Antisense medicinal chemistry, in *Antisense Research and Applications* (Crooke, S. T., ed.), Springer-Verlag, Berlin, pp. 51–101.

19. Cooper, S. R., Taylor, J. K., Miraglia, L. J., and Dean, N. M. (1999) Pharmacology of antisense oligonucleotide inhibitors of protein expression. *Pharmacol. Ther.* **82,** 427–435.

20. Cummins, L. L., Owens, S. R., Risen, L. M., Lesnik, E. A., Freier, S. M., McGee, D., Guinosso, C. J., and Cook, P. D. (1995) Characterization of fully 2'-modified oligoribonucleotide hetero- and homoduplex hybridization and nuclease sensitivity. *Nucleic Acids Res.* **23,** 2019–2024.

21. Bennett, C. F., Chiang, M. Y., Chan, H., Shoemaker, J. E. E., and Mirabelli, C. K. (1992) Cationic lipids enhance cellular uptake and activity of phosphorothioate antisense oligonucleotides. *Mol. Pharmacol.* **41,** 1023–1033.

22. Dean, N. M., McKay, R., Condon, T. P., and Bennett, C. F. (1994) Inhibition of protein kinase C-alpha expression in human A549 cells by antisense oligonucleotides inhibits induction of intercellular adhesion molecule 1 (ICAM-1) mRNA by phorbol esters. *J. Biol. Chem.* **269,** 16,416–16,424.

23. Taylor, J. K., Zhang, Q. Q., Monia, B. P., Marcusson, E. G., and Dean, N. M. (1999) Inhibition of Bcl-xL expression sensitizes normal human keratinocytes and epithelial cells to apoptotic stimuli. *Oncogene* **18,** 4495–4504.

24. Marcusson, E. G., Bhat, B., Manoharan, M., Bennett, C. F., and Dean, N. M. (1998) Phosphorothioate oligodeoxynucleotides dissociate from cationic lipids before entering the nucleus. *Nucleic Acids Res.* **26,** 2016–2023.

25. Bennett, C. F. (1995) Intracellular delivery of oligonucleotides with cationic liposomes, in *Delivery Strategies for Antisense Therapeutics* (Akhtar, S., ed.), CRC Press, Boca Raton, FL, pp. 223–232.

26. Bongartz, J.-P., Aubertin, A.-M., Milhaud, P. G., and Lebleu, B. (1994) Improved biological activity of antisense oligonucleotides conjugated to a fuogenic peptide. *Nucleic Acids Res.* **22,** 4681–4688.

27. Kukowaska-Latallo, J. F., Bielkinska, A. U., Johnson, J., Spindler, R., Tomalin, D. A., and Baker J. R. (1996) Efficient transfer of genetic material into mamma-

lian cells using Starburst polyamidoamine dendrimers. *Proc. Natl. Acad. Sci. USA* **93,** 4897–4902.

28. Boussif, O., Lezoualc'h, F., Zanta, M. A., Mergny, M. D., Scherman, D., Demeneix, B., and Behr, J.-P. (1995) A versatile vector for gene and oligonucle- otide transfer into cells in culture and in vivo: polyethylenimine. *Proc. Natl. Acad. Sci. USA* **92,** 7297–7301.

29. Alahari, S. K., Dean, N. M., Frisher, M. H., Delong, R., Manoharan, M., Tivel, K. L., and Juliano, R. L. (1996) Inhibition of expression of the multidrug resistance- associated P-glycoprotein by phosphorothioate antisense oligonucleotides. *Mol. Pharmacol.* **50,** 808–819.

30. Giles, R. V., Spiller, D. G., Grzybowski, J., Clark, R. E., Nicklin, P., and Tidd, D. M. (1998) Selecting optimal oligonucleotide composition for maximal antisense effect following streptolysin O-mediated delivery into human leukaemia cells. *Nucleic Acids Res.* **26,** 1567–1575.

31. Bergan, R., Connell, Y., Fahmy, B., and Neckers, L. (1993) Electroporation enhances c-myc antisense oligodeoxynucleotide efficacy. *Nucleic Acids Res.* **21,** 3567–3573.

32. McKay, R. A., Cummins, L. L., Graham, M. J., Lesnik, E. A., Owens, S. R., Winniman, M., and Dean, N. M. (1996) enhanced activity of an antisense oligo- nucleotide targeting murine protein kinase C-alpha by the incorporation of 2′-O-propyl modifications. *Nucleic Acids Res.* **24,** 411–417.

33. Stein, C. A. and Kreig, A. M. (1994) Problems in interpretation of data derived from in vitro and in vivo use of antisense oligodeoxynucleotides. *Antisense Rev. Dev.* **4,** 67–69.

34. Woolf, T. M., Melton, D. A., and Jennings, C. G. B. (1992) Specificity of antisense oligonucleotides in vivo. *Proc. Natl. Acad. Sci. USA* **90,** 4665–4669.

II

DIAGNOSIS

7

Genetic Testing in Familial Melanoma

Epidemiologic/Genetic Assessment of Risks and Role of CDKN2A *Analysis*

David Hogg, Ling Liu, and Norman Lassam

1. Introduction

The first description of familial melanoma in the English literature appeared in 1820, when Norris (*1*) reported:

> It is remarkable that this gentleman's father, about thirty years ago, died of a similar disease.... This tumour, I have remarked, originated in a mole, and it is worth mentioning, that not only my patient and his children had many moles on various parts of their bodies, but also his own father and brothers had many of them.... These facts, together with a case that has come under my notice, rather similar, would incline me to believe that this disease is hereditary.

Since then, many families with a predisposition to melanoma have been described worldwide (*2–5*). For purposes of case definition, our laboratory currently defines familial melanoma (FMM) as a family containing ≥2 affected first-degree relatives with melanoma and/or pancreatic carcinoma. According to this definition, about 8–12% of melanoma is inherited as an autosomal dominant trait with variable penetrance. Affected members (AFM) of these FMM kindreds may develop multiple primary melanoma (*6*) and/or pancreatic cancer (*7*) and typically present at an earlier age than do patients with sporadic disease. In a subset of such individuals and kindreds, germline mutations of the *CDKN2A* gene (also known as *p16INK4A* and *MTS1*) cosegregate with cases of melanoma (*2–5*).

We have hypothesized that the identification of mutation carriers may in the future allow us to direct resources to the prevention and surveillance of mela-

From: *Methods in Molecular Medicine, Vol. 61: Melanoma: Methods and Protocols*
Edited by: B. J. Nickoloff © Humana Press Inc., Totowa, NJ

noma in high-risk individuals and families. This chapter provides an overview of melanoma genetics, as well as the indications, drawbacks, and methods of germline *CDKN2A* mutation screening by polymerase chain reaction (PCR) amplification and automated sequencing of genomic DNA.

We have taken care to indicate which clinical definitions we use, because other groups may employ somewhat different criteria to define FMM, dysplastic nevi, and the dysplastic nevus syndrome. As a result, mutation detection rates may differ among groups solely owing to differing disease definitions.

1.1. Genetic Predisposition to Melanoma

Linkage studies of melanoma-predisposed families have identified disease-associated loci on chromosomes *1p36 (8)*, *9p21 (9,10)*, and *6p (11)*. However, only the *9p21* locus has been linked repeatedly to the development of melanoma by multiple groups worldwide. To narrow the critical region containing the putative susceptibility gene, Kamb et al. *(12)* analyzed deletions in melanoma cell lines from sporadic cases of the disease and identified a candidate gene that they designated *MTS1* (now *CDKN2A*). Many groups have since reported that germline coding and noncoding mutations of *CDKN2A* cosegregate with cases of melanoma—and sometimes pancreatic cancer—in families *(2–5,13–17)*. In contrast to the relatively narrow spectrum of malignancy associated with inherited *CDKN2A* alterations, investigators have reported that mutations, deletions, and hypermethylation of *CDKN2A* occur in a large variety of sporadic tumor types. The promiscuous dysfunction of this tumor suppressor gene in human malignancy rivals that of p53 *(12,18)*.

The *CDKN2A* gene is alternatively transcribed from one of two exons designated *E1β* and *E1α*, both of which are spliced to downstream exons 2 and 3. These two transcripts encode two corresponding proteins that utilize different reading frames and are designated p19^{ARF} and p16, respectively (ARF = alternative reading frame) (*see* **Fig. 1**). Both proteins inhibit progression through the cell cycle by entirely different mechanisms: p16 inhibits the phosphorylation of the retinoblastoma protein pRB and thus guards entry into the cell cycle at the G1/S transition, whereas p19^{ARF} blocks degradation of the p53 protein (*see* **Fig. 2**) *(19,20)*. Centromeric to *E1β* lies a second gene, *CDKN2B*, that encodes the p15 protein. Curiously, although p15 appears to play a biochemical role indistinguishable from that of p16, germline mutations of *CDKN2B* have never been observed in cases of FMM *(5)*. Moreover, germline mutations of *CDKN2A* that affect the p19^{ARF} transcript alone have not been observed in melanoma-prone families *(5,21)*, although mice engineered for *E1β* deletions in the germline develop several types of cancer *(22,23)*. Accordingly, p19^{ARF} in humans remains a tumor suppressor in search of a disease. Finally, deletion

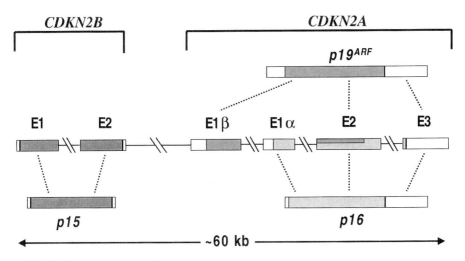

Fig. 1. Gene structure of *MTS2/CDKN2A/p16* and *MTS2/CDKN2B/p15* located at 9p21. The *p15* gene comprises two exons, which are spliced together to form the p15 transcript. Alternate splicing of *CDKN2A* can give rise to two different transcripts: exon 1α, exon 2, and exon 3 produce the *CDKN2A*/p16 transcript, whereas exons 1β, 2, and 3 comprise the p19[ARF] transcript.

studies of other tumor types have suggested that the *9p21* locus contains additional tumor suppressor genes both distal and proximal to *CDKN2A (24–26)*.

Germline coding mutations in *CDKN2A* are not found in all melanoma-prone families, even in kindreds with multiple AFM in whom the disease cosegregates with *9p21* markers. In some families, mutations in noncoding regions of *CDKN2A* alter expression of the protein and predispose to melanoma and/or pancreatic carcinoma *(27)*. In other kindreds and individuals, deletions encompassing the gene may underlie susceptibility to melanoma. Indeed, germline loss in *cis* of both *CDKN2A* and *CDKN2B* has been associated with a familial astrocytoma-melanoma syndrome (MIM no. 155755) *(28)*. Our current PCR/ sequencing protocols will miss such deletions, and we are currently developing additional approaches for mutation detection that include Southern blotting, fluorescence *in situ* hybridization, and the use of chip technology.

1.2. Phenotypes Associated with Germline CDKN2A Mutations and Clinical Implications

In families through which a *CDKN2A* germline mutation is segregating, mutation carriers are at increased risk for melanoma. The lifetime penetrance in carriers appears to be on the order of 50–80%, but this estimate may be biased by the analysis of large kindreds and is subject to revision *(29,30)*. It is

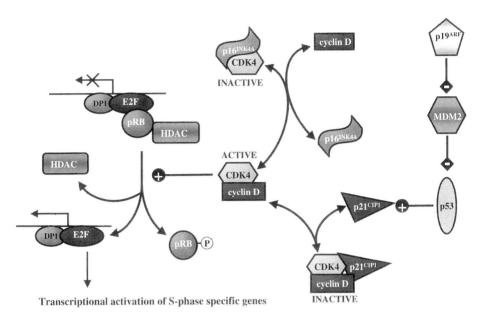

Transcriptional activation of S-phase specific genes

Fig. 2. Control of the restriction point by CIPs, INK4s, and p19^ARF. Phosphorylation of Rb by active cdk4/cyclin D results in the dissociation of the HDAC/Rb/E2F complex. HDAC no longer deacetylates histones surrounding E2F consensus binding sites, thereby rendering these regions transcriptionally active. Two protein families, CIPs (p21, p27, and p57) and INK4s (p15, p16, p18, and p19) can inhibit the activity of cdk4/cyclin D. CIPs bind to both cdk4 and cyclin D, resulting in an inactive trimeric complex. By contrast, INK4s prevent association of the cyclin D regulatory subunit by binding to free cdk4. The alternately spliced transcript of *CDKN2A*, p19^ARF, prevents ubiquitin-dependent degradation of p53 normally brought about by MDM2, an ubiquitin conjugating enzyme. Increased p53 levels can result in cdk4/cyclin D inhibition through a CIP-mediated mechanism.

likely that the risk of melanoma in mutation-bearing individuals may be significantly increased by exposure to ultraviolet (UV) light *(31)*; accordingly, carriers should be counseled to avoid sun exposure and wear protective clothing. At present, it is not clear whether sun blocks provide any degree of protection, but their use seems to be a reasonable precaution.

Melanomas that develop in genetically predisposed individuals are not morphologically different from those observed in sporadic cases, although the familial lesions tend to be shallower *(29)*. Whether this reflects a difference in biologic behavior or is owing to heightened surveillance remains undetermined. It is clear that familial melanoma is just as dangerous as the sporadic disease and carries a high mortality if it is detected at a late stage. Therefore, ongoing surveillance on a 6-mo basis of mutation-bearing individuals seems reasonable

Table 1
Estimated Mutation Detection Frequencies[a]

Criteria	MDF (95% CI)
All families	31 (17–46)
2 AFM	18 (6–30)
3+ AFM	57 (40–73)
Multiple primary	14 (3–25)

[a]Probability of detecting a germline *CDKN2A* mutation. Criteria refers to the selection criteria employed prior to testing: All families, ≥2 AFM, who may be first- or second-degree relatives; multiple primary, patients with 2 or more primary melanomas. MDF, mutation detection frequency. Note that a family with one or more members with multiple primary melanomas or one or more cases of pancreatic carcinoma may have a somewhat higher probability of carrying a germline *CDKN2A* mutation.

(*see* **Subheading 1.6.**). *CDKN2A* mutation carriers may also develop pancreatic carcinoma (relative risk 22X) *(7)*, albeit at a considerably lower frequency than melanoma. At this time, we cannot offer any recommendations for surveillance of this disease. The risk of additional malignancies, such as breast, colon, and respiratory cancers, is so far indeterminate. Both of these areas of question will best be addressed by a large multicenter study.

Individuals with two or more primary melanomas *(6)*, or those who present with a combination of melanoma and pancreatic cancer *(43)*, may also possess a germline *CDKN2A* mutation even in the absence of a family history of either disease. The identification of such a mutation may prompt further examination of the proband's family, with identification of other carriers or affected individuals.

1.3. Mutation Detection Frequencies

The estimates for mutation frequency in typical clinical scenarios (*see* **Table 1**) are based on our analysis of individuals and families with melanoma in Toronto and from other referral centers in North America. Our melanoma-prone patient population described herein is largely of European origin; we do not yet know the impact of germline *CDKN2A* mutations in a population of African origin.

We caution that mutation detection frequencies may differ significantly among different laboratories for the following reasons. First, our analyses are performed using PCR-sequencing of exons 1α and 2 of the *CDKN2A* gene (exon 3 encodes only three amino acids and we do not sequence it at this time), and laboratories that utilize methods such as single-strand conformation polymorphism may miss significantly more mutations *(6)*. Second, our current protocol will not detect medium to large (>100 bp to >1 megabase) deletions.

Third, the frequency of mutations or the type of mutation (missense vs deletion) may vary considerably among different ethnic groups. Fourth, a high lifetime risk of sporadic melanoma in the population under study (e.g., 1/14 in Queensland, Australia *(32)* vs 1/110 in Canada) will result in a considerable number of phenocopies that may confound the selection criteria for mutation analysis.

1.4. Other Genes That Predispose to Melanoma

In ~30% of high-risk melanoma-prone families (≥3 AFM), germline mutations of *CDKN2A* have not been detected. Moreover, some of these kindreds do not demonstrate linkage of the disease to *9p21* makers *(33)*. Therefore, it is highly likely that another major locus or loci predisposes to the disease. Investigators have described three families that bear germline coding mutations in the *CDK4* gene (chromosome *12q14*) and are identical in clinical presentation to kindreds that bear *CDKN2A* mutations *(34,35)*. The aberrant *CDK4* proteins bear mutations at amino acid 24 that abrogate binding to p16. In Toronto, to date, we have not detected any melanoma-prone family with a *CDK4* mutation in a survey of more than 60 kindreds; moreover, we have not identified analogous mutations in the orthologous *CDK6* gene *(44)*. Germline mutations of the *RB* gene (which encodes the target of the *CDK4* kinase and maps to chromosome *13q14.1–q14.2*) predispose to retinoblastoma and osteosarcoma. *RB* mutations are also associated with a 10-fold increase in melanoma risk in adult life *(36)*. Finally, mutations of the *BRCA2* breast cancer gene also predispose to melanoma *(37)*. In conclusion, mutations of genes other than *CDKN2A* (including but not restricted to members of the retinoblastoma pathway) may predispose carriers to melanoma. However, families segregating such mutations are relatively rare and cannot account for all kindreds that are unlinked to *9p21*. Thus, it seems likely that another major melanoma susceptibility gene or genes will be described in the future.

1.5. Dysplastic Nevus Syndrome

Patients with dysplastic nevus syndrome (DNS) may develop melanoma that typically arises in dysplastic nevi (abnormal moles). We define patients with DNS as those individuals who possess ≥100 nevi in addition to at least 2 dysplastic nevi (this is the current definition used by the International Melanoma Consortium). We define dysplastic nevi as nevi ≥8 mm in diameter that often have an irregular border and variegated pigmentation. Numerous epidemiologic studies have consistently demonstrated substantial risk of melanoma associated with dysplastic nevi. For example, Tucker et al. *(38)* studied 716 patients with nevi and reported that 1 clinically dysplastic nevus was associated with a 2-fold risk of melanoma (95% confidence interval [CI], 1.4–3.6), whereas 10 or more conferred a 12-fold increased risk (95% CI, 4.4–31).

DNS may segregate through families or may occur sporadically. The locus or gene that predisposes to familial DNS is unknown but probably segregates independently of *CDKN2A* in families with FMM *(39,40)*. Notably, germline mutations of *CDKN2A* do not appear to predispose to DNS, although they may affect the expressivity or penetrance of this syndrome *(39)*. However, in patients possessing both DNS and a *CDKN2A* germline mutation, the relative risk of melanoma is extremely high and its penetrance may approach 100%. More important, DNS is associated with other malignancies, including Hodgkin and non-Hodgkin lymphoma *(41)* and testicular germ cell cancer (GCT) *(42)*. Therefore, the identification of the DNS gene or genes would have a profound effect on our understanding of melanoma predisposition, and possibly lymphomas and GCT as well.

1.6. Current Roles and Drawbacks of CDKN2A Mutation Analysis

Surveillance of families with both FMM and DNS may decrease mortality, even in the absence of genetic testing *(29)*. Mutation analysis of the *CDKN2A* gene in melanoma-prone individuals and families is still a research tool. The clinical utility of such testing will not be known until two questions are addressed: (1) Do mutation carriers within a family develop cancer at a much higher rate than do noncarriers? and (2) Does surveillance of mutation carriers—combined with curative biopsies of suspicious lesions—prevent morbidity and mortality. Data on the first question should be available in the near future, but it may take years to determine the impact of mutation testing on survival and quality of life.

Currently, we counsel both carriers and noncarriers identically in families segregating *CDKN2A* mutations. In part, this is because we suspect that genes other than *CDKN2A* may modify melanoma susceptibility in both the presence and absence of *CDKN2A* mutations. If we are correct, the risk of melanoma in a noncarrier is not necessarily the same as that of the general population. Moreover, if a melanoma-prone family is found not to bear a germline *CDKN2A* mutation, this does not mean that their risk is less than that of a mutation-positive kindred. Rather, a *CDKN2A* mutation may not be detected by our current protocol, or another melanoma susceptibility gene may underlie the predisposition to melanoma observed in this family.

2. Materials

2.1. Genomic DNA

1. Genomic DNA dissolved in water or TE (10 m*M* Tris-HCl, pH 7.5, 1 m*M* EDTA) at a concentration of 50 ng/μL.

Table 2
PCR Primers

Exon	Name	Sequence
1	880F[a]	5′-TCC TTC CTT GCC AAC GCT GGC TC
	1590R	5′-TTC GAG AGA TCT GTA CGC GCG TG
2	E2FBF	5′-GGC TCA CAC AAG CTT CCT TTC CG
	E2RBR	5′-CGG GCT GAA CTT TCT GTG CTG G

[a]F, sense/forward sequence; R, antisense or reverse sequence.

2.2. Polymerase Chain Reaction

1. PCR thermocycler (we use a Perkin-Elmer 2400 or 9600).
2. Microtubes (0.2 mL), pipet for 1 to 20-μL vol, plastic pipet tips.
3. PCR reagents: 10X PCR buffer (200 mM Tris-HCl, pH 8.4, 500 mM KCl); 50 mM MgCl$_2$; 2.0 mM of each: dATP, dCTP, dGTP and dTTP; *Taq* DNA polymerase; deionized dimethyl sulfoxide (DMSO); and ddH$_2$O.
4. PCR primers (*see* **Table 2**).
5. Electrophoresis apparatus for small agarose gel; agarose; ethidium bromide; 10X loading buffer (50% glycerol, 1% bromophenol blue), and a molecular weight marker suitable for a size range of 50–1000 bp. (We use the 100-bp ladder marker from Pharmacia Canada.)
6. UV transilluminator, camera, and films (for recording image from agarose gel).

2.3. Automatic Sequencing

1. Automated sequencer: Micro Gene Blaster (Visible Genetics, Toronto, Canada) and ancillary equipment and reagents (gel cartridge and gel plates, gel Toaster, color printer to record electropherograms).
2. GeneObjects™ software (Visible Genetics) to analyze sequences.
3. Sequencing reagents: 10X sequencing buffer I (200 mM Tris-HCl, pH 8.3, 39 mM MgCl$_2$); 32 U/μL Thermo Sequenase (Amersham); Thermo Sequenase dilution buffer (100 mM Tris-HCl, pH 8.0, 1 mM 2-mercaptoethanol, 0.5% [v/v] Tween-20, 0.5% [v/v] NP-40); deionized DMSO; termination mix (750 μM of each: dATP, dCTP, dGTP, and dTTP and 2.5 μM of each: terminators ddATP, ddCTP, ddGTP, ddTTP [300:1 ratio of dNTP to ddNTP]). All of these reagents are provided in the Cy™5/Cy5.5 Day Primer Cycle Sequencing Kit (Visible Genetics).
4. Cy5.5 labeled primers (*see* **Table 3**).

3. Methods

3.1. PCR Amplification of CDKN2A Exons 1 and 2

1. Amplify exon 1 and 5′ untranslated sequences (5′UTR): In a 0.2-mL microtube on ice, add the following reagents: 1.5 μL of 10X buffer (Gibco), 0.6 μL of 50 mM

Table 3
Sequencing Primers

Exon	Name	Sequence	T_a (°C)	Purpose
1	E1-CF[a]	5'-ACT TCA GGG GTG CCA CAT TCG CT	60	5'-UTR and E1 coding
	E1-FF	5'-CAC CAG AGG GTG GGG CGG AC	64	E1 coding and splice donor
	E1-RR	5'-AAA CTT TCG TCC TCC AGA GTC GCC C	64	E1 coding and some 5' UTR
2	E2-FF	5'-GCT TCC TTT CCG TCA TGC CG	58	E2 coding and splice sites
	E2-RR	5'-TGC TGG AAA ATG AAT GCT CTG AG	60	E2 coding and splice sites

[a]F, sense/forward sequence; R, antisense or reverse sequence.

MgCl$_2$, 1.5 µL of 2.0 m*M* dNTP, 0.75 µL of DMSO, 0.6 µL of primer 880F (10 pmol/µL), 0.6 µL of primer 1590R (10 pmol/µL), 1.0 µL of DNA (50 ng/µL), 0.1 µL of *Taq* (Gibco), 8.35 µL of ddH$_2$O, for a total volume of 15 µL. Place the tube(s) in a thermocycler and amplify using the following program: 3 min at 95°C; 35 cycles of 30 s at 95°C, 30 s at 64°C, 60 s at 72°C; 5 min at 72°C; hold at 4°C.

2. Amplify exon 2: In a 0.2-mL microtube on ice, add the following reagents: 1.5 µL of 10X buffer (Gibco), 0.5 µL of 50 m*M* MgCl$_2$, 1.5 µL of 2.0 m*M* dNTP, 1.5 µL of DMSO, 0.6 µL of primer E2FBF (10 pmol/µL), 0.6 µL of primer E2RBR (10 pmol/µL), 1.0 µL of DNA (50 ng/µL), 0.1 µL of *Taq* (Gibco), 7.7 µL of ddH$_2$O, for a total volume of 15 µL. Place the tube(s) in a thermocycler and amplify using the following program: 3 min at 95°C; 35 cycles of 30 s at 95°C, 30 s at 62°C, 60 s at 72°C; 5 min at 72°C; hold at 4°C.

3. Check the PCR products: Load 4 µL of PCR products and 4 µL of 1:10 diluted molecular weight marker (final concentration of 0.1 µg/µL) on a 1% agarose gel. The bands corresponding to the PCR products should migrate at the expected sizes (E1 is 800 and E2 is 465 bp) and there should be little remaining oligonucleotide or primer dimer (*see* **Fig. 3**). If the products appear clean and bright, they may be sequenced directly.

3.2. Cycle Sequencing

1. Prepare the master mix: In a 0.2-mL microtube on ice, add the following reagents (scale up to sequence additional amplifications): 2.5 µL of VGI buffer, 0.75 µL of DMSO, 1.0 µL of specific primer (*see* **Table 3**), 2.5 µL of Sequenase (diluted 1:10), 6.25 µL of ddH$_2$O, for a total volume of 13 µL.

2. Prepare individual terminator mixes: Label four tubes A, C, G, and T. Add 3 µL of the master mix to each tube, and then add an equal volume of termination mix to each tube.

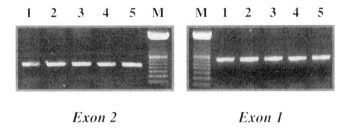

Fig. 3. PCR products from amplification of exons 1 and 2 of *CDKN2A*. Lanes 1–5 are separate amplifications of genomic DNA samples; M, is the molecular mass marker (100-bp ladder; Pharmacia). Note the equal intensity of each band and the lack of contaminating amplimers.

3. Add the PCR product to the terminator mixes: Dilute the PCR product to 5 ng/µL and add 2 µL of product (10 ng total) to the tubes labeled A, C, G, and T from **step 2**. Layer 8 µL of clear mineral oil on top (even on thermocyclers with heated lids).

4. Place the tube(s) in a thermocycler and amplify using the following program: 3 min at 95°C, 35 cycles of 30 s at 95°C, 30 s at T_a (*see* **Table 3**), 60 s at 72°C; 5 min at 72°C; hold at 4°C.

5. Analyze the sequencing reactions: Add 6 µL of loading dye (Provided in the Cy5/Cy5.5 Day Primer Cycle Sequencing Kit) to each tube and denature at 95°C for 2 min. Load 2 µL of each sample per lane on the Micro Gene Blaster automated sequencer (Visible Genetics) and run for 35 min at 50°C and 1300 V. Analyze the sequence using GeneObjects software (Visible Genetics) (*see* **Fig. 4**).

4. Notes

1. We have optimized our PCR conditions for the Perkin-Elmer thermocycler models 2400 and 9600. Because of the very high G:C content in and around the *CDKN2* locus, these conditions may have to be optimized for other thermocyclers.

2. We have optimized our protocol for the Cy5.5 chemistry protocol, for the Dye Primer Cycle Sequencing Kit and the Micro Gene Blaster automated sequencer (Visible Genetics). While these protocols should be easily adapted to other chemistries and sequencers, a few cautionary notes are in order. First, we recommend that dye primer, rather than dye terminator, technologies be used. The more even peak heights achieved with dye primers allow more accurate detection of heterozygous mutations in missense mutations. Similarly, we do not recommend using manual sequencing (i.e., ^{35}S-labeled primers) owing to the difficulty of detecting subtle mutations.

3. Because of the high G:C content in and around the *CDKN2* locus, compressions, or "stops," in the sequence are sometimes observed. Such artifacts mandate the use of at least two sequencing primers (the -FF and -RR series in **Table 3**), so that

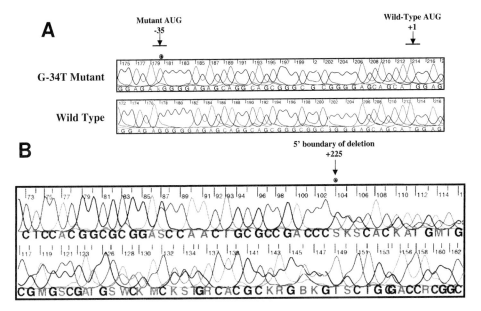

Fig. 4. (**A**) Example of a *CDKN2A* 5′ missense mutation detected by sequencing. This electropherogram demonstrates a noncoding mutation in the 5′UTR, designated G-34T, that gives rise to a novel initiation codon out of frame with the wild-type AUG. We sequenced genomic DNA samples from a mutation carrier (upper electropherogram: heterozygous for the wild-type and G-34T nucleotides) and a normal control (lower electropherogram). Horizontal bands above the electropherograms show the location of the mutant (–35) and the wild-type (+1) ATG codons. The arrow indicates the mutation at nucleotide –34. (**B**) Example of a *CDKN2A* deletion detected by sequencing. This electropherogram demonstrates a deletion in exon 2 at position +74 (position +225 of the corresponding mRNA, as indicated by the arrow). Note the sudden appearance of ambiguous sequence, owing to a frameshift in the mutant allele that leads to a sequence divergence in the PCR fragment sequencing reaction. This sequence results from the use of the forward primer (E2-FF); comparing the sequence derived from the reverse primer (E2-RR) reveals the 3′ boundary of the deletion.

sequence is derived from both strands. In addition, we recommend the use of the E1-CF primer to better visualize the 5′UTR of exon 1 (*see* **Fig. 4**).
4. Many *CDKN2A* germline mutations have been observed in melanoma-prone families worldwide, providing strong evidence that these specific mutations are indeed associated with the disease. Several mutations encode proteins that are deficient in binding to the *CDK4/6* kinases, providing a biologic marker of clinical behavior. (The sole but important exception to this rule is a 24-bp insertion or deletion at the beginning of the coding region of exon 1. Despite binding to *CDK4* as easily as the wild-type protein, this mutant clearly predisposes to melanoma.) Intragenic deletions, especially those that lead to a frameshift, abrogate the func-

tion of the protein. A recent review of *CDKN2A* biology and a compendium of mutations has been published by Ruas and Peters *(45)*. Novel mutations should be genetically and functionally defined before any conclusions can be drawn about their impact on p16 function.

5. Unless *CDKN2A* mutation analysis is conducted on anonymous specimens, we insist that genetic counseling be offered to patients prior to and following genetic testing. A genetic counselor, clinical geneticist, or physician who is expert in the field of general and cancer genetics should provide this counseling.

References

1. Norris, W. (1820) A case of fungoid disease. *Edinburgh Med. Surg. J.* **16,** 562.
2. Hussussian, C. J., et al. (1994) Germline p16 mutations in familial melanoma. *Nat. Genet.* **8,** 15–21.
3. Kamb, A., et al. (1994) Analysis of the p16 gene (CDKN2) as a candidate for the chromosome 9p melanoma susceptibility locus. *Nat. Genet.* **8,** 23–26.
4. FitzGerald, M. G., et al. (1996) Prevalence of germ-line mutations in p16, p19ARF, and CDK4 in familial melanoma: analysis of a clinic-based population. *Proc. Natl. Acad. Sci. USA* **93,** 8541–8545.
5. Liu, L., et al. (1997) Affected members of melanoma-prone families with linkage to 9p21 but lacking mutations in CDKN2A do not harbor mutations in the coding regions of either CDKN2B or p19ARF. *Genes Chromosomes Cancer* **19,** 52–54.
6. Monzon, J., et al. (1998) CDKN2A mutations in multiple primary melanomas. *N. Engl. J. Med.* **338,** 879–887.
7. Goldstein, A. M., et al. (1995) Increased risk of pancreatic cancer in melanoma-prone kindreds with p16INK4 mutations. *N. Engl. J. Med.* **333,** 970–974.
8. Bale, S. J., et al. (1989) Mapping the gene for hereditary cutaneous malignant melanoma-dysplastic nevus to chromosome 1p. *N. Engl. J. Med.* **320,** 1367–1372.
9. Cannon-Albright, L. A., et al. (1992) Assignment of a locus for familial melanoma, MLM, to chromosome 9p13-p22. *Science* **258,** 1148–1152.
10. Cannon-Albright, L. A., et al. (1994) Localization of the 9p melanoma susceptibility locus (MLM) to a 2-cM region between D9S736 and D9S171. *Genomics* **23,** 265–268.
11. Walker, G. J., et al. (1994) Linkage analysis in familial melanoma kindreds to markers on chromosome 6p. *Int. J. Cancer* **59,** 771–775.
12. Kamb, A., et al. (1994) A cell cycle regulator potentially involved in genesis of many tumor types. *Science* **264,** 436–440.
13. Bergman, W., Gruis, N. A., Sandkuijl, L. A., and Frants, R. R. (1994) Genetics of seven Dutch familial atypical multiple mole-melanoma syndrome families: a review of linkage results including chromosomes 1 and 9. *J. Invest. Dermatol.* **103,** 122S–125S.
14. Parry, D. and Peters, G. (1996) Temperature-sensitive mutants of p16CDKN2 associated with familial melanoma. *Mol. Cell. Biol.* **16,** 3844–3852.

15. Smith-Sorensen, B., and Hovig, E. (1996) CDKN2A (p16INK4A) somatic and germline mutations. *Hum. Mutat.* **7,** 294–303.
16. Holland, E. A., et al. (1995) Analysis of the p16 gene, CDKN2, in 17 Australian melanoma kindreds. *Oncogene* **11,** 2289–2294.
17. Walker, G. J., et al. (1995) Mutations of the CDKN2/p16INK4 gene in Australian melanoma kindreds. *Hum. Mol. Genet.* **4,** 1845–1852.
18. Kamb, A. (1995) Cell-cycle regulators and cancer. *Trends Genet.* **11,** 136–140.
19. Sherr, C. J. and Roberts, J. M. (1999) CDK inhibitors: positive and negative regulators of G1-phase progression. *Genes Dev.* **13,** 1501–1512.
20. Sherr, C. J. (1998) Tumor surveillance via the ARF-p53 pathway. *Genes Dev.* **12,** 2984–2991.
21. Stone, S., et al. (1995) Complex structure and regulation of the P16 (MTS1) locus. *Cancer Res.* **55,** 2988–2994.
22. Kamijo, T., Bodner, S., van de Kamp, E., Randle, D. H., and Sherr, C. J. (1999) Tumor spectrum in ARF-deficient mice. *Cancer Res.* **59,** 2217–2222.
23. Kamijo, T., et al. (1997) Tumor suppression at the mouse INK4a locus mediated by the alternative reading frame product p19ARF. *Cell* **91,** 649–659.
24. Watson, J. E, et al. (1999) Identification and characterization of a homozygous deletion found in ovarian ascites by representational difference analysis. *Genome Res.* **9,** 226–233.
25. Czerniak, B., et al. (1999) Superimposed histologic and genetic mapping of chromosome 9 in progression of human urinary bladder neoplasia: implications for a genetic model of multistep urothelial carcinogenesis and early detection of urinary bladder cancer. *Oncogene* **18,** 1185–1196.
26. Farrell, W. E., et al. (1997) Chromosome 9p deletions in invasive and noninvasive nonfunctional pituitary adenomas: the deleted region involves markers outside of the MTS1 and MTS2 genes. *Cancer Res.* **57,** 2703–2709.
27. Liu, L., et al. (1999) Mutation of the CDKN2A 5′ UTR creates an aberrant initiation codon and predisposes to melanoma. *Nat. Genet.* **21,** 128–132.
28. Bahuau, M., et al. (1998) Germ-line deletion involving the INK4 locus in familial proneness to melanoma and nervous system tumors. *Cancer Res.* **58,** 2298–2303.
29. Tucker, M. A., et al. (1993) Risk of melanoma and other cancers in melanoma-prone families. *J. Invest. Dermatol.* **100,** 350S–355S.
30. Goldstein, A. M. and Tucker, M. A. (1995) Genetic epidemiology of familial melanoma. *Dermatol. Clin.* **13,** 605–612.
31. Battistutta, D., et al. (1994) Incidence of familial melanoma and MLM2 gene. *Lancet* **344,** 1607–1608.
32. MacLennan, R., Green, A. C., McLeod, G. R., and Martin, N. G. (1992) Increasing incidence of cutaneous melanoma in Queensland, Australia. *J. Natl. Cancer Inst.* **84,** 1427–1432.
33. Goldstein, A. M., et al. (1994) Linkage of cutaneous malignant melanoma/dysplastic nevi to chromosome 9p, and evidence for genetic heterogeneity. *Am. J. Hum. Genet.* **54,** 489–496.

34. Soufir, N., et al. (1998) Prevalence of p16 and CDK4 germline mutations in 48 melanoma-prone families in France. The French Familial Melanoma Study Group. *Hum. Mol. Genet.* **7,** 209–216 (published erratum appears in *Hum. Mol. Genet.* 1998;7[5]:941).

35. Zuo, L., et al. (1996) Germline mutations in the p16INK4a binding domain of CDK4 in familial melanoma. *Nat. Genet.* **12,** 97–99.

36. Traboulsi, E. I., Zimmerman, L. E., and Manz, H. J. (1988) Cutaneous malignant melanoma in survivors of heritable retinoblastoma. *Arch. Ophthalmol.* **106,** 1059–1061.

37. Consortium, T. B. C. L. (1999) Cancer risks in BRCA2 mutation carriers. *J. Natl. Cancer Inst.* **91,** 1310–1316.

38. Tucker, M. A., et al. (1997) Clinically recognized dysplastic nevi: a central risk factor for cutaneous melanoma. *JAMA* **277,** 1439–1444.

39. Greene, M. H. (1997) Genetics of cutaneous melanoma and nevi. *Mayo Clin. Proc.* **72,** 467–474.

40. Hashemi, J., Linder, S., Platz, A., and Hansson, J. (1999) Melanoma development in relation to non-functional p16/INK4A protein and dysplastic naevus syndrome in Swedish melanoma kindreds. *Melanoma Res.* **9,** 21–30.

41. Tucker, M. A., Misfeldt, D., Coleman, C. N., Clark, W. H. Jr., and Rosenberg, S. A. (1985) Cutaneous malignant melanoma after Hodgkin's disease. *Ann. Intern. Med.* **102,** 37–41.

42. Raghavan, D., et al. (1994) Multiple atypical nevi: a cutaneous marker of germ cell tumors. *J. Clin. Oncol.* **12,** 2284–2287.

43. Lal, G., et al. (2000) Patients with both pancretic adenocarcinoma and melanoma may harbor germline CDKN2A mutations. *Genes, Chromosomes, Cancer* **27,** 358–361.

44. Shennan, M. G., et al. (2000) Lack of germline *CDK6* mutations in familial melanoma. *Oncogene* **19,** 1849–1852.

45. Ruas, M. and Peters, G. (1998) The *p16INK4a/CDKN2A* tumor suppressor and its relatives. *Biochim. Biophys. Acta.* **1378,** F115–F177.

8

Role of Molecular Biology in Diagnostic Pathology of Melanoma

Andrzej Slominski, Andrew Carlson, Jacobo Wortsman, and Martin C. Mihm

1. Introduction

Cutaneous melanoma is the most rapidly increasing malignancy in the white European population; its clinical significance is enhanced because it can affect younger individuals *(1–3)*. The high mortality rate among melanoma patients, second to lung cancer, is related to melanoma's resistance to therapy once the metastastic process has started *(4–6)*. The tumor derives from epidermal melanocytes, either activated or genetically altered; thus, important precursors include activated melanocytes present within solar lentigo or forming premalignant lesions such as lentigo maligna *(7–10)*. Melanoma can also arise from relatively benign or atypical nevomelanocyte lesions *(7–10)*. Benign lesions that can nevertheless result in melanoma include congenital melanocytic nevus, nevus of Ota, nevus of Ito, and cellular blue nevus. The atypical lesions with the same possible outcome are represented by acquired dysplastic melanocytic nevus, melanocytic dysplasia on the acral or mucosal surface, spindle cell and/or atypical epithelioid melanocytic nevus (Spitz nevus), and dysplastic and/or congenital nevus spilus *(7–10)*.

The standard tool for the diagnosis of pigmented lesions is the histologic examination, which allows assessment of the level of dysplasia, separation of premalignant from malignant lesions, and prediction of the behavior of melanoma *(6–15)*. In this regard, determination of the presence of well-defined histopathologic features and assessment of clinical variables contribute significantly to establish terminal prognosis and optimal management by helping in the design and implementation of specific therapeutic strategies *(6–15)*.

From: *Methods in Molecular Medicine, Vol. 61: Melanoma: Methods and Protocols*
Edited by: B. J. Nickoloff © Humana Press Inc., Totowa, NJ

For example, melanomas recognized early, at the radial growth phase (RGP), when the disease is still localized and restricted to the skin, can be cured by proper surgical excision. Conversely, the appearance within a primary lesion of a new cell population with metastatic capability is recorded histologically as vertical growth phase (VGP). This stage has a fundamental impact on the clinical course of the disease, because it conveys a marked decrease in life expectancy and requires additional therapeutic efforts (7–15).

Recent advances in the genetics, molecular biology, and immunology of melanoma have provided the background for the development of new markers to predict tumor behavior and metastatic potential (16–20). Furthermore, novel immunotherapy and gene therapy protocols have raised hopes that metastatic melanoma may eventually become curable (21–28). Indeed, the current challenge for both academic and practicing pathologists is to determine which of the new molecular tests should become part of a standard pathology report, and in what context they should be included. The objective of the supplementary information added to the standard clinical and histologic descriptions is to increase significantly the accuracy of melanoma diagnosis and prognosis and, thus, contribute to the design of the optimal therapy. It is therefore important to become familiar with the rapidly growing knowledge of the biology of melanoma to determine its proper clinical and pathologic context. The present review includes current as well as accepted concepts on melanoma. It emphasizes what, in our opinion, represents the most promising areas of clinical and diagnostic value, while attempting to predict future therapeutic strategies based on the new information. Areas where rigorous testing of new data are yet to be performed or that are openly controversial have been purposefully left out of this presentation.

2. Dermatopathologic Criteria for Diagnosis of Melanoma

The American Joint Committee on Cancer recommends a four-stage system for the classification of melanoma: stages I and II, with tumor thickness <4 mm, indicate localized growth; stage III, with tumor thickness >4 mm, presence of satellite lesions within 2 cm, or involvement of regional lymph nodes, indicates regional involvement; and stage IV indicates distant metastases (4–10). In stages I and II, survival depends on the level of invasion according to the classification of Clark, the measured tumor thickness defined by Breslow, the type of growth, and the dermatopathologic and clinical criteria listed in **Table 1**. Most of these criteria are considered as independent variables, and as such they directly affect patient survival (7–15).

In melanoma, one of the most important criteria for prognosis is the type of growth, i.e., *in situ* pattern or a radial or VGP (**Figs. 1–3**). RGP melanomas

Table 1
Melanoma Profile

Histologic and Clinical Variables

1. Body sites[a]
2. Sex[a]
3. Age[a]
4. Classification
5. Clark's level[a]
6. Breslow's depth[a]
7. Tumor-infiltrating lymphocyte response[a]
8. Regression[a]
9. Dermal mitoses[a]
10. Radial growth phase[a]
11. Vertical growth phase[a]
12. Satellitosis[a]
13. Ulceration[a]
14. Angiolymphatic spread
15. Neurotropism
16. Margins[a]
17. Cell phenotype
18. Coexisting nevus

[a]Independent variables predicting survival of melanoma patient *(9,11,12,15)*.

typically exhibit an admixture of brown/tan or pink/white coloration. At this stage, melanoma cells may be either confined almost exclusively to the intraepidermal compartment (*in situ* RGP) (**Fig. 1**) or invade the papillary dermis (invasive RGP) in the form of single cells or small nests of melanocytes similar in size and number (no more than 5–10 melanoma cells) (**Fig. 2**). These melanocytes are deposited along the dermal epidermal junction, replacing the basilar region, and/or in a pagetoid spread but with similar cytology. Mitoses are frequently seen in the epidermis but rarely present in the papillary dermal component. The nest aggregates do not become expansile. An inflammatory response by lymphocytes is commonly elicited in the papillary dermis. Occasionally, single cells may infiltrate into the upper reticular dermis. On initial biopsy, the thickness at RGP is <0.76 mm in 97% of melanomas with tissue invasion at level II in 93% of them. Of note, the RGP melanoma is associated with a long metastasis-free survival—according to some investigators at least 13.7 yr *(12–14)*.

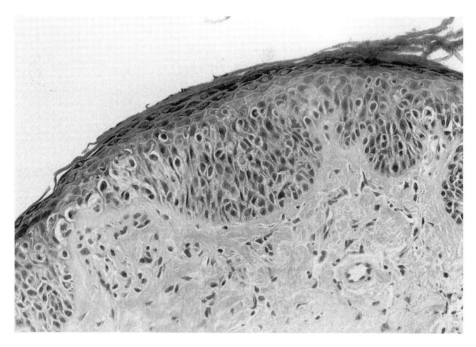

Fig. 1. Melanoma *in situ*.

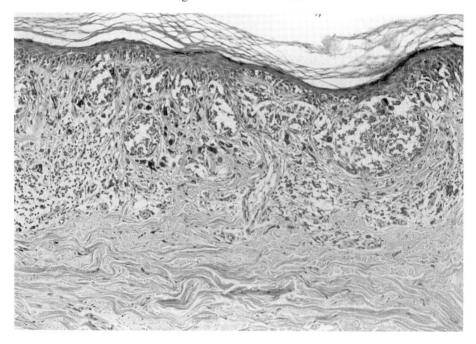

Fig. 2. RGP of invasive superficial spreading melanoma.

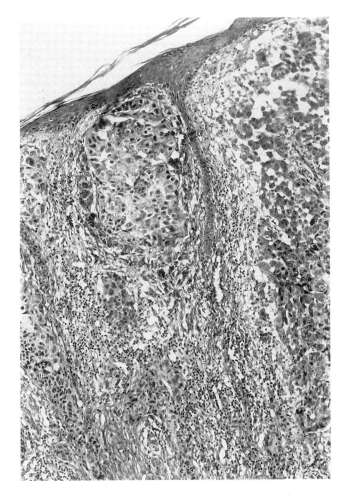

Fig. 3. VGP of invasive superficial spreading melanoma.

The VGP is classified as early and late (developed). In the early VGP, a small papulonodule supervenes in an RGP lesion, usually of a darker coloration or blue/black. In in the papillary dermis, early VGP appears as small expansile cell aggregates of a type different from that of RGP, and in larger numbers (often 20–25); mitotic figure may also be seen. In the developed VGP melanoma (**Fig. 3**), the cells grow in the form of expansile nodules in the dermis, whose cytology is frequently different from the melanoma cells in the overlying epidermis. For example, the intraepidermal melanocytes may be of epitheliod shape with very fine melanin granularity, whereas the corresponding dermal nodules may consist of spindle cells, small epitheliod cells, or a mixed pattern. Mitotic figures are variably present and melanoma cells may extend into the reticular dermis or even subcutaneous fat. In the VGP, epidermal nodules are larger than those of the RGP intraepidermal nests. Survival in the VGP is related directly to the measured depth of invasion; it is also influenced by the presence of a regression, of a tumor-infiltrating lymphocyte response, dermal mitotic activity, ulceration, and satellitosis. Additional prognostic factors include gender, age, and anatomic site. In general, when reaching the VGP, melanoma cells gain metastatic competence.

The prognosis for stage I and II disease also correlates with the more traditional melanoma subtypes with better prognosis for lentigo maligna melanoma (LMM) and superficial spreading melanoma (SSM) than for nodular melanoma or acral-lentiginous melanoma (ALM) *(4–10)*. LMM is limited to the most sun-exposed areas of the skin and is characterized by a prolonged period of intraepidermal or radial growth (long RGP). At this stage the melanoma is composed of pleomorphic melanocytes confined to the basal region of a markedly atrophic epidermis above the dermal changes consisting of marked solar elastosis and the presence of a chronic inflammatory infiltrate. In SSM, the malignant melanocytes proliferating in the epidermis have monotonous morphologic features with prominent nuclei and variable cytoplasm filled with fine melanin granules. This intraepidermal growth phase is generally of shorter duration than in LMM. ALM is the most common form of melanoma in dark-skinned persons; it has an RPG and involves the palms, soles, and nail beds (**Fig. 4**). Similar to LMM, in ALM atypical melanocytes are confined to the dermal-epidermal junction, but the epidermis is usually hyperplastic. Melanocytes are large and uniformly atypical with prominent dendrites surrounded by a striking clear space. ALM has more aggressive behavior than LMM. While still at RGP, LMM, SSM, and ALM can be completely cured by surgical removal, because it is at the VGP that tumors acquire a potential for metastases. Nodular melanoma exhibits a pure VGP, and the disease cannot be detected at the intraepidermal growth phase or RGP.

Once the VGP stage has been reached, the appearance of a new cell population with metastatic capability decides the clinical course of the disease *(12–15)*. The process of melanoma metastasis is composed of several well-defined and interrelated steps whose temporal sequence is determined by the intrinsic biologic behavior of melanoma cells and the host response *(29)*. These steps comprise extensive vascularization of the tumor mass, local invasion of stroma including invasion by lymphatic and hematogenous capillaries, interactions with blood cell components, and formation of small cell aggregates. These melanoma cell aggregates can survive in the circulation and potentially arrest

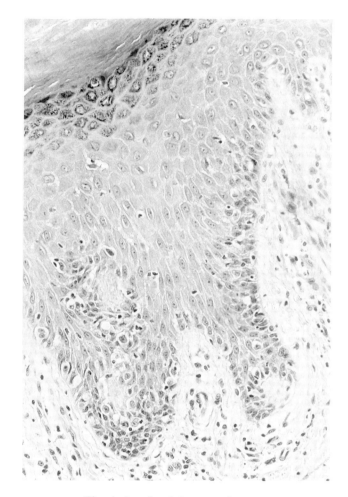

Fig. 4. Acrolentiginous melanoma.

in target organs, through adhering to capillary endothelial cells or to the subendothelial basement membrane. Following cellular extravasation and establishment of the proper microenvironment for growth and proliferation in the parenchyma of the target organ, a tumor vascular network develops and there is continued evasion of the host immune system. To produce clinically detectable metastasis, again, melanoma cells must complete all these processes *(29)*.

Metastatic disease causes a dramatic decrease in the survival of patients with stage III and IV melanomas *(4–12)*. When the regional lymph nodes are involved, survival time decreases to approx 30–40% at 5 yr, with worsening of the prognosis as the number of involved lymph nodes increases, extranodal disease becomes apparent, and the primary tumor increases in thickness and ulcerates *(4–15)*. The prognosis is also worse for primary tumors localized in the trunk vs extremities. Once distant metastases are present, the disease is almost incurable and median survival is approx 6 mo *(4–11)*. Other factors predicting unfavorable prognosis are an increased number of metastases, involvement of visceral sites, and shorter duration of remission. In addition, gender may influence the course of the disease, with worse prognosis for males than females.

3. Role of Constitutional and Environmental Factors in Etiology of Melanoma

Genetic, constitutional, and environmental factors interact in the etiology and pathogenesis of melanoma *(1–9,16–19,30–32)*. Thus, familial incidence of melanoma, skin type, and history of sun exposure result in specific impacts on the etiology, pathogenesis, and progression of pigmented lesion, respectively. Clinical information on these variables as well as racial groups, gender, age, number of pigmented nevi, and number of large nevi are therefore all important for the diagnosis and prognosis of pigmented lesions. Overall, approx 10% of patients with cutaneous melanomas have a family history and are associated with the familial atypical multiple mole melanoma (FAMMM) syndrome *(4,17,18)*. In these cases, studies on chromosomes and gene aberrations are advisable and should be reported by a pathologist when available (for rationale *see* Chapter 9).

There is a close relationship between racial group and incidence of cutaneous melanoma; the highest incidence is found in white European and the lowest frequencies in black African, dark Asian, and East Oriental populations *(1–10)*. The effect of racial groups is further emphasized by the relatively higher incidence of melanoma on acral sites with a less favorable course of the disease among African-American and Asian populations. Another factor that correlates with racial and ethnic background is skin type *(1–10)*. Thus, there is an inverse correlation between skin type and a probability of melanoma, which is the highest in the photosensitive skin of type I and lowest in the tanning-prone skin of type IV. Finally, individuals with red or blond hair and blue eyes are more susceptible to develop melanomas.

In general, women with melanomas have a better rate of survival than men *(4)*. This has been rationalized by a potential suppressive effect of estrogens acting directly on melanocytes or through the local or systemic immune stimulation. It is known that melanocytes and immune cells express receptors for estrogen and androgens; thus, they are potentially able to modify melanocyte function and modulate local and systemic immunity *(33,34)*. We recently reported that cultured human melanoma cells can metabolize progesterone, and that the intermediate products of this metabolism include biologically active steroids such as deoxycorticosterone, corticosterone, and 18OHDOC *(35)*.

Patient age also influences the risk of melanoma and the clinical type of potential malignant pigmented lesions. Thus, the risk of developing melanoma is higher in individuals older than 15 yr than in younger children *(1–4)*. This observation implies a role for endocrine factors on melanocyte fuction and skin environment that results in more permissive conditions for melanocyte carcinogenesis after puberty. Some premalignant or malignant pigmented lesions such as lentigo maligna or melanoma of lentigo maligna type are in fact characteristic of older age *(4,8,9)*. Other constitutional factors, inherited or environmental, that may affect clinical expression are the number, size, and type of melanocytic nevi *(1–9)*. For example, the risk of developing a melanoma in patients having 50 nevi >2 mm, 12 nevi >5 mm, 5 nevi >7 mm, and 5 nevi >5 mm increases by factors of 64, 41, 16, and 10, respectively, over the risk in the average population *(4–6)*. Lesions with a relatively lesser risk include benign or atypical nevomelanocytic lesions such as nevus of Ota and Ito, congenital nevus, cellular blue nevus, dysplastic and/ or congenital nevus spilus, atypical Spitz nevus, and acquired dysplastic nevus *(1–10)*.

4. Role of Inherited and Acquired Genetic Alterations in Melanoma

4.1. Chromosomal Aberrations

Benign nevi demonstrate a normal karyotype, whereas dysplastic nevi or atypical nevi of patients with FAMMM syndrome usually show chromosomal abnormalities (reviewed in **refs. *1*, *4*, *16–19***, and ***30***). The FAMMM syndrome is of particular interest because the recurrent chromosomal abnormalities detected in the atypical nevi have also been found in fibroblasts and lymphocytes (cf. **refs. *4*** and ***18***). Several studies have demonstrated a linkage of the FAMMM syndrome to 9p21 with p16 being the most frequently mutated gene (*see* below) *(1,4,16–19,30)*. An earlier study showed a linkage to chromosome 1p36 *(17,18)*.

Benign melanocytic tumors with abnormal karyotype are diploid or pseudodiploid without recurrent chromosomal aberration. Sporadic dysplastic nevi have shown a significant rate of loss of heterozygosity (LOH) in chromosomes 1p and 9q *(36)*. Furthermore, studies in dysplastic melanocytic nevi showed a predominant allelic deletion at chromosome 9p21 (p16 locus), accompanied in some cases by allelic deletion in 17p13 (p53 locus); none of these changes were seen in benign nevi *(37)*. Cytogenetic heterogeneity has also been reported in some Spitz nevus *(38)*. These observations support the hypothesis that there is a genetic predisposition for progression to melanoma in some melanocytes of dysplastic nevi. Telomerase activity, a potential tumoral marker, is higher in dysplastic than in benign common melanocytic nevi and increases further during progression to melanoma *(39)*.

Chromosomes 1, 6, 7, 9, and 10 are most commonly affected in melanoma *(1,4,6–9,16–18,30–32,40–44)*. In chromosome 1, frequent structural rearrangements include translocations or deletions of 1p12-22 (cf. **ref. *17***), LOH in 1p *(17,45,46)*, and deletion of 1p36 *(17,47)*. A putative tumor suppressor gene is located on 1p36 and deletion of 1p36 is frequently found in nodular melanoma; this deletion is also more frequent at the higher Clark levels *(17,47)*. Concerning chromosome 6, the most commonly noted changes have been nonreciprocal translocations or deletions involving 6q11-6q24 *(16,17,31,32,43,46)* and increased frequency of LOH in 6q *(48–50)*. Chromosome 6 may contain a tumor supressor gene for malignant melanoma *(51,52)*. The abnormalities in chromosome 7 include the loss or gain of this chromosome *(30,43,46,47,53)*. Gain of chromosome 7 may be associated with increased expression of epidermal growth factor receptor (EGF-R) located at 7p12-13 *(54)*. It is also interesting and potentially important that the human homolog of a platyfish and swordfish tumor suppressor gene, *Tu*, maps to 7p11-13 (cf. **ref. *17***). Regarding chromosome 10, its loss is frequently associated with progression of melanoma *(17,30,53,55,56)*, and the *nma* gene, a potential inhibitor of metastatic potential, is located in chromosome 10p11.2-p12.3 *(57,58)*. Additional studies on the relationship between melanoma karyotype and clinical progression have demonstrated that abnormalities in chromosomes 7 and 11 are linked to shorter survival of melanoma patients.

The cytogenetic changes of chromosome 9 deserve special attention because of strong evidence that a defect in chromosome 9p21 may play an important role in the development of melanoma *(1,4,16–19,30,41,42,46,59–66)*. Thus, it has been proposed that this region encodes tumor suppressor genes *(59–66)*. For example, the tumor suppressor gene p16[INK4] that maps to chromosome 9p13-22 contains the putative locus of familial melanoma *(17,18,59–64)*. Moreover, melanomas frequently carry nonsense, missense, frameshift, or p16[INK4] deletion mutations *(18,59,60,62–64)*. The p15[INK4B] tumor suppressor gene, is also located on chromosome 9p21, and its possible role in melanoma progression is emphasized by the recent finding of homozygous deletion of p15[INK4B] in some melanomas despite retention and expression of p16[INK4] *(67)*.

4.2. Mutations in Tumor Suppressor Genes and Oncogenes

The product of the cyclin-dependent kinase (CDK) p16, which acts at the G1/S checkpoint of the cell cycle, is considered the tumor suppressor gene most important in the development of melanoma *(16–18,59–66)*. Mutations, LOH, and deletion in the p16 locus have been frequently reported in sporadic and familial melanomas, and the decreased expression of p16 was reported to correlate positively with more aggressive melanoma behavior *(16–18,59–66)*. However, mutations at p16 locus were also detected in normal melanocytes and in benign compound nevi lacking signs of clinical or histologic atypia *(68)*; a high frequency of p16 deletions was seen in primary and metastatic tumoral cell lines but not in metastatic melanoma specimens *(69)*. This suggests that the loss of p16 gene may not represent an initiating event in human melanocytic transformation and progression *(68)*. In addition, analysis of familial melanomas from Australia suggests that mutation of other genes closely linked to p16 on chromosome 9p may be involved in some hereditary melanoma kindreds *(62)*. It has been suggested that germline p16 mutation explains most, if not all, 9p21-linked familiar melanomas, whereas the genetic basis of non-9p21-linked melanoma kindreds remains to be identified *(70)*. Analysis of melanoma kindreds that do not carry germline p16 mutations has shown specific mutations in the p16 binding domain of CDK4 that generate a dominant ocogene resistant to normal physiologic inhibition by p16 *(70)*. Recent immunocytochemical studies on expression of p16[INK4] and CDK4 proteins showed characteristic overexpression of CDK4 in malignant melanoma *(69)*. Thus, although p16 is still the best candidate for tumor suppressor gene in melanoma, further studies on its role and that of other cell-cycle regulatory proteins are necessary to define their participation in the progression of melanoma. Among important issues that need clarification is whether the frequent inactivation of the p16[INK4] gene in melanoma lines reflects a tissue culture artifact or whether it is operative in vivo *(66)*.

Other genes coding proteins regulating cell cycle and potentially involved in melanocyte transformation include p15 and p19, which are located on chromosome 9p *(17,41,59,63,67)*. Genes that may inhibit melanoma metastatic potential and therefore represent potential candidates for tumor suppressors include nm23, nmb, and nma *(17,40,46,57,58)*. Specifically, expression of nm23 correlates inversely with tumor progression *(18,46)*. An additional candidate for melanoma tumor suppressor gene is p53, the most commonly mutated gene that has been implicated in the etiology of many neoplastic disorders. To date, the correlations between p53 gene rearrangement or altered expression of p53 protein and progression of melanocytic lesion has not been significant *(71)*. This is in contrast to epidermal skin cancers in which a high frequency of mutation at p53 locus has been noted *(72)*. Nevertheless, some investigators suggest that p53 could still have a pathogenic role in melanoma, albeit in a more complex relationship. Thus, p53 could act on downstream effector genes as MDM2, GADD45, and CIP1/WAF1, an effect detected in human melanoma cell lines *(73)*. It is also postulated that modulation of p53 expression may change the response of melanoma cells to chemotherapeutic agents *(74)*. Thus, further studies on the role of p53-activated pathways in melanoma biology are warranted *(75)*.

Expression of the Ha-, Ki-, and N-ras protooncogenes in melanoma cells has been reported *(17,40,46)*. Cultured metastatic melanomas expressing mutated N- and Ki-ras displayed high expression of EGF-R and dedifferentiated phenotype *(17,40,46)*. The mutated ras genes were detected in approx 5–6% of melanoma specimens *(46)*, and mutation in N-ras has been found most frequently at sun-exposed areas *(17,19)*. The Ki-ras mutation has also been found in benign nevi besides primary and metastatic melanomas *(46)*. Although ras may play a role in proliferation of melanoma cells, its function in the development of melanoma remains to be clarified.

Altered expression of nuclear oncogenes c-*myb*, c-*myc*, c-*fos*, and c-*jun* was reported in cultured melanoma cells *(17,40,46,76)*. However, the random character of these changes and lack of clear-cut relation to defined stage of progression of melanocytic lesion do not support their use as prognostic markers. Similarly, the expression of c-*src*, a nonreceptor membrane-associated tyrosine kinase, did not reveal significant differences between cultured melanocytes and melanoma cells *(17,46)*. The c-*kit* protooncogene encodes the transmembrane tyrosine kinase receptor KIT/SCF-R *(77)*. The KIT receptor plays an important role in the migration and differentiation of melanoblasts toward melanocytes *(77)*. The KIT receptor acts as a regulator of melanocyte proliferation and differentiation, but its potential role in the development of melanoma remains unclear.

5. Growth Factors, Cytokines, and Their Receptors

Several growth factor transduction systems can regulate melanocyte phenotype, including basic fibroblast growth factor (bFGF), mast cell growth factor (MGF), hepatocyte growth factor (HGF), transforming growth factor-α (TGF-α), insulin growth factor-1 (IGF-1), neuron growth factor (NGF), and endothelins *(78–84)*. bFGF acts as a growth-stimulating factor and plays a central role as a growth regulator in normal melanocytes *(78,79)*. Melanoma cells cultured in vitro do not require exogenous bFGF because of autocrine stimulation by endogenously produced bFGF *(78,79)*. Accordingly, both antisense deoxynucleotide against bFGF and anti-bFGF antibodies inhibit the growth of melanoma cells *(46,79)*. Moreover, *in situ* studies show that bFGF expression is absent in epidermal melanocytes but easily detectable during progression of melanocytic lesion *(85)*. Because bFGF lacks the signal peptide necessary for extracellular secretion, the autocrine role of bFGF in the development of melanoma has been questioned *(46,80)*. However, a mechanism for the secretion of peptide hormones lacking signal peptide has been described recently *(86)*.

HGF and MGF stimulate melanocyte growth similar to bFGF, through activation of membrane-bound receptors that have intrinsic tyrosine kinase activity *(17,40,46,79,80)*. HGF operates on the c-met receptor and MGF via the protein product of the c-*kit* protooncogene. The c-*kit* encodes the Kit/stem cell factor receptor (SCF-R) of 145 kDa that regulates proliferation and differentiation of melanocytes. Endothelins can also regulate proliferation, motility, and differentiation of melanocytes *(17,81)*.

Other hormones that can modify the phenotype of normal and malignant melanocytes include insulin *(87–89)* and melatonin *(90,91)*. Insulin can stimulate the growth of some melanoma cells, both in vivo and in vitro. Studies performed by Kahn et al. *(87)* have provided evidence that insulin can also inhibit the proliferation of melanoma cells depending on the genotype of the target cells. In several mutant melanoma lines, insulin inhibited growth, similar to its effects in wild-type melanocytes; however, other mutant lines were stimulated by insulin or were resistant to the hormone *(87,89,89)*. The common thread in the lines responsive to insulin was the presence of a specific protein of approx 85–90 kDa (pp90) in the phosphorylated state *(93,94)*. The insulin-resistant lines were characterized by decreases or loss of pp90 and defects in the α- and β-subunits of the insulin receptor *(89,94)*. It was then suggested that the β-subunit of the insulin receptor underwent adenosine triphosphate–dependent partial proteolysis in the mutant lines, making the cells resistant to the antiproliferative action of the insulin *(89)*. Such inactivation of signal transduction would allow the tumor cells to escape growth-regulatory control by insulin.

Melatonin is a pineal gland hormone, first isolated and characterized by Lerner et el. *(95)*, whose pharmacologic concentrations can inhibit melanogenesis in normal follicular melanocytes and in cultured melanoma cells *(90,91)*. Binding sites for melatonin have been detected in membrane preparation of rodent skin and in membrane fraction and purified nuclei from melanoma cells *(90,91)*. These targets become interesting when considering that mammalian skin has the potential to synthesize and metabolize melatonin *(96)*. It has been proposed further that defective melatonin receptors may participate in the development of vitiligo *(97)*.

The cytokines tumor necrosis factor-α (TNF-α), interleukin-1 (IL-1), and IL-6 can inhibit melanocyte proliferation and melanogenesis *(98)*. In addition, TNF-α, IL-1, IL-6, IL-7, interferon-γ (IFN-γ), and TNF-β can upregulate the expression of intercellular adhesion molecule-1 and major histocompatibility complex (MHC) class II molecules on melanocytes *(17,40,46,79,80,99,100)*.

Eicosanoids can stimulate growth (LTC_4 and LTD_4), cell motility (LTC_4), and stimulate (LTB_4) or inhibit (LTB_4) melanogenesis *(80,100)*. Melanocytes can also produce and secrete various peptide hormones, cytokines, eicosanoids, and extracellular matrix components *(79,80,100)*. These include proopto-melanocortin (POMC)-derived adrenocorticotropic hormone (ACTH), melano-cyte stimulating hormone (MSH), and β-endorphin *(101)*; IL-1, IL-3, IL-6, and IL-8; granulocyte macrophage colony-stimulating factor (GM-CSF); TGF-α and TGF-β; TNF-α; MCAF; 12-HETE; 12-HHT; LTB_4; fibronectin; laminin; thrombospondin; and plasminogen activator *(17,40,46,79,80,100)*.

Of interest for prognostic purposes, *in situ* analyses of the expression and localization of several receptors, including NGF, transferrin, and EGF *(102–104)* and of growth factors such as TGF-α *(105)*, TGF-β *(106–108)*, and IGF-1 *(109)*, may correlate with stage of development of melanocytic lesion. Thus, *in situ* analyses demonstrate increased expression of TGF-β in advanced stages of development of melanoma in comparison to low levels of expression in benign lesions *(106–108)*. However, the progression of melanoma does not change in parallel with TGF-β receptor expression, although there may be some correlation between the progression of melanoma and increased expression of IGF-1 or EGF-R *(104,109)*. Recent studies have shown the production rate of TGF-α by dysplastic nevi to be higher than in benign nevi, supporting the previous hypothesis that the TGF-α/EGF-R system could play a role in the evolution of melanocytic lesions *(104,105)*.

Melanomas produce several additional growth factors and cytokines and express their corresponding receptors. These include keratinocyte growth factor (KGF), platelet-derived growth factor-α (PDGF-α), PDGF-β, SCF, MGSA/gro, IL-1α, IL-1β, IL-6, IL-7, IL-8, IL-10, IL-12, GM-CSF, G-CSF, TNF-α, IFNγ, and IFN-β *(17,40,46,78–81,101,110–115)*. Many of these factors can potentially act as regulators of melanoma cell proliferation, differentiation, and motility. They can also stimulate angiogenesis and induce expression of major histocompatability antigens, cell adhesion molecules, integrins, nonintegrin matrix adhesion receptors, and extracellular matrix proteins on melanocytes and surrounding cells. Simultaneously, many of these factors can modify further the local immune system after being produced within the tumor by cells other than malignant melanocytes. The complexity of the interactions suggests that testing for single factor expression with costly assays may be of limited diagnostic value. In this context, it is important to note that expression of multicytokine resistance and multi–growth factor autonomy owing to autocrine stimulatory mechanisms are characteristic for advanced stages of melanoma *(113)*. It has been suggested that, in contrast to VGP, RGP melanomas are deficient inducers of angiogenesis, are highly sensistive to several cytokines and growth factors, and are more sensitive to undergoing apoptosis under a variety of growth conditions *(111)*.

6. Melanocortin System

The POMC-derived neuropeptides MSH and ACTH can modify the phenotype of normal and malignant melanocytes *(17,17,82,100,101,116–122)*. Both ACTH and MSH stimulate proliferation, melanogenesis, and dendrite formation through interaction with specific cell-surface receptors *(82,100,101,116–120)*. Transduction of the melanotropic signal in melanocytes starts with the activation of cell-surface receptors coupled to the G-stimulatory protein complex and involves stimulation of adenylate cyclase with cyclic adenosine monophosphate (cAMP) production *(82,100,101,116–122)*. In some melanomas, the signaling pathway proceeds through the activation of phospholipase C with changes in intracellular concentration of Ca^{2+} (cf. **ref. 82**). In melanoma cells, the expression and activity of MSH receptors can be stimulated by UV light, dbcAMP, and MSH itself, and phosphorylated isomers of L-DOPA, L-tyrosine, retinoic acid, IL-1, IFN-α, IFN-β, and IFN-γ *(123–132)*. The transduction of the α-MSH or ACTH signals in melanocytes is associated with activation of the MC1 receptor (MC1-R) subclass *(117–122)*. The possibility of expression of other MC receptors, e.g., MC2–MC5, on pigment cells should be the subject of future studies. A possible role of MC1-R in the development of melanoma is emphasized by finding that mutations at the MC1-R locus that lead to the red hair phenotype are also present in melanoma *(133,134)*.

Melanoma cells have been shown to express the gene for POMC that encodes the peptides ACTH, MSH, and β-endorphin *(100,101,135–139)*. ACTH, MSH, and β-endorphin were found below the limit of detectability by immunocytochemistry in normal skin melanocytes and in benign blue nevi *(136,137)*. By contrast, common and dysplastic melanocytic nevi showed weak positivity for α-MSH, ACTH, and β-endorphin antigens, with a tendency for higher expression levels in dysplastic nevi *(137)*. In melanoma, POMC antigens were easily detectable in a large number of cases, and the stain was also more intense and diffuse in the VGP of melanoma *(136,137)*. Direct measurement of α-MSH with radioimmunoassay found detectable concentrations of the peptide in skin with melanoma (0.21–2.32 pmol/g of wt) and in lymph nodes with metastases (0.31–4.25 pmol/g of wt), which contrasted with very low (<0.2 pmol/g of wt) or undetectable levels of the peptide in normal skin *(138)*. Even the serum levels of α-MSH-IR are increased in melanoma patients and are positively correlated with the more advanced clinical stage or level of invasion *(139)*. Thus, local expression of POMC peptides such as MSH and ACTH could directly alter melanoma cell phenotype through auto-, intra-, or paracrine mechanisms; alternatively, the peptide may act indirectly by affecting surrounding tissues such as immune elements or the vascular system *(101,116,130,139,140)*. The end result would be further promotion of tumor growth and metastatic cascade. UV light (a positive punitive melanocyte carcinogen) can also stimulate the production of MSH and ACTH as well as the expression of corresponding receptors *(101,129–131,139)*.

7. Melanogenesis

An important diagnostic tool to separate melanoma from other tumors is the use of their ability to synthesize melanin and to express enzymatic and structural proteins involved in this process. Melanin synthesis is initiated with the hydroxylation of L-tyrosine to L-dihydroxyphenylalanine (L-DOPA) and oxidation of L-DOPA to DOPAquinone *(122,141–146)*. Both reactions are catalyzed by tyrosinase, the product of c locus *(143)*. The limiting step of melanogenesis is tyrosine hydroxylation, and the velocity of the pathway depends on DOPA oxidation *(122,141–146)*. The subsequent transformation of DOPAquinone to melanin can occur spontaneously; it is, however, accelerated by metal cations *(147)*. Depending on the genotype and cellular environment, melanogenesis generates the black pigment eumelanin, the reddish to yellow pigment pheomelanin, or mixed melanin that contains both components *(122,147–149)*. The biochemical cascade leading to the formation of eumelanin starts with the transformation of DOPAquinone to leukoDOPAchrome, followed by a series of oxidoreduction reactions catalyzed by post-DOPA oxidase regulators *(122,141–149)*. A second pathway involved in the synthesis of pheomelanin starts with the conjugation of DOPAquinone with cysteine or glutathione yielding cysteinylDOPA and glutathionylDOPA, which are then transformed into pheomelanin through a series of chemical reactions *(147,148)*. Eumelanogenesis is controlled by multiple identical gene products *(122,143–149)*, whereas the biochemical regulators of pheomelanogenesis are yet to be determined. Eumelanin differs from pheomelanin in chemical composition, structure, and physical properties *(147,148)*. For example, eumelanin is characterized by the presence of paramagnetic centers that are solely of the semiquinone type, whereas pheomelanin contains additional unpaired electrons near the nucleus of [14]N *(150,151)*. These properties allow the identification and quantification of melanin type by electron paramagnetic spectroscopy *(150–155)*.

The enzymatic and structural elements of melanosomes are processed and assembled in different membrane compartments *(117,122,156)*. The stage I premelanosomes are formed by a smooth membrane outpouching from the rough endoplasmic reticulum *(157)*. In the eumelanogenic pathway, a fibrillar matrix is formed in stage II melanosomes, which are devoid of melanin. After delivery of tyrosinase via vesicles from the *trans* Golgi reticulum, melanin synthesis begins and III melanosomes are formed. Stage IV melanosomes are represented by organelles filled with electron-dense melanin. Thus, tyrosinase is present only in stage II–IV but not in stage I melanosomes, and the tyrosine-related protein-1 (TRP-1) is delivered already from the endosomal/lysosomal pathway to melanosome stage I and II (cf. **refs. *117*** and ***158***). The timing of incorporation or melanosome development stage for other melanosome-related proteins such as TRP-2, Pmel17, and p protein is still unclear. The mechanism of formation of pheomelanosomes is less precisely defined. Briefly, vesiculoglobular bodies are incorporated into stage I melanosomes. At stage II melanosomes, a vesiculoglobular matrix can be seen, on which pheomelanin is deposited. The process of pheomelanogenesis depends on the availability of cysteine to conjugate with DOPAquinone and form cysteinylDOPA, the precursor to pheomelanin *(147,148)*. Under pathologic conditions, as in melanoma, this orderly process becomes defective: tyrosinase is incorporated and activated at stage I of melanosome formation and melanin is deposited within organelles of "grandular type" that do not contain either fibrillar or vesiculoglobular matrix *(159,160)*. Melanosomes contain a proton pump that allows regulation of intramelanosomal pH and can incorporate cell-surface MSH receptors via the endocytic pathway *(117)*. Those properties, together with the incorporation of lysosomal enzymes such as acid phosphatase and of lysosomal protective protein of LAMP, support the view that lysosomes and melanosomes share a common pathway of organellogenesis *(117,161)*.

Melanosomes are metabolically active organelles, and as such they may affect and regulate metabolic status and function of the host melanocyte or keratinocyte (cf. **refs. *100*** and ***162***). In this manner, melanosomes modify the energy-yielding metabolism by switching the oxidative catabolism to anaerobic glycolysis *(163)*, altering the intracellular NAD/NADH and NADP/NADPH ratio *(164)*, or stimulating the pentose phosphate pathway *(165)*. The presence of pigment granules may also affect the function of the host cell by buffering calcium ions, or by reversibly binding bioregulatory compounds such as catecholamines, serotonin, and prostaglandins (cf. *166*).

The gene coding for tyrosinase, the crucial enzyme of melanogenesis, is approx 70 kb long, contains five exons, and maps to chromosome 11q *(82,122,167,168)*. Although there are several alternatively spliced products of the c-locus, only one expresses tyrosinase activity *(169)*. It has been sugested that the different products of alternatively spliced tyrosinase mRNA may serve as receptors for L-tyrosine and L-DOPA, and may possibly act as positive regulators of differentiated functions of melanocytes *(162,170)*. Newly synthesized tyrosinase is a protein of a molecular weight of 55 kDa that is glycosylated in the Golgi complex, increasing in size to 65–72 kDa, although forms with higher molecular weight have also been described *(146,171–175)*. It has been suggested that tyrosinase can act as a regulatory protein by controlling intracellular levels of L-DOPA *(176)*; L-DOPA is a potential intracrine regulator of gene expression *(170,176–180)*. Other members of the tyrosinase gene family encode two other TRPs: TRP-1 (gp75 or b-locus protein) and TRP-2 (homolog of slaty locus in mice). These are cysteine-rich membrane-bound proteins with two copper binding sites and share about 40% amino acid homology *(181–187)*. The promoter region of the TRP family contains an M box, which binds microphtalmia gene product, a transcription factor of the basic helix-loop-helix family *(188,189)*. The TRP-1 gene is 15–18 kb long, contains eight exons separated by seven introns and is located on chromosome 9. TRP-1 acts as a 5,6-dihydroxyindole carboxylic acid (DHICA) oxidase generating indole-5,6-quinone-carboxylic acid *(182,183)*. Its activity appears to be important in the pathway for eumelanogenesis, as opposed to pheomelanogenesis *(173,190)*. The TRP-2 gene, which contains eight exons, is located on chromosome 13 *(185–187)*. TRP-2 protein acts as dopachrome tautomerase *(191)*, which catalyzes the enzymatic transformation of dopachrome to DHICA *(145)*. Of interest, TRPs contain sequences that can interact to form multimeric complexes of 200–700 kDa *(175,184)*. These sequences are homologous to EGF, supporting a role as regulators of melanocyte-differentiated functions for TRPs, in addition to their mechanistic action as enzymes *(162,170)*.

Other melanogenesis-related proteins (MRPs) include protein Pmel 17, which maps to chromosome 12 and is homologous to silver locus in mice *(192,193)* (**Table 2**). Pmel 17 is a glycoprotein recognized by the HMB45 monoclonal antibodies; it is located in the matrix of the melanosomes and contains cysteine- and histidine-rich regions *(194–196)*. Alternate names for this protein are gp100 and HMB50. Pmel 17 catalyzes the polymerization of DHICA to melanin *(197)*. A recently cloned p gene located on chromosome 15 encodes a membrane-bound proteins with certain homology to bacterial transporter for tyrosine *(198,199)*. Mutations at the p-locus can result in type II oculocutaneous albinism. Melanosomes also contain the lysosome-associated membrane proteins (LAMPs) which protect the lysosomal membrane from soluble hydroxylases *(161,200)*. As mentioned above, the presence of LAMP-1, -2, and -3 proteins in melanosomes supports a common ancestral origin for melanosomes and lysosomes *(200)*. It has been suggested that LAMP-1 may protect melanosomal integrity by acting as a scavenger of free radicals produced during melanogenesis *(200)*. The membrane-bound calcium-binding protein calnexin (p90) of 90 kDa may also be associated with the regulation of tyrosinase enzyme *(200)*.

Table 2
Melanogenesis-Related Proteins

Protein[a]	Function	Clinical use
Tyrosinase	Tyrosine hydroxylase, DOPA oxidase	Differentiation marker, target for immunotherapy
TRP-1	DHICA oxidase	Differentiation marker, target for immunotherapy
TRP-2	DOPAchrome tautomerase	Differentiation marker, target for immunotherapy
Pmel-17 (gp75)	Converts DHICA to melanin	Differentiation marker, target for immunotherapy
Mart-1/Melan-A	Melanosomal protein	Differentiation marker, target for immunotherapy
P protein	Melanosomal protein[b]	Differentiation marker
LAMP (1-3)	Membrane-associated proteins	Not determined
Calnexin (p90)	Protein chaperone	Not determined
MITF	Transcriptional regulator	Differentiation marker

[a]TRP-1, tyrosine-related protein-1; TRP-2, tyrosine-related protein-2; LAMP, lysosome-associated membrane proteins; MITF, microphtalmia-associated transcription factor.

[b]Unclear: regulatory protein, probably ion exchange protein [*J. Invest. Dermatol.* (2000) **115,** 607–613].

8. Markers of Melanogenesis in Diagnosis of Melanoma
8.1. Melanin

The finding of melanin is one of the most important markers to differentiate melanoma from other tumors. Melanin can be detected with standard histology techniques or with the histochemical Fontana-Masson method. Melanin concentration as well as identification of its type (eu-melanin or pheomelanin) can be conveniently measured by electron paramagnetic spectroscopy spectroscopy from paraffin blocks or fresh tissue *(152–155)*. The detection and quantification of melanin also provide information about possible therapeutic options and outcome. Thus, melanin can attenuate radio-, photo-, or chemotherapy (cf. **refs.** *100*, *152*, *166*, *201*), whereas intermediate products of melanogenesis can suppress immune response *(201–206)*. It is therefore likely that the presence of melanogenesis products or melanin itself is responsible for unsatisfactory outcome to therapy with the exception of surgically removing localized lesions. Furthermore, uncontrolled melanogenesis by generating an oxidative environment and producing genotoxic and mutagenic intermediates *(207–209)* can destabilize tumor cells and their microenvironment *(97,201)*, resulting in the progression of melanoma *(97,201)*, which is further amplified by the immunosuppressive effect of melanin precursors *(201)*. The cytotoxicity of melanogenesis has also led to an experimental therapeutic strategy. This involves upregulation of melanogenesis with intratumoral delivery of potentially cytotoxic false precursors of melanin *(210,211)*.

8.2. Ultrastructure

The ultrastructural marker of melanoma is the presence of melanosomes that are frequently abnormal in malignant lesions *(212)*. A defect in melanosomal structure can cause the leakage of melanogenesis-related cytotoxic and potentially mutagenic products into other cellular compartments *(159,212– 214)*. Thus, electron microscopy can be used for the diagnosis of melanoma and also to predict behavior of the pigment cell on the basis of degree and type of melanosomal defect.

8.3. Immunocytochemistry

The S-100 antigen, although found in the majority of melanomas and thus having high sensitivity, is not a specific tool for the detection of melanoma because it is also expressed in other nonmelanocytic cells. Among the currently used melanogenic markers, the HMB45 melanosomal antigen is less sensitive but highly specific for pigmented cells *(194–196)*. Another melanosomal protein, MART-1/Melan-A, may also serve as a promising tool in the diagnosis of melanoma *(215)*. Tyrosinase enzyme represents a powerful marker of melanoma, because expression of tyrosinase gene is restricted to cells of melanocytic origin. In fact, tyrosinase protein or its mRNA can be detected even in undifferentiated amelanotic melanomas *(116,159,173,216,217)*, including those in which lack of premelanosomes has been documented on the ultrastructural level *(159)*. Most recently, tyrosinase expression has been detected in selected cases of desmoplastic melanoma. Therefore, we strongly recommend determination of tyrosinase as a powerful marker for the diagnosis of melanoma. In addition, the relative abundance of mRNA for tyrosinase in some undifferentiated amelanotic melanomas *(173)* allows the use of *in situ* hybridization as a valuable diagnostic option. The same can be applied to the determination of TRP-1, which is recognized by a commercially available antibody MEL-5, and TRP-2, which acts as dopachrome tautomerase. Expression of these genes and proteins is restricted to cells of melanocytic lineage. Thus, investigation of the melanosomal proteins, tyrosinase, TRP-1, and TRP-2, collectively called MRPs, should provide highly specific and sensitive (tyrosinase) tools for the separation of melanoma from other tumors.

One of the most important issues in the management of melanoma is the identification of melanoma cells in the sentinel lymph node (SLN). This becomes a problem when the SLN is negative for overt melanoma cells on hematoxylin and eosin sections. To detect metastatic disease, HMB-45 immunocytochemistry frequently lacks sensitivity, and S-100 immunocytochemistry is nonspecific; for example, it also stains cells of nonmelanocytic origin. The last property introduces a high degree of subjectivity in final diagnosis, because it would be based on detection of atypia in immunopositive cells. In such a setting the use of antibodies against MART-1, tyrosinase, TRP-1, and TRP-2 could help in the identification of true melanoma cells. These immunocytochemistry tests could be complemented by molecular analyses (see below).

8.4. Molecular Biology

One of the most important problems in the management of melanoma is the development of a highly sensitive method to detect a metastatic process that influences markedly the staging of the disease. In this regard, it is important that the mRNA for MRP can be abundant even in amelanotic melanoma cells *(173)*. Therefore, detection of mRNA for tyrosinase, TRP-1, TRP-2, MART-1, and Pmel 17 by means of Northern blotting or reverse transcriptase polymerase chain reaction (RT-PCR) provides a significant help in the differential diagnosis of melanoma or in the detection of metastatic disease and should probably become the standard tool. The successful detection of mRNA for tyrosinase and other MRPs using RT-PCR in blood or bone marrow demonstrates that this method can detect circulating metastatic cells before their presence can be assessed clinically *(218–225)*. Significant effort has also gone into the use of RT-PCR for the detection of MRP in SLN *(220,224,225)*. It has thus been found that many SLNs that have been histologically and immunocytochemically negative for melanoma cells become positive after RT-PCR for tyrosinase mRNA *(220,224,225)*. Therefore, amplification of cDNA encoding MRP should be used in conjuction with histology for detection of metastatic disease in SLN; regular histology would exclude false positive signals generated by a possible presence of a benign melanocytic nevus in the lymph node.

8.5. Biochemical Markers of Melanoma

Serum levels of tyrosinase and of melanin precursors can correlate with the progression of melanoma *(226–230)*. Thus, patients with advanced melanoma show increased plasma or urine levels of the melanin precursors DOPA, 5-*S*-cysteinyldopa (5-*S*-CD), DHI, its carboxylic form (DHICA), and *O*-methyl derivatives of DHI and DHICA *(227–230)*. More selective staging is also possible; for example, high plasma levels of 6-hydroxy-5-methoxyindole-2-carboxylic acid are correlated with a tumor thickness >3.0 mm independently of the presence or absence of metastasis. In thinner melanomas, the same abnormality is seen only when metastases are present *(227)*. In addition, serum levels of 5-*S*-CD increase during the progression of melanoma *(228–230)*. Therefore, body fluid levels of MRP or concentration of melanogenic products provides valuable information on progression, regression, or recurrence of the disease. Changes in their levels could then help in detecting occult melanoma. Serum tyrosinase can be detected with assays for enzyme activity (tyrosine hydroxylase) or directly with radioimmunoassay *(231–233)*. From the therapeutic point of view, it must be emphasized that intermediates of melanogenesis can act as potent immunosuppressors *(201)*, and tyrosinase may amplify this process through continous oxidation of tyrosine and DOPA with generation of lymphocytotoxic precursors of melanogenesis *(234)*. Therefore, increased serum levels of intermediates of melanogenesis and of tyrosinase activity may also serve as indicators of potential impairment in the host immune response to melanoma.

9. Immune Markers for Melanoma Therapy

Tyrosinase, TRP-1, TRP-2, Pmel17, and melanocyte-specific MART 1 can be classified as MHC class I–restricted tumor antigens *(20–23,26–28,235–238)*, suggesting that their expression in relation to specific human haplotypes could be used as a guide for potential immunotherapy. The continuously growing family of MHC class I–restricted melanoma antigens also includes the MAGE proteins, which are expressed on melanoma cells but not melanocytes *(239)*. The diagnostic usefulness of detecting melanocyte-specific proteins derives from the fact that they generate specific peptides that become antigens when presented to CD8[+] cytotoxic T-cells (cytotoxic T-lymphocytes) and HLA-A2 molecules. This in turn would activate T-lymphocyte response against melanoma cells. The T-cell immune response may be highly heterogeneous because tyrosinase-derived peptides may be recognized by T-cells in association with HLA-A2, HLA-A24, HLA-B44, HLA-A1, HLA-DR4, and HLA-DR15 *(20–23,235–238)*. Immunization with purified tyrosinase enzyme has also been suggested as an adjuvant therapeutic strategy for malignant melanoma *(234)*. Because melanogenesis can have mutagenic and immunosuppressive effects, optimal immunotherapy strategy should comprise a differential upregulation of MRP with inhibition of melanogenesis *(201)*.

Stimulation of the humoral response against cell-surface antigens represents another immunotherapeutic approach for treatment of melanoma. Gangliosides are good candidates as substrates for antimelanoma vaccines *(24–26,240–244)*. However, the pattern of ganglioside expression changes during progression of melanocytic lesions, from increased expression of GD3, GD2, and GM2 to the appearance of GT3 and 9-0-Ac-GD3 *(240,241,245,246)*. In animal models of melanoma, a low level of GM3 and increased concentrations of GD3 and 0-acetyl-GD3 correlate with fast growth and undifferentiated phenotype *(247,248)*. Conversely, a slow growth rate and melanoma differentiation correlate with decreased expression of GD3 and 0-acetyl-GD3 and increased expression of GM3 *(247)*. In either localized or metastatic lesions, the expression of gangliosides is heterogeneous and their proper identification requires specialized analyses such as high-performance thin-layer chromatography *(249)*. While ganglioside pattern cannot be used as a diagnostic marker of melanoma progression, the analysis for the presence of a particular fraction of gangliosides (e.g., GD2, GD3, 0-Ac-GD3, or GM2) is valuable in the context of immunotherapy with antiganglioside antibodies or with ganglioside containing antimelanoma vaccine. In a similar fashion, high molecular weight melanoma-associated antigens (HMWMAA) have also been proposed as targets in a specific antimelanoma therapy *(21,22,24,26–29,250–252)*. Therefore, in specialized centers, the expression of specific ganglioside fraction or of HMWMAA should be a part of the dermatopathology report when considering those antigens as a target for immunotherapy.

10. Conclusion

To summarize, melanin can impair radiotherapy and phototherapy (cf. **refs. *201*, *152*, *253***, and ***254***). Intermediates of melanogenesis can suppress immune responses, and, therefore, ongoing active melanogenesis may reduce the effectiveness of immunotherapy (cf. **ref. *201***). Furthermore, uncontrolled melanogenesis that generates an oxidative environment and produces geneotoxic and mutagenic intermediates can destabilize tumor cells and their microenvironment, triggering the progression of melanoma (cf. **ref. *201***). This is further amplified by the immunosuppressive effect of melanogenesis itself (cf. **ref *201***). Therefore, the ideal melanoma therapy should combine differential upregulation of MRP expression, antigen-specific immunization, and inhibition of melanogenesis (cf. **refs. *201* and *234***). Inhibition of melanogenesis could play an adjuvant role when preparation of a vaccine from nonmelanogenic antigens, e.g., gangliosides, is considered in the therapy of melanoma.

Acknowledgment

This work was supported in part by a grant to A. S. from the American Cancer Society, IL Division (no. 99-51), and by the internal funding at the Department of Pathology, University of Tennessee.

References

1. Elder, D. E. (1995) Skin cancer. *Cancer* **75,** 245–256.
2. Glass, A. G. and Hoover, R. N. (1989) The emerging epidemic of melanoma and squamous cell skin cancer. *JAMA* **262,** 2097–2100.

3. Marks, R. (1989) Freckles, moles, melanoma and the ozone layer: a tale of the relationship between humans and their environment. *Med. J. Aust.* **151,** 611–613.
4. Lejeune, F. J., Chaudhuri, P. K., and Das Gupta, P. K. (1994) *Malignant Melanoma: Medical and Surgical Management*, McGraw-Hill, New York.
5. Johnson, T. M., Smith, J. W., Nelson, B. R., and Chang, A. (1995) Current therapy for cutaneous melanoma. *J. Am. Acad. Dermatol.* **32,** 689–707.
6. Rossi, C. R., Foletto, M., Vecchiato, A., Alessio, S., Menin, N., and Lise, M. (1997) Management of cutaneous melanoma M0: state of the art and trends. *Eur. J. Cancer* **33,** 2302–2312.
7. Slominski, A., Ross, J., and Mihm, M. (1995) Cutaneous melanoma: pathology, relevant prognostic indicators and progression. *Br. Med. Bull.* **51,** 548–569.
8. Mihm, M. C., Murphy, G. F., and Kaufman, N. (1988) *Pathobiology and Recognition of Malignant Melanoma*, Williams & Wilkins, Baltimore.
9. Balch, C. M., Houghton, A. N., Milton, G. W., Sober, A. J., and Song, S.-J. (1992). *Cutaneous Melanoma*, JB Lippincott, Philadelphia.
10. Elenitsas, R. and Schuchter, L. M. (1998) The role of the pathologist in the diagnosis of melanoma. *Curr. Opin. Oncol.* **10,** 162–169.
11. Eton, M., Legha, S. S., Moon, T. E., Buzaid, A. C., Papadopoulos, N. E., Plager, C., Burgess, A. M., Bedikian, A. Y., Ring, S., Dong, Q. Glassman, A. B., Balch, C. M., and Benjamin, R. S. (1998) Prognostic factors for survival of patients treated systemically for disseminated melanoma. *J. Clin. Oncol.* **16,** 1103–1111.
12. Clark, W. H. Jr., Elder, D. E., Guerry D. P. IV, Braitman, L. E., Trock, B. J., Schultz, D., Synnestvedt, M., and Halpern, A. C. (1989) Model predicting survival in stage I melanoma based on tumor progression. *J. Natl. Cancer. Inst.* **81,** 1893–1904.
13. Clark, W. H. Jr., Elder, D. E., Guerry D. P. IV, Epstein, M. N., Greene, M. H., and Van Horn, M. (1984) A study of tumor progression: the precursor lesions of superficial spreading and nodular melanoma. *Hum. Pathol.* **15,** 1147–1165.
14. Guerry D. P. IV, Synnestvedt, M., Elder, D. E., and Schultz, D. (1993) Lessons from tumor progression: the invasive radial growth phase of melanoma is common, incapable of metastasis, and indolent. *J. Invest. Dermatol.* **100,** 342S–345S.
15. Haffner, A. C., Garbe, C., Burg, G., Buttner, P., Orfanos, C. E., and Rassner, G. (1992) The prognosis of primary and metastasizing melanoma: an evaluation of the TNM classification in 2,495 patients. *Br. J. Cancer* **66,** 856–861.
16. Slominski, A., Wortsman, J., Nickoloff, B., McClatchey, K., Mihm, M., and Ross, J. S. (1998) Molecular pathology of malignant melanoma. *Am. J. Clin. Pathol.* **110,** 788–794.
17. Sauter, E. R. and Herlyn, M. (1998) Molecular biology of human melanoma development and progression. *Mol. Carcinog.* **23,** 132–143.
18. Halpern, A. C. and Altman, J. F. (1999) Genetic predisposition to skin cancer. *Curr. Opin. Oncol.* **11,** 132–138.
19. Bilchrest, B. A., Eller, M. S., Geller, A. C., and Yaar, M. (1999) The pathogenesis of melanoma induced by ultraviolet radiation. *N. Engl. J. Med.* **340,** 1341–1348.

20. Sakai, C., Kawakami, Y., Law, L. W., Furumura, M., and Hearing, V. J. (1997) Melanosomal proteins as melanoma-specific immune targets. *Melanoma Res.* **7,** 83–95.

21. Durrant, L. G. (1997) Cancer vaccines. *Anticancer Drugs* **8,** 727–733.

22. Demiere, M.-F. and Koh, H. K. (1997) Adjuvant therapy for cutaneous malignant melanoma. *J. Am. Acad. Dermatol.* **36,** 747–764.

23. Rosenbers, S. A. (1996) The immunotherapy of solid cancers based on cloning the genes encoding tumor-rejection antigens. *Annu. Rev. Med.* **47,** 481–491.

24. Livingtston, P. O. and Ragupathi, G. (1997) Carbohydrate vaccines that induce antibodies against cancer. 2. Previous experience and future plans. *Cancer Immunol. Immunother.* **45,** 10–19.

25. Ravindranath, M. H. and Morton, D. L. (1997) Immunogenicity of membrane-bound gangliosides in viable whole-cell vaccines. *Cancer Invest.* **15,** 491–499.

26. Scott, A. M. and Cebon, J. (1997) Clinical promise of tumor immunology. *Lancet* **349,** 19–22.

27. Schadendorf, D. (1997) Cytokines, autologous cell immunostimulatory, and gene therapy for cancer treatment, in *The Skin Immune System* (Bos, J. D., ed.), CRC Press, Boca Raton, FL, pp. 657–659.

28. Bonnekoh, B., Bickenbach, J. R., and Roop, D. R. (1997) Immunological gene therapy approaches for malignant melanoma. 2. Preclinical studies and clinical strategies. *Skin Pharmacol.* **10,** 105–125.

29. Fidler, I. (1996) Critical determinants of melanoma metastasis. *J. Invest. Dermatol. Symp. Proc.* **1,** 203–208.

30. Parmiter, R. H. and Nowell, P. C. (1993) Cytogenetics of melanocytic tumors. *J. Invest. Dermatol.* **100,** 254S–258S.

31. Su, Y. A. and Trent, J. M. (1995) Genetics of cutaneous malignant melanoma. *Cancer Control* **2,** 392–397.

32. Fountain, J. W., Bale, S. J., Housman, D. E., and Dracopoli, N. C. (1990) Genetics of melanoma. *Cancer Surv.* **9,** 645–671.

33. Jee, S.-H., Lee, S.-Y., Chiu, H.-C., Chang, C.-C., and Cheng, T. J. (1994) Effects of estrogen and estrogen receptor in normal human melanocytes. *Biochem. Biophys. Res. Commun.* **199,** 1407–1412.

34. Beattie, C. W., Roman, S. G., and Amoss, M. S. Jr. (1991) Estrogens influence the natural history of Sinclair swine cutaneous melanoma. *Cancer Res.* **51,** 2025–2028.

35. Slominski, A., Gomez-Sanchez, Celso., Foecking, M. F., and Wortsman, J. (1999) Metabolism of progesterone to DOC, corticosterone and 18OHDOC in cultured human melanoma cells. *FEBS Lett.* **445,** 364–366.

36. Boni, R. and Zhuang, Z. (1998) Loss of heterozygosity detected on 1 p and 9q in microdissected atypical nevi. *Arch. Dermatol.* **134,** 882–883.

37. Park, W.-S., Vortmeyer, A. O., Pack, S., Duray, P. H., Boni, R., Guerami, A. A., Emmert-buck, M. R., Liotta, L. A., and Zhuang, Z. (1997) Allelic deletion at chromosome 9p21 (p16) and 17p13(p53) in microdissected sporadic dysplastic nevus. *Hum. Pathol.* **29,** 127–130.

38. Bastian, B. C., Wesselmann, U., Pinkel, D., and LeBoit, P. E. (1999) Molecular cytogenetic analysis of Spitz nevi shows clear differences to melanoma. *J. Invest. Dermatol.* **113,** 1065–1069.

39. Glaessl, A., Bosserhoff, A. K., Buettner, R., Hohenleutner, U., Landthaler, M., and Stolz, W. (1999) Increase in telomerase activity during progression of melanocytic cells from melanocytic naevi to malignant melanomas. *Arch. Dermatol. Res.* **291,** 81–87.

40. Weterman, M. A. J., Van Muije, G. N. P., Bloemers, H. P. J., and Ruiter, D. (1994) Biology of disease: molecular markers of melanocytic tumor progression. *Lab. Invest.* **70,** 593–608.

41. Flores, J. F., Walker, G. J., Glendening, J. M., Haluska, F. G., Castresana, J. S., Rubio, M. P., Pastorfide, G. C., Boyer, L. A., Kao, W. H., Bulyk, M. L., Barnhill, R. L., Hayward, N. K., Housman, D. E., and Fountain, J. W. (1996) Loss of the p16^{INK4a} and p15^{INK4b} genes as well as neighboring 9p21 markers, in sporadic melanoma. *Cancer Res.* **56,** 5023–5032.

42. Holland, E. A., Beaton, S. C., Edwards, B. G., Kefford, R. F., and Mann, G. J. (1994) Loss of heterozygosity and homozygous deletions on 9q21-22 in melanoma. *Oncogene* **9,** 1361–1365.

43. Thompson, F. H., Emerson, J., Olson, S., et al. (1995) Cytogenetics in 158 patients with regional or disseminated melanoma: subset analysis of near-diploid and simple karyotype. *Cytogenet. Cell Genet.* **83,** 93–104.

44. Robertson, G., Coleman, A., and Lugo, T. G. (1996) A malignant melanoma tumor suppressor on human chromosome 11. *Cancer Res.* **56,** 487–4492.

45. Dracopoli, N. C., Houghton, A. N., and Old, L. J. (1985) Loss of polymorphic restriction fragments in malignant melanoma: implications for tumor heterogeneity. *Proc. Natl. Acad. Sci. USA* **82,** 1470–1474.

46. Herlyn, M., (1993) *Molecular and Cellular Biology of Melanoma,* RG Landes, Austin, TX.

47. Poetsch, M., Woenckhaus, C., Dittberner, T., Pambor, M., Lorenz, G., and Herrmann, F. H. (1998) Differences in chromosomal aberrations between nodular and superficial spreading malignant melanoma detected by interphase cytogenetics. *Lab. Invest.* **78,** 883–887.

48. Millikin, D., Meese, E., Vogelstein, B., et al. (1991) Loss of heterozygosity for loci on the long arm of chromosome 6 in human malignant melanoma. *Cancer Res.* **51,** 5449–5443.

49. Walker, G. J., Palmer, J. M., Walters, M. K., Nancarrow, D. J., Parsons, P. G., and Hayward, N. K. (1994) Simple tandem repeat allelic deletions confirm the preferential loss of distal chromosome 6q in melanoma. *Int. J. Cancer* **58,** 203–206.

50. Robertson, G. P., Coleman, A. B., and Lugo, T. G. (1996) Mechanisms of human melanoma cell growth and tumor suppression by chromosome 6. *Cancer Res.* **56,** 1635–1641.

51. Trent, J. M., Stanbridge, E. J., McBride, H. L., Meese, E. U., Casey, G., Araujo, D. E., Witkowski, C. M., and Nagle, R. B. (1990) Tumorigenicity in human melanoma cell lines controlled by introduction of human chromosome 6. *Science* **247,** 568–571.

52. Ray, M. E., Su, Y. A., Meltzer, P. S., and Trent, J. M. (1996) Isolation and characterization of genes associated with chromosome-6 mediated tumor suppression in human malignant melanoma. *Oncogene* **12**, 2527–2533.

53. Bastian, B. C., LeBoit, P. E., Hamm, H., Brocker, E., and Pinkel, D. (1998) Chromosomal gains and losses in primary cutaneous melanomas detected by comparative genomic hybridization. *Cancer Res.* **58**, 2170–2175.

54. Koprowski, H., Herlyn, M., Balaban, G., Parmiter, A., Ross, A., and Nowell, P. (1985) Expression of the receptor for epidermal growth factor correlates with increased dosage of chromosome 7 in malignant melanoma. *Somatic Cell Mol. Genet.* **11**, 297–302.

55. Robertson, G. P., Herbst, R. A., Nagane, M., Huang, H.-J., and Cavenee, W. K. (1999) The chromosome 10 monosomy common in human melanomas results from the loss of two separate tumor suppressor loci. *Cancer Res.* **59**, 3596–3601.

56. Isshiki, K., Elder, D. E., Guerry, D. P., and Linnenbach, A. J. (1993) Chromosome 10 allelic loss in malignant melanoma gene chromosomes. *Cancer* **8**, 178–184.

57. Degen, W. G. J., Weterman, A. A. J., VanGroningen, J. J.. Cornelissen, I. M., Lemmers, J. P., Agterbos, M. A., Geurts van Kessel, A., Swart, G. W., and Bloemers, H. P. (1996) Expression of nma, a novel gene, inversely correlates with the metastatic potential of human melanoma cell lines and xenografts. *Int. J. Cancer* **65**, 460–465.

58. Easty, D. J., Maung, K., Lascu, I., Veron, M., Fallowfield, M. E., Hart, I. R., and Bennett, D. C. (1996) Expression of NM23 in human melanoma progression and metastasis. *Br. J. Cancer* **74**, 109–114.

59. Naylor, M. F. and Everett, M. A. (1996) Involvement of the p16INK4 (CDKN2) gene in familial melanoma. *Melanoma Res.* **6**, 139–145.

60. Borg, A., Johansson, U., Hakansson, O., Westerdahl, J., Masback, A., Olsson, H., and Ingvar, C. (1996) Novel germline p16 mutation in familial melanoma in southern Sweden. *Cancer Res.* **56**, 2497–2500.

61. Ohta, M., Berd, D., Shimizu, M., et al. (1996) Deletion mapping of chromosome region 9p21-p22 surrounding the CDKN2 locus in melanoma. *Int. J. Cancer* **65**, 762–767.

62. Holland, E. A., Beaton, S. C., Becker, T. M., Grulet, O. M., Peters, B. A., Rizos, H., Kefford, R. F., and Mann, G. J. (1995) Analysis of the p16 gene, CDKN2, in 17 Australian melanoma kindreds. *Oncogene* **11**, 2289–2294.

63. Fitzgerald, M. G., Harkin, D. P., Silva-Arrieta, S., MacDonald, D. J., Lucchina, L. C., Unsal, H., O'Neill, E., Koh, J., Finkelstein, D. M., Isselbacher, K. J., Sober, A. J., and Haber, D. A. (1996) Prevalence of germ-line mutations in p16, p19ARF, and CDK4 in familial melanoma: analysis of a clinic-based population. *Proc. Natl. Acad. Sci. USA* **93**, 8541–8545.

64. Kamb, A., Gruis, N. A., Weaver-Feldhaus, J., Liu, Q., Harshman, K., Tavtigian, S. V., Stockert, E., Day, R. S., Johnson, B. E., and Skolnick, M. H. (1994) A cell cycle regulator potentially involved in genesis of many tumor types. *Science* **264**, 436–440.

65. Reed, J. A., Loganzo, F. Jr., Shea, C. R., et al. (1995) Loss of expression of the p16/cyclin-dependent kinase inhibitor 2 tumor suppressor gene in melanocytic

lesions correlates with invasive stage of tumor progression. *Cancer Res.* **55,** 2713–2718.

66. Ohta, M., Nagai, H., Shimizu, M., et al. (1994) Rarity of somatic and germline mutations of the cyclin-dependent kinase 4 inhibitor gene, CDK41, in melanoma. *Cancer Res.* **54,** 5269–5272.

67. Glendening, J. M., Flores, J. F., Walker, G. J., Stone, S., Albino, A. P., and Fountain, J. W. (1995) Homozygous loss of the p15^{INK4B} gene (and not the p16^{INK4} gene) during tumors progression in sporadic melanoma patients. *Cancer Res.* **55,** 5531–5535.

68. Wang, Y. and Becker, D. (1996) Differential expression of the cyclin-dependent kinase inhibitors p16 and p21 in the human melanocytic system. *Oncogene* **12,** 1069–1075.

69. Wang, Y.-L., Uhara, H., Yamazaki, Y., Nikaido, T., and Saida, T. (1996) Immunocytochemical detection of CDK4 and p16^{INK4} proteins in cutaneous malignant melanoma. *Br. J. Dermatol.* **134,** 269–275.

70. Zuo, L., Weger, J., Yang, Q., Goldstein, A. M., Tucker, M. A., Walker, G. J., Hayward, N., and Dracopoli, N. C. (1996) Germline mutations in the p16^{INK4a} binding domain of CDK4 in familial melanoma. *Nat. Genet.* **12,** 97–99.

71. Harris, C. C. (1996) P53: at the crossroads of molecular carcinogenesis and molecular epidemiology. *J. Invest. Dermatol. Symp. Proc.* **1,** 115–118.

72. Matsumura, Y., Sato, M., Nishigori, C., Zghal, M., Yagi, T., Imamura, S., and Takebe, H. (1995) High prevalence of mutations in the p53 gene in poorly differentiated squamous cell carcinomas in xeroderma pigmentosum patients. *J. Invest. Dermatol.* **105,** 399–401.

73. Bae, I., Smith, M. L., Sheikh, M. S., Zhan, Q., Scudiero, D. A., Friend, S. H., O'Connor, P. M., and Fornace, A. J. Jr. (1996) An abnormality in the p53 pathway following 8-irradiation in many wild-type p53 human melanoma lines. *Cancer Res.* **56,** 840–847.

74. Davol, P. A., Goulette, F. A., Frackelton, A. R. Jr., and Darnowski, J. W. (1996) Modulation of p53 expression by human recombinant interferon-α2a correlates with abrogation of cisplastin resistance in a human melanoma cell line. *Cancer Res.* **56,** 2522–2526.

75. Hartmann, A., Blaszyk, H., Cunningham, J. S., McGovern, R. M., Schroeder, J. S., Helander, S. D., Pittelkow, M. R., Sommer, S. S., and Kovach, J. S. (1996) Overexpression and mutations of p53 in metastatic malignant melanomas. *Int. J. Cancer* **67,** 313–320.

76. Yamanishi, D. T., Buckmeier, J. A., and Meyskens, F. L. (1991) Expression of c-jun, jun-B, and c-fos proto-oncogenes in human primary melanocytes and metastatic melanomas. *J. Invest. Dermatol.* **97,** 349–353.

77. Manova, K. and Bachvarova, R. F. (1991) Expression of c-kit encoded at the W locus of mice in developing embryonic germ cells and presumptive melanoblasts. *Dev. Biol.* **146,** 312–324.

78. Halaban, R., Kwon, B. S., Ghosh, S., Delli Bovi, P., and Baird, A. (1988) bFGF as an autocrine growth factor for human melanomas. *Oncogene Res.* **3,** 177–186.

79. Halaban, R. (1991) Growth factors and tyrosine protein kinases in normal and malignant melanocytes. *Cancer Met. Rev.* **10,** 129–140.

80. Halaban, R., Rubin, J. S., Funasaka, Y., et al. (1992) Met and hepatocyte growth factor/scatter factor signal transduction in normal melanocytes and melanoma cells. *Oncogene* **7,** 2195–2206.

81. Yaar, M. and Gilchrest, B. (1991) Human melanocyte growth and differentiation: a decade of new data. *J. Invest. Dermatol.* **97,** 611–617.

82. Thody, A. J. (1995) Epidermal melanocytes: their regulation and role in skin pigmentation. *Eur. J. Dermatol.* **5,** 558–565.

83. Imokawa, G., Yada, Y., and Kimura, M. (1996) Signalling mechanisms of endothelin-induced mitogenesis and melanogenesis in human melanocytes. *Biochem. J.* **314,** 305–312.

84. Spritz, R. A. (1994) Molecular basis of human piebaldism. *J. Invest. Dermatol.* **103,** 137S–140S.

85. Scott, G., Stoler, M., Sarkar, S., and Halaban, R. (1991) Localization of basic fibroblast growth factor mRNA in melanocytic lesions by in situ hybridization. *J. Invest. Dermatol.* **96,** 318–322.

86. Kuchler, K. and Thomer, J. (1992) Secretion of peptides lacking hydrophobic signal sequence: the role of adenosine triphosphate-driven membranes translocators. *Endocr. Rev.* **13,** 499–514.

87. Kahn, R., Murray, M., and Pawelek, J. (1980) Inhibition of proliferation of Cloudman S91 melanoma cells by insulin and characterization of some insulin-resistant variants. *J. Cell. Physiol.* **103,** 109–119.

88. Bregman, M. D., Abdel Malek, Z. A., and Meykens, F. L. (1985) Anchorage-independent growth of murine melanoma in serum-less media is dependent on insulin or melanocyte-stimulating hormone. *Exp. Cell Res.* **157,** 419–428.

89. Slominski, A., McNeely, T., and Pawelek, J. (1992) Insulin receptor proteolysis in insulin resistant variants of Cloudman S91 melanoma cells. *Melanoma Res.* **2,** 115–122.

90. Slominski, A., Chassalerris, N., Mazurkiewicz, J., and Paus, R. (1994) Murine skin as a target for melatonin bioregulation. *Exp. Dermatol.* **3,** 45–40.

91. Slominski, A. and Pruski, D. (1993) Melatonin inhibits proliferation and melanogenesis in rodent melanoma cells. *Exp. Cell Res.* **206,** 189–294.

92. Pawelek , J., Murray, M., and Fleischman, R. D. (1982) Genetic studies of insulin action in Cloudman melanoma cells. *Cold Spring Harb. Conf. Cell. Prolif.* **9,** 911–919.

93. Fleischmann, R. D. and Pawelek, J. M. (1985) Evidence that a 90-kDa phosphoprotein, an associated kinase, and a specific phosphatase are involved in the regulation of Cloudman melanoma cell proliferation by insulin. *Proc. Natl. Acad. Sci. USA* **82,** 1007–1011.

94. McNeely, T., Slominski, A., Bomirski, A., and Pawelek, J. (1986) Phosphorylation of protein of approximately 90 K daltons is a factor in the regulation of melanoma cell growth by insulin and the expression of high affinity receptors for insulin, in *Advances in Gene Technology: Molecular Biology of the Endocrine System* ICSU Short Reports (Puet, D., et al., eds.), University Press, Cambridge, MA, p. 55.

95. Lerner, A., Case, J. D., Takahashi, Y., et al. (1958) Isolation of melatonin, the pineal gland factor that lightens melanocytes. *J. Am. Chem. Soc.* **80,** 2857–2860.

96. Slominski, A., Baker, J., Rosano, T., Guisti, L. W., Ermak, G., Grande, M., and Gaudet, S. J. (1996) Metabolism of serotonin to N-acetylserotonin, melatonin and 5-hydroxytryptamine in hamster skin culture. *J. Biol. Chem.* **271,** 12,281–12,286.

97. Slominski, A., Paus, R., and Bomirski, A. (1989) Hypothesis: a possible role of the melatonin receptor in vitiligo. *J. R. Soc. Med.* **82,** 539–541.

98. Swope, V. B., Abdel-Malek, Z., Kassem, L. M., and Nordlund, J. J. (1991) Interleukins 1α and 6 and tumor necrosis factor-α are paracrine inhibitors of human melanocyte proliferation and melanogenesis. *J. Invest. Dermatol.* **96,** 180–185.

99. Krasagakis, K., Garbe, C., and Orfanos, C. E. (1993) Cytokines in human melanoma cells: synthesis, autocrine stimulation and regulatory functions-an overview. *Melanoma Res.* **3,** 425–433.

100. Slominski, A., Paus, R., and Schanderdorf, D. (1993) Melanocytes as sensory and regulatory cells in the epidermis. *J. Theor. Biol.* **164,** 103–120.

101. Slominski, A., Paus, R., and Wortsman, J. (1993) On the potential role of proopiomelanocortin in skin physiology and pathology. *Mol. Cell. Endocrinol.* **93,** C1–C6.

102. Elder, D. E., Rodeck, U., Thurin, J., Cardillo, F., Clark, W. H., Stewart, R., and Herlyn, M. (1989) Antigenic profile of tumor progression stages in human melanocytic nevi and melanomas. *Cancer Res.* **49,** 5091–5096.

103. Carrel, S., Dore, J. F., Ruiter, D. J., Prade, M., Lejeune, F. J., Kleeberg, U. R., Rumke, P., and Brocker, E. B. (1991) The EORTC melanoma group exchange program: evaluation of a multicenter monoclonal antibody study. *Int. J. Cancer* **48,** 836–847.

104. Ellis, D. L., King, L. E., and Nanney, L. B. (1992) Increased epidermal growth factor receptors in melanocytic lesions. *J. Am. Acad. Dermatol.* **27,** 539–546.

105. Nanney, L. B., Coffey, R. J., and Ellis, D. L. (1994) Expression and distribution of transforming growth factor-α within melanocytic lesions. *J. Invest. Dermatol.* **103,** 707–714.

106. Reed, J. A., McNutt, N. S., Prieto, V. G., and Albino, A. P. (1994) Expression of transforming growth factor-β2 in malignant melanoma correlates with the depth of tumor invasion. *Am. J. Pathol.* **145,** 97–104.

107. Schmid, P., Itin, P., and Rufli, T. (1995) In situ analysis of transforming growth factors-βs (TGF-β1, TGF-β2, TGF-β3), and TGF-β type II receptor expression in malignant melanoma. *Carcinogenesis* **16,** 1499–1503.

108. Van Belle, P., Rodeck, U., Nuamah, I., Halpern, A. C., and Elder, D. E. (1996) Melanoma-associated expression of transforming growth factor-β isoforms. *Am. J. Pathol.* **148,** 1887–1894.

109. Fleming, M. G., Howe, S. F., and Graf, L. H. (1994) Expression of insulin-like growth factor I (IGF-I) in nevi and melanomas. *Am. J. Dermatopathol.* **16,** 383–391.

110. Lattime, E. C., Mastrangelo, M. J., Bagasra, O., Li, W., and Berd, D. (1995) Expression of cytokine mRNA in human melanoma tissues. *Cancer Immunol. Immunother.* **41,** 151–156.

111. Kerbel, R. S., Kobayashi, H., Graham, C. H., and Lu, C. (1996) Analysis and significance of the malignant 'eclipse' during the progression of primary cutaneous human melanomas. *J. Invest. Dermatol. Symp. Proc.* **1,** 183–187.

112. Moretti, S., Pinzi, C., Spallanzani, A., Berti, E., Chiarugi, A., Mazzoli, S., Fabiani, M., Vallecchi, C., and Herlyn, M. (1999) Immunohistochemical evidence of cytokine networks during progression of human melanocytic lesions. *Int. J. Cancer* **20,** 160–168.

113. Kerbel, R. S. (1992) Expression of multi-cytokine resistance and multi-growth factor independence in advanced stage metastatic cancer. *Am. J. Pathol.* **141,** 519–524.

114. Armstrong, C. A., Botella, R., Galloway, T. H., Murray, N., Kramp, J. M, Song, I. S., and Ansel, J. C. (1996) Antitumor effects of granulocyte-macrophage colony-stimulating factor production by melanoma cells. *Cancer Res.* **56,** 2191–2198.

115. Dummer, W., Bastian, B. C., Ernst, N., Schanzle, C., Schwaaf, A., and Brocker, E. B. (1996). Interleukin-10 production in malignant melanoma: preferential detection of IL-10-secreting tumor cells in metastatic lesions. *Int. J. Cancer* **66,** 607–610.

116. Slominski, A. and Paus, R. (1993) Bomirski melanomas: a versatile and powerful model for pigment cell and melanoma research. *Int. J. Oncol.* **2,** 221–228.

117. Moellmann, G., Slominski, A., Kuklinska, E., and Lerner, A. B. (1988) Regulation of melanogenesis in melanocytes. *Pigment Cell Res.* **(Suppl. 1),** 79–87.

118. Hunt, G. (1995) Melanocyte-stimulating hormone: a regulator of human melanocyte physiology. *Pathobiology* **63,** 12–21.

119. Eberle, A. N., (1988) *The Melanotropins: Chemistry, Physiology and Mechanism of Action,* S Karger, New York.

120. Nordlund, J. J., Boissy, R. E., Hearing, V. J., King, R. A., and Ortonne, J. P. (1988) *The Pigmentary System. Physiology and Pathophysiology,* Oxford University Press, New York.

121. Mountjoy, K. G., Robbins, L. S., Mortrud, M., and Cone, R. D. (1992) The cloning of a family genes that encode melanocortin receptors. *Science* **257,** 1248–1251.

122. Cone, R. and Mountjoy, K. G. (1993) Molecular genetics of the ACTH and melanocyte-stimulating hormone receptors. *Trends Endocrinol. Metab.* **4,** 242–247.

123. Dipasquale, A., McGuire, J., and Varga, J. M. (1977) The number or receptors for β-melanocyte stimulating hormone in Cloudman melanoma cells is increased by dibutyryl adenosine 3′:5′-cyclic monophosphate or cholera toxin. *Proc. Natl. Acad. Sci. USA* **74**, 601–605.

124. Chakraborty, A. K. and Pawelek, J. (1992) Up-regulation of MSH receptors by MSH in Cloudman melanoma cells. *Biochem. Biophys. Res. Commun.* **188**, 1325–1331.

125. McLane, J., Osber, M., and Pawelek, J. (1987) Phosphorylated isomers of L-dopa stimulate MSH binding capacity and responsiveness to MSH in cultured melanoma cells. *Biochem. Biophys. Res. Commun.* **145**, 719–725.

126. Slominski, A. and Pawelek, J. (1987) MSH binding in Bomirski amelanotic melanoma cells is stimulated by L-tyrosine. *Biosci. Rep.* **7**, 949–954.

127. Slominski, A., Jastreboff, P., and Pawelek, J. (1989) L-tyrosine stimulates induction of tyrosinase activity by MSH and reduces cooperative interactions between MSH receptors in hamster melanoma cells. *Biosci. Rep.* **9**, 579–587.

128. Chakraborty, A. K., Orlow, S. J., and Pawelek, J. (1990) Stimulation of melanocyte-stimulating hormone receptors by retinoic acid. *FEBS Lett.* **276**, 205–208.

129. Chakraborty, A., Pawelek, J. M., Bolognia, J., Funasaka, Y., and Slominski, A. (1999) UV light and MSH receptors. *Ann. NY Acad. Sci.* **885**, 100–116.

130. Slominski, A. and Pawelek, J. (1998) Animals under the sun: effects of UV radiation on mammalian skin. *Clin. Dermatol.* **16**, 503–515.

131. Chakraborty, A., Slominski, A., Ermak, G., Hwang, J., and Pawelek, J. (1995) Ultraviolet and melanocyte-stimulating hormone (MSH) stimulate mRNA production of αMSH receptors and proopiomelanocortin-derived peptides in mouse melanoma cells and transformed keratinocytes. *J. Invest. Dermatol.* **105**, 655–659.

132. Kameyama, K., Tanaka, S., Ishida, Y., and Hearing, V. J. (1989) Interferons modulate the expression of hormone receptors on the surface of murine melanoma cells. *J. Clin. Invest.* **83**, 213–221.

133. Valverde, P., Healy, E., Jackson, I., Rees, J. L., and Thody, A. J. (1995) Variants of the melanocyte-stimulating hormone receptor gene are associated with red hair and fair skin in humans. *Nat. Genet.* **11**, 328–330.

134. Valverde, P., Healy, E., Sikkink, S., Haldane, F., Thody, A. J., Carothers, A., Jackson, I. J., and Rees, J. L. (1996) The Asp84Glu variant of the melanocortin 1 receptor (MC1R) is associated with melanoma. *Hum. Mol. Genet.* **5**, 1663–1666.

135. Slominski, A. (1991) POMC gene expression in mouse and hamster melanoma cells. *FEBS Lett.* **291**, 165–168.

136. Slominski, A., Wortsman, J., Mazurkiewicz, J., Matsuoka, L., Lawrence, K., and Paus, R. (1993) Detection of the proopiomelanocortin derived-antigens in normal and pathologic human skin. *J. Lab. Clin. Med.* **122**, 658–656.

137. Nagahama, M., Funasaka, Y., Fernandez-Frez, M. L., Ohashi, A., Chakraborty, A. K., Ueda, M., and Ichihashi, M. Immunoreactivity of α-melanocyte-stimulating hormone, adrenocorticotrophic hormone and β-endorphin in cutaneous malignant melanoma and benign melanocytic naevi. *Br. J. Dermatol.* **138**, 981–985.

138. Loir, B., Bouchard, B., Morandini, R., Del Marmol, V., Deraemaecker, R., Garcia-Borron, J. C., and Ghanem, G. (1997) Immunoreactive α-melanotropin as an autocrine effector in human melanoma cells. *Eur. J. Biochem.* **244,** 923–930.

139. Ghanem, G., Lienard, D., Hanson, P., Lejeune, F., and Fruhling, J. (1986) Increased serum α-melanocyte stimulating hormone (α-MSH) in human malignant melanoma. *Eur. J. Cancer Clin. Oncol.* **22,** 535,536.

140. Luger, T. A., Scholzen, T., Brzoska, T., Becher, E., Slominski, A., and Paus, R. (1998) Cutaneous immunomodulation and coordination of skin stress responses by alpha-melanocyte-stimulating hormone. *Ann. NY Acad. Sci.* **840,** 381–394.

141. Raper, H. S. (1928) The aerobic oxidases. *Physiol. Rev.* **8,** 245–282.

142. Lerner, A. B. and Fitzpatrick, T. B. (1950) Biochemistry of melanin formation. *Physiol. Rev.* **30,** 91–126.

143. Pawelek, J. and Korner, A. (1982) The biosynthesis of mammalian melanin. *Am. Sci.* **70,** 136–145.

144. Korner, A. M. and Pawelek, J. M. (1982) Mammalian tyrosinase catalyzed three reactions in the biosynthesis of melanin. *Science* **217,** 1163–1165.

145. Pawelek, J. (1991) After Dopachrome? Pigment. *Cell. Res.* **4,** 53–62.

146. Hearing, V. J. and Tsukamato, K. (1991) Enzymatic control of pigmentation in mammals. *FASEB J.* **5,** 2902–2909.

147. Prota, G. (1988) Progress in the chemistry of melanins and related metabolites. *Med. Res. Rev.* **8,** 525–556.

148. Prota, G. (1995) The chemistry of melanins and melanogenesis. *Fortsch. Chem. Organ. Natur.* **64,** 93–148.

149. Silvers, W. K., (1979) *The Coat Colors of Mice: A Model for Mammalian Gene Action and Interaction*, Springer Verlag, New York.

150. Sealy, R. C., Hyde, J. S., Felix, C. C., Menon, I. A., Prota, G., Swartz, H. M., Persad, S., and Haberman, H. F. (1982) Novel free radicals in synthetic and natural pheomelanins: distinction between dopa melanins and cysteinyldopa melanins by ESR spectroscopy. *Proc. Natl. Acad. Sci. USA* **79,** 2885–2889.

151. Sealy, R. C., Hyde, J. S., Felix, C. C., Menon, I. A., and Prota, G. (1982) Eumelanins and pheomelanins: characterization by electron spin resonance spectroscopy. *Science* **217,** 545–547.

152. Lukiewicz, S. (1976) Interference with endogenous radioprotectors as a method of radiosensitization, in *IAEA's Modification of Radiosensitivity of Biological Systems*, Proc. Advisory Group Meeting, International Atomic Energy Agency, Vienna, pp. 61–76.

153. Slominski, A. (1985) Some properties of Bomirski Ab amelanotic melanoma cells, which underwent spontaneous melanization in primary cell culture: growth kinetics, cell morphology, melanin content and tumorogenicity. *J. Cancer Res. Clin. Oncol.* **109,** 29–37.

154. Slominski, A., Paus, R., Plonka, P., Chakraborty, A., Maurer, M., Pruski, D., and Lukiewicz, S. (1994) Melanogenesis during the anagen-catagen-telogen transformation of the murine hair cycle. *J. Invest. Dermatol.* **102,** 862–869.

155. Slominski, A., Paus, R., Plonka, P., Handjiski, B., Maurer, M., Chakraborty, A., and Mihm, M. C. Jr. (1996) Pharmacological disruption of hair follicle pigmentation as a model for studying the melanocyte response to and recovery from cytotoxic damage in situ. *J. Invest. Dermatol.* **106,** 1203–1211.

156. Seiji, M. (1967) Subcellular particles and melanin formation in melanocytes. *Adv. Biol. Skin* **8,** 189–222.

157. Stanka, P., Kinzel, V., and Mohr, U. (1969) Elektronenmikroskopische Untersuchung uber die Pramelanosomenentstehung an Melanomzellen in vitro. *Virchows Arch. Abt. B. Zellpath.* **2,** 91–102.

158. Orlow, S., Boissy, R. E., Moran, D. J., and Pifko-Hirst, S. (1993) Subcellular distribution of tyrosinase and tyrosinase-related protein-1: implications for melanosomal biogenesis. *J. Invest. Dermatol.* **100,** 55–64.

159. Bomirski, A., Slominski, A., and Bigda, J. (1988) The natural history of a family of transplantable melanomas in hamsters. *Cancer Met. Rev.* **7,** 95–119.

160. Jimbow, K., Miyake, Y., Homma, K., Yasuda, K., Izumi, Y., Tsutsumi, A., and Ito, S. (1984) Characterization of melanogenesis and morphogenesis of melanosomes by physicochemical properties of melanin and melanosomes in malignant melanoma. *Cancer Res.* **44,** 1128–1134.

161. Orlow, S. J. (1995) Melanosomes are specialized members of lysosomal lineage of organelles. *J. Invest. Dermatol.* **105,** 3–7.

162. Slominski, A. and Paus, R. (1990) Are L-tyrosine and L-dopa hormone-like bioregulators. *J. Theor. Biol.* **143,** 123–138.

163. Scislowski, P. W. D., Slominski, A., and Bomirski, A. (1984) Biochemical characterization of three hamster melanoma variants. II. Glycolysis and oxygen consumption. *Int. J. Biochem.* **16,** 327–331.

164. Scislowski, P. W. D. and Slominski, A. (1983) The role of NADP-dependent dehydrogenases in hydroxylation of tyrosine in hamster melanoma. *Neoplasma* **30,** 239–243.

165. Scislowski, P. W. D., Slominski, A., Bomirski, A., and Zydowo, M. (1985) Metabolic characterization of three hamster melanoma variants. *Neoplasma* **32,** 593–598.

166. Drager, U. C. and Balkema, G. W. (1987) Does melanin do more than protect from light? *Neurosci. Res. Suppl.* **6,** S75–S86.

167. Kwon, B. S., Haq, A. K., Pomerantz, S. H., and Halaban, R. (1987) Isolation and sequencing of a cDNA clone for human tyrosinase that maps at the mouse c-albino locus. *Proc. Natl. Acad. Sci. USA* **84,** 7473–7477.

168. Shibahara, S., Tomita, Y., Tagami, H., Muller, R. M., and Cohen, T. (1988) Molecular basis for the heterogeneity of human tyrosinase. *Tohoku J. Exp. Med.* **156,** 403–414.

169. Ruppert, S., Muller, G., Kwon, B., and Schultz, G. (1988) Multiple transcripts of the mouse tyrosinase gene are generated by alternative splicing. *EMBO J.* **7,** 2715–2722.

170. Slominski, A. and Paus, R. (1994) Towards defining receptors for L-tyrosine and L-DOPA. *Mol. Cell. Endocrinol.* **99,** C7–C11.

171. DelMarmol, V. and Beermann, F. (1996) Tyrosinase and related proteins in mammalian pigmentation. *FEBS Lett.* **381,** 165–168.
172. Sanchez-Ferrer, A., Rodriguez-Lopez, J. P., Garcia-Canovas, F., and Garcia-Carmona, F. (1995) Tyrosinase: a comprehensive review of its mechanism. *Biochim. Biophys. Acta.* **1247,** 1–11.
173. Slominski, A., Costantino, R., Howe, J., and Moellmann, G. (1991) Molecular mechanism governing melanogenesis in hamster melanomas: relative abundance of tyrosinase and catalase-B (gp 75). *Anticancer Res.* **11,** 257–263.
174. Slominski, A., Paus, R., and Costantino, R. (1991) Differential expression and activity of melanogenesis-related proteins during induced hair growth in mice. *J. Invest. Dermatol.* **96,** 172–179.
175. Orlow, S. J., Zhou, B. K., Chakraborty, A. K., Drucker, M., Pifko-Hirst, S., and Pawelek, J. M. (1994) High molecular weight forms of tyrosinase and the tyrosinase-related proteins: evidence for a melanogenic complex. *J. Invest. Dermatol.* **103,** 196–201.
176. Slominski, A., Moellmann, G., and Kuklinska, E. (1989) L-tyrosine, L-dopa and tyrosinase as positive regulators of the subcellular apparatus of melanogenesis in Bomirski Ab amelanotic melanoma. *Pigment Cell Res.* **2,** 109–116.
177. Slominski, A., Moellmann, G., Kuklinska, E., Bomirski, A., and Pawelek, J. (1988) Positive regulation of melanin pigmentation by two key substrates of the melanogenic pathway: L-tyrosine and L-dopa. *J. Cell Sci.* **89,** 287–296.
178. Slominski, A. and Costantino, R. (1991) Molecular mechanism of tyrosinase regulation by L-DOPA. *Life Sci.* **48,** 2075–2079.
179. Slominski, A. and Friedrich, T. (1992) L-DOPA inhibits in vitro phosphorylation of melanoma glycoproteins. *Pigment Cell Res* **5,** 396–400.
180. Slominski, A. and Pruski, D. (1992) L-DOPA binding sites in rodent melanoma cells. *Biochim. Biophys. Acta.* **1139,** 324–328.
181. Cohen, T., Muller, R. M., Tomita, Y., and Shibahara, S. (1990) Nucleotide sequence of the cDNA encoding human tyrosinase-related protein. *Nucl. Acid Res.* **18,** 2807,2808.
182. Jackson, I. J., Chambers, D. M., Budd, P. S., and Johnson, R. (1991) The tyrosinase-related protein-1 gene has a structure and promoter sequence very different from tyrosinase. *Nucl. Acid Res.* **19,** 3799–3804.
183. Kobayashi, T., Urabe, K., Winder, A., Jimenez-Cervantes, C., Imokawa, G., Brewington, T., Solano, F., Garcia-Borron, J. C., and Hearing, V. J. (1994) Tyrosinase related protein 1 (TRP1) functions as a DHICA oxidase in melanin biosynthesis. *EMBO J.* **13,** 5818–5825.
184. Jackson, I. J., Chambers, D. M., Tsukamato, K., Copeland, N. G., Gilbert, D. J., Jenkins, N. A., and Hearing, V. (1992) A second tyrosinase related protein, TRP2, maps to and is mutated at the mouse slaty locus. *EMBO J.* **11,** 527–535.
185. Yokoyama, K., Yasumoto, K.-I., Suzuki, H., and Shibahara, S. (1994) Cloning of the human DOPAchrome tautomerase/tyrosinase-related protein 2 gene and

identification of two regulatory regions required for its pigment cell-specific expression. *J. Biol. Chem.* **269,** 27,080–27,087.

186. Bouchard, B., DelMarmol, V., Jackson, I. J., Cherif, D., and Dubertret, L. (1994) Molecular characterization of human tyrosinase-related-protein-2 cDNA. Patterns of expression in melanocytic cells. *Eur. J. Biochem.* **219,** 127–134.

187. Yokoyama, K., Suzuki, H., Yasumoto, K., Tomita, Y., and Shibahara, S. (1994) Molecular cloning and functional analysis of a cDNA coding for human DOPAchrome tautomerase/tyrosinase related protein-2. *Biochim. Biophys. Acta.* **1217,** 317–321.

188. Yavuzer, U., Keenan, E., Lowings, P., Vachtenheim, J., Currie, G., and Goding, C. R. (1995) The microphtalmia gene product interacts with the retinoblastoma protein in vitro and is a target for deregulation of melanocyte-specific transcription. *Oncogene* **10,** 123–134.

189. Yasumoto, K.-I., Mhalingam, H., Suzuki, H., Yoshizawa, M., and Yokoyama, K. (1995) Transcriptional activation of the melanocyte-specific genes by the human homolog of the mouse microphthalmia protein. *J. Biochem.* **118,** 874–881.

190. DelMarmol, V., Ito, S., Jackson, I., Vachtenheim, J., Berr, P., Ghanem, G., Morandini, R., Wakamatsu, K., and Huez, G. (1993) TRP-1 expression correlates with eumelanogenesis in human pigment cells in culture. *FEBS Lett.* **327,** 307–310.

191. Tsukamato, K., Jackson, I. J., Urabe, K., Monatague, P. P., and Hearing, V. (1992) A second tyrosinase-related protein, TRP-2, is a melanogenic enzyme termed DOPAchrome tautomerase. *EMBO J.* **11,** 5219–5526.

192. Kwon, B. S., Chintamanemi, C., Kozak, C. A., Copeland, N. G., Gilbert, D. J., Jenkins, N., Barton, D., Francke, U., Kobayashi, Y., and Kim, K. K. (1991) A melanocyte-specific gene, Pmel17 maps near the silver coat color locus on mouse chromosome and is in synthetic region on human chromosome 12. *Proc. Natl. Acad. Sci. USA* **88,** 9228–9232.

193. Kwon, B. S. (1993) Pigmentation genes: the tyrosinase gene family and the Pmel17 gene family. *J. Invest. Dermatol.* **100,** 134S–140S.

194. Adema, G. J., deBoer, A. J., van't Hullenaar, R., Denijn, M., Ruiter, D. J., Vogel, A. M., and Figdor, C. G. (1993) Melanocyte lineage-specific antigens recognized by monoclonal antibodies NKI-beteb, HMB-50, and HMB-45 are encoded by a single cDNA. *Am. J. Pathol.* **143,** 1579–1585.

195. Wagner, S. N., Wagner, C., Hofler, F. H., Atkinson, M. J., and Goos, M. (1995) Expression cloning of the cDNA encoding a melanoma-associated Ag recognized by mAb HMB-45: identification as melanocyte-specific Pmel17 cDNA. *Lab. Invest.* **73,** 229–235.

196. Adema, G. J., deBoer, A. J., Vogel, A. M., Loenen, W. A., and Figdor, C. G. (1994) Molecular characterization of the melanocyte lineagespecific antigen gp 100. *J. Biol. Chem.* **269,** 20,126–20,133.

197. Chakraborty, A. K., Platt, J. L., Kwon, B. S., Bennett, D. C., and Pawelek, J. M. (1996) Polymerization of 5,6-dihydroxyindole 2-carboxylic acid to melanin by the PMEL17/silver locus. *Eur. J. Biochem.* **236,** 180–188.

198. Rinchik, E. M., Bultman, S. J., Horstlemke, B., Lee, S. T., Strunk, K. M., Spritz, R. A., Avidano, K. M., Jong, M. T., and Nicholls, R. D. (1993) A gene for the mouse pink-eyed dilution locus and for human type II oculocutaneous albinism. *Nature* **361,** 72–76.

199. Gardner, J. M., Nakatsu, Y., Gondo, Y., Lee, S., Lyon, M. F., King, R. A., and Brilliant, M. H. (1992) The mouse pink-eyed dilution gene: association with human Prader-Willi and Angelman syndromes. *Science* **257,** 1121–1124.

200. Salopek, T. G. and Jimbow, K. (1996) Induction of melanogenesis during the various melanoma growth phases and the role of tyrosinase, lysosome-associated membrane proteins, and p90 calnexin in the melanogensis cascade. *J. Invest. Dermatol.* **1,** 195–202.

201. Slominski, A., Paus, R., and Mihm, M. C. (1998) Inhibition ofmelanogenesis as an adjuvant strategy in the treatment of melanotic melanomas: selective review and hypothesis. *Anticancer Res.* **18,** 3709–3716.

202. Slominski, A. and Goodman-Snitkoff, G. (1992) DOPA inhibits induced proliferative activity of murine and human lymphocytes. *Anticancer Res.* **12,** 753–756.

203. Wick, M. (1983) The chemotherapy of malignant melanoma. *J. Invest. Dermatol.* **80,** 61S–62S.

204. Josefsson, E., Bergquist, J., Ekman, R., and Tarkowski, A. (1996) Catecholamines are synthesized by mouse lymphocytes and regulate function of these cells by induction of apoptosis. *Immunology* **88,** 140–146.

205. Berquist, J., Tarkowski, A., Ekman, R., and Ewing, A. (1994) Discovery of endogenous catecholamines in lymphocytes and evidence for catecholamine regulation of lymphocyte function via an autocrine loop. *Proc. Natl. Acad. Sci. USA* **91,** 12,912–12,916.

206. Huffnagle, G. B., Chen, G.-H., Curtis, J. L., McDonald, R. A., Strieter, R. M., and Toews, G. B. (1995) Down-regulation of the afferent phase of T cell-mediated pulmonary inflamation and immunity by a high melanin-producing strain of Cryptococcus neoformans. *J. Immunol.* **155,** 3507–3516.

207. Miranda, M., Ligas, C., Amicarelli, F., Dalessandro, E., Brisdelli, F., Zarivi, O., and Poma, A. (1997) Sister chromatid exchange (SCE) rates in human melanoma cells as an index of mutagenesis. *Mutagenesis* **12,** 233–236.

208. Miranda, M., Botti, D., and Di Cola, M. (1984) Possible genotoxicity of melanin synthesis intermediates: tyrosinase reaction products interact with DNA *in vitro*. *Mol. Gen. Genet.* **193,** 395–399.

209. Miranda, M., Poma, A. A., Ragnelli, A. M., Scirri, C., Aimola, P. p., Masciocco, L., Bonfigli, A., and Zarivi, O. (1994). Cyto-genotoxic species leakage with human melanoma melanosomes, molecular-morphological correlation. *Biochem. Mol. Biol. Int.* **32,** 913–922.

210. Alena, F., Jimbow, K., and Ito, S. (1990) Melanocytotoxicity and antimelanoma effects of phenolic amine compounds in mice *in vivo*. *Cancer Res.* **50,** 3743–3747.

211. Riley, P. A. (1991) Melanogenesis: a realistic target for antimelanoma therapy? *Eur. J. Cancer* **27,** 1172–1177.

212. Ortega, V. V., Diaz, F. M., Romero, C. C., Pacheco, G. O., Jordan, M. C., and Rubiales, F. C. (1995) Abnormal melanosomes: ultrastructural markers of melanocytic atypia. *Ultrastruct. Pathol.* **19,** 119–128.

213. Bomirski, A., Wrzolkowa, T., Arendarczyk, M., Bomirska, M., Kuklinska, E., Slominski, A., and Moellmann, G. (1987) Pathology and ultrastructural characteristics of a hypomelanotic variant of transplantable hamster melanoma with high tyrosinase activity. *J. Invest. Dermatol.* **89,** 469–473.

214. Borovansky, J., Mirejovsky, P., and Riley, P. A. (1991) Possible relationship between abnormal melanosome structure and cytotoxic phenomena in malignant melanoma. *Neoplasma* **38,** 393–400.

215. Hofbauer, G. F. L., Kamarashev, J., Geertsen, R., Boni, R., and Dummer, R. (1998) Melan A/MART-1 immunoreactivity in formalin-fixed paraffin-embedded primary and metastatic melanoma: frequency and distribution. *Melanoma Res.* **8,** 337–343.

216. Guo, J., Cheng, L., Wen, D. R., and Cochran, A. J. (1998) Detection of tyrosinase mRNA in formalin-fixed, paraffin-embedded archival sections of melanoma, using the reverse transcriptase in situ polymerase chain reaction. *Diagn. Mol. Pathol.* **7,** 10–15.

217. Hofbauer, G. G. L., Kamarashev, J., Geertsen, R., Boni, R., and Dummer, R. (1998) Tyrosinase immunoreactivity in formalin-fixed, paraffin-embedded primary and metastatic melanoma: frequency and distribution. *J. Cutan. Pathol.* **25,** 204–209.

218. Brossart, P., Keilholz, U., Willhauck, M., Scheibenbogen, C., Mohler, T., and Hunstein, W. (1993) Hematogenous spread of malignant melanoma cells in different stages of disease. *J. Invest. Dermatol.* **101,** 887–889.

219. Hoon, D. S. B., Wang, Y., Dale, P. S., Conrad, A. J., Schmid, P., Garrison, D., Kuo, C., Foshag, L. J., Nizze, A. J., and Morton, D. L. (1995) Detection of occult melanoma cells in blood with multiple-marker polymerase chain reaction assay. *J. Clin. Oncol.* **13,** 2109–2116.

220. Shivers, S. C., Wang, X., Li, W., Joseph, E., Messina, J., Glass, F., DeConti, R., Cruse, W., Berman, C., Fenske, N. A., Lyman, G. H., and Reintgen, D. S. (1998) Molecular staging of malignant melanoma. *JAMA* **280,** 1410–1415.

221. Ghossein, R. A., Bhattacharya, S., and Rosai, J. (1999) Molecular detection of micrometastases and circulating tumor cells in solid tumors. *Clin. Cancer Res.* **5,** 1950–1960, 1999.

222. Curry, B. J., Myers, K., and Hersey, P. (1998) Polymerase chain reaction detection of melanoma cells in the circulation: relation to clinical stage, surgical treatment, and recurrence from melanoma. *J. Clin. Oncol.* **16,** 1760–1769.

223. Ghossein, R. A., Coit, D., Brennan, M., Zhang, Z. F., Wang, Y., Bhattacharya, S., Houghton, A., and Rosai, J. (1998) Prognostic significance of peripheral blood and bone marrow tyrosinase messenger RNA in malignant melanoma. *Clin. Cancer Res.* **4,** 419–428.

224. Goydos, J. S., Ravikumar, T. S., Germino, F. J., Yudd, A., and Bancila, E. (1998) Minimally invasive staging of patients sith melanoma-sentinel lymphadenec-

tomy and detection of the melanoma-specific proteins MART-1 and tyrosinase by reverse transcriptase polymerase chain reaction. *J. Am. Coll. Surg.* **187,** 182–188.

225. Blaheta, H. J., Schittek, B., Breuniger, H., Maczey, E., Kroeber, S., Sotlar, K., Ellwanger, U., Thelen, M. H., Rassner, G., Bultmann, B., and Garbe, C. (1998) Lymph node micrometastases of cutaneous melanoma: increased sensitivity of molecular diagnosis in comparison to immunohistochemistry. *Int. J. Cancer* **21,** 318–323.

226. Rorsman, H., Agrup, G., Hansson, C., and Rosengren, E. (1983) Biochemical recorders of malignant melanoma. *Pigment Cell* **6,** 93–115.

227. Hara, H., Walsh, N., Yamada, K., and Jimbow, K. (1994) High plasma levels of a eumelanin precursor, 6-hydroxy-5-methoxyindole-2-carboxylic acid as a prognostic marker for malignant melanoma. *J. Invest. Dermatol.* **102,** 501–505.

228. Horikoshi, T., Ito, S., Wakamatsu, K., Onodera, H., and Eguchi, H. (1994) Evaluation of melanin-related metabolites as markers of melanoma progression. *Cancer* **73,** 629–636.

229. Karnell, R., Vonschoultz, E., Hansson, L. O., Nilsson, B., Arstrand, K., and Kagedal, B. (1997) S100B protein, 5-S-cysteinyldopa and 6-hydroxy-5-methoxyindole-2-carboxylic acid as biochemical markers for survival prognosis in patients with malignant melanoma. *Melanoma Res.* **7,** 393–399.

230. Wimmer, I., Meyer, J. C., Seifert, B., Dummer, R., Flace, A., and Burg, G. (1997) Prognostic value of serum 5-S-cysteinyldopa for monitoring human metastatic melanoma during immunochemotherapy. *Cancer Res.* **57,** 5073–5076.

231. Agrup, P., Carstam, R., Wittbjer, A., Rorsman, H., and Rosengren, E. (1989) Tyrosinase activity in serum from patients with malignant melanoma. *Acta. Derm. Venereol. (Stockh.)* **69,** 120–124.

232. Sonesson, B., Elde, S., Ringborg, U., Rorsman, H., and Rosengren, E. (1995) Tyrosinase activity in the serum of patients with malignant melanoma. *Melanoma Res.* **5,** 113–116.

233. Rosbullon, M. R., Sanchezpedreno, P., and Martinezliarte, J. H. (1998) Serum tyrosine hydroxylase activity is increased in melanoma patients—an ROC curve analysis. *Cancer Lett.* **129,** 151–155.

234. Slominski, A. and Paus, R. (1995) Inhibition of melanogenesis for melanoma therapy? *J. Invest. Dermatol.* **103,** 742.

235. Brichard, V., Van Pel, A., Wolfel, T., Wolfel, C., De Plaen, E., Lethe, B., Coulie, P., and Boon, T. (1993) The tyrosinase gene codes for an antigen recognized by autologous cytolytic T lymphocytes on HLA-A2 melanoma. *J. Exp. Med.* **178,** 489–495.

236. Bakker, A. B. H., Schreurs, M. W. J., DeBoer, A. J., Kawakami, Y., Rosenberg, S. A., Adema, G. J., and Figdor, C. G. (1994) Melanocyte lineage-specific antigen gp100 is recognized by melanoma-derived tumor-infiltrating lymphocytes. *J. Exp. Med.* **179,** 1005–1009.

237. Cox, A. L., Skipper, J., Chen, Y., Henderson, R. A., Darrow, T. L., Shabanowitz, J., Engelhard, V. H., Hunt, D. F., and Slingluff, C. L. Jr. (1994) Identification of a peptide recognized by five melanoma-specific human cytotoxic T cell lines. *Science* **264,** 716–719.

238. Kawakami, Y., Eliyahu, S., Sakaguchi, K., Robbins, P. F., Rivoltini, L., Yannelli, J. R., Appella, E., and Rosenberg, S. A. (1994) Identification of the immuno-dominant peptides of the MART-1 human melanoma antigen recognized by the majority of HLA-A2-restricted tumor infiltrating lymphocytes. *J. Exp. Med.* **180,** 347–352.

239. Celis, E., Tsai, V., Crimi, C., DeMars, R., Wentworth, P. A., Chesnut, R. W., Grey, H. M., Sette, A., and Serra, H. M. (1994) Induction of anti-tumor cyto-toxic T lymphocytes in normal humans using primary cultures and synthetic peptide epitopes. *Proc. Natl. Acad. Sci. USA* **91,** 2105–2109.

240. Ravindranath, M. H. and Irie, R. F. (1988) Gangliosides as antigens of human melanoma, in *Malignant Melanoma: Biology, Diagnosis, and Therapy* (Nathason, L., ed.) Kluwer Academic, Boston, pp. 17–43.

241. Ritter, G., Ritter-Boosfeld, E., Adluri, R., Calves, M., Ren, S., Yu, R. K., Oettgen, H. F., Old, L. J., and Livingston, P. O. (1995) Analysis of the antibody response to immunization with purified 0-acetyl GD3 gangliosides in patients with malignant melanoma. *Int. J. Cancer* **62,** 668–672.

242. Livingston, P. O., Wong, G. Y. C., Adluri, S., et al. (1994) Improved survival in stage III melanoma patients with GM2 antibodies: a randomized trial of adju-vant vaccination with GM2 ganglioside. *J. Clin. Oncol.* **12,** 1036–1044.

243. Portoukalian, J., Carrel, S., Dore, J. F., and Rumke, P. (1991) Humoral immune response in disease-free advanced melanoma patients after vaccination with melanoma-associated gangliosides. *Int. J. Cancer* **49,** 893–899.

244. Houghton, A. N. (1995) On course for a cancer vaccine. *Lancet* **345,** 1384–1385.

245. Hamilton, W. B., Helling, F., Llloyd, K. O., and Livingston, P. (1993) Ganglio-side expression on human malignant melanoma assessed by quantitative immune thin-layer chromatography. *Int. J. Cancer* **53,** 566–573.

246. Ravidranath, M. H., Tsuchida, T., Morton, D. L., and Irie, R. F. (1991) Ganglio-side GM3:GD3 ratio as an index for the management of melanoma. *Cancer* **67,** 3029–3035.

247. Ren, S., Slominski, A., and Yu, R. (1989) Glycosphingolipids in Bomirski trans-plantable hamster melanomas. *Cancer Res.* **49,** 7051–7056.

248. Ren, S. L., Ariga, T., Scarsdale, J. N., Zhang, Y., Slominski, A., Livingston, P. O., Ritter, G., Kushi, Y., and Yu, R. K. (1993) Characterization of a hamster mela-noma associated ganglioside antigen as 7-0-acetylated disialoglanglioside GD3. *J. Lipid Res.* **34,** 1565–1572.

249. Tsuchida, T., Saxton, R. E., Morton, D. L., and Irie, R. F. (1987) Gangliosides of human melanoma. *J. Natl. Cancer. Inst.* **78,** 45–54.

250. Carrel, S. and Rimoldi, D. (1993) Melanoma-associated antigens. *Eur. J. Cancer* **29A,** 1903–1907.

251. Kageshita, T., Nakamura, T., Yamada, M., Kuriya, N., Arao, T., and Ferrone, S. (1991) Differential expression of melanoma associated antigens in acral lenti-ginous melanoma and in nodular melanoma lesions. *Cancer Res.* **51,** 1726–1732.

252. Kageshita, T., Kuriya, N., Ono, T., Horikoshi, T., Takahashi, M., Wong, G. Y., and Ferrone, S. (1993) Association of high molecular weight melanoma-

associated antigen expression in primary acral lentiginous melanoma lesions with poor prognosis. *Cancer Res.* **53,** 2830–2833.

253. Favilla, I., Favilla, M. L., Gosbell, A. D., Barry, W. R., Ellims, P., Hill, J. S., and Byrne, J. R. (1995) Photodynamic therapy: a 5-year study of its effectiveness in the treatment of posterior uveal melanoma, and evaluation of haematoporphyrin uptake and photocytotoxicity of melanoma cells in tissue culture. *Melanoma Res.* **5,** 355–364.

254. Zygulska-Mach, H., Maciejewski, Z., Lukiewicz, S., Iwasiow, B., and Link, E. (1979) Clinical trials on chemical radiosensitization of malignant melanoma of the chorid. *Ophthalmologica* **178,** 194–197.

9

Identification of Altered Gene Expression Associated with Pigmentary Lesions by Differential Display Analysis

I. Caroline Le Poole and Thomas L. Brown

1. Introduction

Identification of alterations in gene expression is an important step in understanding the development and progression of human disease. For pigmentary disorders with an unresolved hereditary component, genetic and epigenetic changes that alter the expression of genes as a direct or indirect consequence can be investigated by expression analysis. This can be of particular importance in conditions in which multiple genes are involved, as in melanoma or vitiligo *(1,2)*. Differential display analysis is a technique that is widely used and entails semiquantitative polymerase chain reaction (PCR) amplification of 3' ends of messenger RNA (mRNA) *(3–6)*. The primer sets used hybridize to the poly-A tail of mRNA on one end, and to an arbitrary countersequence on the other. Each set of primers is designed to amplify some 150 messages present in the RNA under study. These messages are subsequently separated by polyacrylamide gel electrophoresis. Using a labeled nucleotide in the PCR reaction, the intensity of each band can subsequently be compared in samples of interest. Following reamplification, confirmation, cloning, and sequencing, the fragments of interest are further analyzed. **Figure 1** outlines this sequence of events. Although the length of the fragments amplified usually excludes coding regions, the 3' noncoding regions are unique and can serve to identify the gene of interest, provided the fragment belongs to a gene or an expressed sequence tag (EST) that has previously been submitted to GenBank *(7)*. For other fragments, underlying genes can be further characterized by screening a cDNA library or by a 5'RACE extension of the fragment *(8–10)*.

From: *Methods in Molecular Medicine, Vol. 61: Melanoma: Methods and Protocols*
Edited by: B. J. Nickoloff © Humana Press Inc., Totowa, NJ

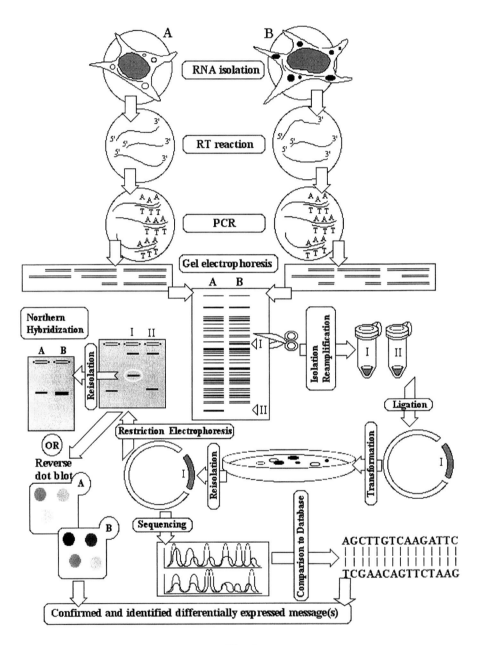

Fig. 1

By using the PCR reaction, the sensitivity of detection is greatly improved when compared to earlier methods of expression analysis, such as subtractive hybridization and some applications of the more novel microarray techniques discussed in Chapter 2 *(11,12)*. The amplification step also has extended the use of this technique to samples in which very little RNA substrate is available, such as in vitiligo research *(13)*.

In pigmentation research, the control cells for any comparison to be made cannot be isolated as compact tissue, because melanocytes are sparsely distributed throughout the skin in vivo. For this reason, the application of differential display analysis has been limited to purified cells propagated in vitro. In spite of this limitation, differential display has been used extensively to understand further the process of malignant transformation of melanocytes. Making use of unlimited resources, melanoma cell behavior has often been investigated using B16 mouse tumors *(14)*. Normal pigment cells from the hair shafts of the mouse can be used for comparison, and subclones of varying metastatic potential have been used as well *(15,16)*. Such comparisons have revealed many genes now associated with malignant transformation *(17–22)*. Similarly, gene expression in stable melanoma cell lines has been compared with that of benign melanocytes from separate control donors. When nonsyngeneic cells are compared, care must be taken to eliminate fragments related to donor-to-donor variation from the comparison, because these are not relevant to the process under study *(23)*.

Apart from comparing cultured cells under baseline conditions, the technique can be used to explore the effect of environmental conditions on gene

---

Fig. 1. *(previous page)* Differential display analysis. RNA is isolated from samples A and B and reverse transcribed (RT reaction). The cDNA is amplified in presence of a radiolabeled nucleotide (PCR) and resulting fragments are displayed on a gel (Gel electrophoresis). Bands of interest, representing messages upregulated (I) or downregulated (II) in sample B are isolated from the gel and reamplified (Isolation, Reamplification). Such fragments are ligated into a T-vector (Ligation) and used to transform bacteria (Transformation). Following amplification in bacteria, the plasmid is reisolated (Reisolation). The size of the inserted fragment is checked by restriction analysis (Restriction, Electrophoresis) and the inserted band is reisolated from gel (Reisolation). RNA from original samples A and B is then probed with the fragment in a Northern (Northern Hybridization) or fragments are blotted onto membranes and probed with labeled amplification products representing samples A and B (Reverse dot blot). Both methods are suited to confirm differential expression. Meanwhile, plasmids are used to sequence the cloned cDNA fragments of interest (Sequencing). Next, such sequences are compared to the sequence database, which can result in the identification of differentially expressed messages (Comparison to database, Confirmed and identified differentially expressed messages).

expression. For example, the involvement of ultraviolet (UV) irradiation, cytokines, growth factors, and melanogenic effectors in melanoma genesis has been analyzed by comparing gene expression in exposed and nonexposed cells *(24,25)*. In general, the differential display technique has provided and will continue to provide major insights into the process of malignant transformation in melanoma.

2. Materials

1. Diethylpyrocarbonate (DEPC) water: Stir 0.1% DEPC into ddH_2O and maintain in clean glassware overnight. Autoclave to inactivate the DEPC.
2. 2 *M* NaOAc, pH 4.0. Store at room temperature.
3. Chloroform:isoamyl alcohol (24:1). Store at room temperature.
4. Solution D: 4 *M* guanidinium isothiocyanate; 100 m*M* Tris-HCl, pH 7.6; 0.5% Sarkosyl; 50 m*M* EDTA. Store at room temperature. Add 36 µL of 2-mercaptoethanol/10 mL of Solution D just before use.
5. Phenol saturated with Tris-HCl to pH 8.0. Store refrigerated.
6. 70% Ethanol prepared with 0.1% DEPC-treated water.
7. 5X DNase I buffer: 50 m*M* Tris-HCl, pH 8.3, 250 m*M* KCl, 6 m*M* $MgCl_2$ in DEPC-treated H_2O. Store at –20°C.
8. 5X first-strand RT buffer: 250 m*M* Tris-HCl, pH 8.3, 375 m*M* KCl; 15 m*M* $MgCl_2$. Store at –20°C.
9. 5X PCR buffer: 250 m*M* KCl, 5 m*M* Tris-HCl, pH 8.0, 12.5 m*M* $MgCl_2$. Store at –20°C.
10. 40% Acrylamide solution: 380 g/L of acrylamide and 20 g/L of *N,N*′-methylenebisacrylamide, filtered and stored at room temperature in the dark.
11. TBE buffer: Combine 10.8 g of Trizma base, 5.5 g of boric acid, and 4 mL of 0.5 *M* EDTA (pH 8.0) and add H_2O to a total volume of 1 L. Store as 10X stock at room temperature.
12. 10X Exchange buffer: 0.5 *M* imidizole-Cl, pH 6.6, 0.1 *M* $MgCl_2$, 50 m*M* dithiothreitol (DTT), 1 m*M* spermidine, 1 m*M* EDTA.
13. TAE buffer: Combine 4.84 g of Trizma base, 1,142 µL of glacial acetic acid, and 2 mL of 0.5 *M* EDTA (pH 8.0) and add H_2O to a total volume of 1 L. Store as 50X stock at room temperature.
14. 5X Ligase buffer: 150 m*M* Tris-HCl, pH 7.8, 50 m*M* $MgCl_2$, 50 m*M* DTT, 5 m*M* adenosine triphosphate (ATP).
15. Luria broth (LB): 10 g/L of bacto-tryptone, 5 g/L of bacto-yeast extract, 5 g/L of NaCl. Adjust pH to 7.5 and autoclave. Store refrigerated.
16. TE buffer: 1 m*M* EDTA, 10 m*M* Tris-HCl, pH 8.0. Store at room temperature.
17. 5X MESA running buffer: 0.1 *M* 3-*N*-morpholino-propanesulfonic acid, pH 7.0; 40 m*M* NaOAc, 5 m*M* EDTA, pH 8.0. Prepare with DEPC-treated water and sterilize by filtration. On autoclaving or prolonged storage the solution will darken; discard if darker than straw-colored.

18. 10X Northern loading dye: 50% glycerol, 1 mM EDTA, pH 8.0, 0.25% bromophenol blue, 0.25% xylene cyanol FF prepared with DEPC water. Store refrigerated.
19. Hybridization solution: 6X saline sodium citrate (SSC), 0.5% sodium dodecyl sulfate (SDS), 100 µg/mL of denatured salmon sperm DNA, 50% formamide. Store at –20°C.
20. SSC: Prepare 20X stock solution as 3 M NaCl and 0.3 M sodium citrate, pH 7.0.
21. Klenow 10X buffer: 100 mM Tris-HCl, pH 7.5; 500 mM NaCl.
22. Klenow nucleotide mixes: Every mix contains 1.66 µM of the deoxynucleotide for which the mix is named and 33 µM of other dioxynucleotides except dATP, together with the dideoxynucleotide for which the mix is named at 16.7 µM ddCTP, 100 µM dATP, 117 µM dTTP, or 16.7 µM ddGTP. In addition, every mix contains 10 mM Tris-HCl, pH 7.5, 50 mM NaCl, 10 mM MgCl$_2$, and 1 mM DTT.
23. Sequencing chase solution: 34 mM Tris-HCl, pH 8.3, 50 mM NaCl, 6 mM MgCl$_2$, 5 mM DDT; 2 mM of each dNTP.
24. Sequencing stop solution: 98% formamide; 10 mM EDTA, pH 8.0, 0.1% xylene cyanol FF, 0.1% bromophenol blue. Store refrigerated.

3. Methods

3.1. Total RNA Isolation from Cultured Adherent Cells.

1. Rinse cells with phosphate-buffered saline, add 700 µL of Solution D per 100-cm^2 dish, agitate, and transfer to microfuge tubes (*see* **Notes 1** and **2**).
2. Add sequentially and mix thoroughly after each addition the following: 1/10 vol of 2 M NaOAc, pH 4.0 (70 µL); 1 vol of phenol (700 µL); 2/10 vol of chloroform : isoamyl alcohol (24 : 1) (140 µL). Shake final suspension vigorously for 10 s.
3. Cool on ice for 15 min and spin at 14,000g in a microfuge at 4°C for 15 min.
4. Transfer the upper aqueous phase to a new tube and add 1 vol of isopropanol (750 µL).
5. Precipitate for at least 1 h at –20°C.
6. Centrifuge for 15 min at 4°C, 14,000g and resuspend the pellet in 0.3 vol of initial Solution D (210 µL); precipitate with 1 vol of isopropanol for 1 h at –20°C.
7. Centrifuge for 15 min at 4°C and wash the pellet in 70% ethanol.
8. Remove the ethanol and dry the pellet.
9. Resuspend in 1–200 µL of DEPC water, measure the concentration spectrophotometrically at 260/280 nm, and store at –70°C.

3.2 Removal of Chromosomal DNA

1. Combine the following: 38 µL of 50 µg of total RNA in DEPC water, 10 µL of 5X DNase I buffer, 1 µL of H placental RNase Inhibitor (40 U), 1 µL of RNase-free DNase I (10 U), for a total of 50 µL.
2. Incubate at 37°C for 30 min.

3. Adjust the volume to 500 µL with DEPC water.
4. Extract once with Tris-saturated phenol, pH 8.0.
5. Extract once with chloroform : isoamyl alcohol (24 : 1).
6. Precipitate with 2.5 vol of ethanol and 1/10 vol of 3 *M* NaOAc, pH 5.2, overnight at –20°C.
7. Spin 15K, 15 min at 4°C, and discard the supernatant.
8. Wash the pellet one time with 75% ethanol, and dry in a speedvac.
9. Resuspend in DEPC water and measure the concentration spectrophotometrically, check for degradation on 1.2% gel before use, and dilute to 0.05 µg/µL.

3.3. Reverse Transcription

1. Combine the following for 10 PCR reactions: 5 µL of DEPC-treated water, 4 µL of DNase-treated RNA (0.05 µg/µL), 2 µL of 200 µ*M* dNTPs, 4 µL of 5X first-strand RT buffer, 2 µL of 0.1 *M* DTT, 2 µL of 25 µ*M* dT$_{11}$V$\underline{N}$ anchor primer (V = equimolar mixture of A, C, G, and T; N = either A, C, G, or T—one N/tube [*see* **Note 3**]), 1 µL of reverse transcriptase (50–100 U/0.2 µg of RNA (RT II, RNaseH⁻ or AMV), for a total volume of 20 µL.
2. Mix and quick spin.
3. Incubate at 37°C 1 h.
4. Stop the reaction at 95°C for 5 min.

3.4. Polymerase Chain Reaction

1. Combine the following: 7 µL of sterile water, 4 µL of 5X PCR buffer, 2 µL of RT mix, 2 µL of 25 µ*M* dT$_{11}$VN (appropriate anchor primer, also used for RT), 1 µL of 5 µ*M* of arbitrary primer— 10mer (one/tube) (*see* **Note 4**), 1 µL of 20 µ*M* dNTPs, 2 µL α-³²P-dCTP (0.5 µCi/µL) (*see* **Note 5**), 1 µL of *Taq* polymerase (1 U), for a total volume of 20 µL.
2. Quick spin.
3. Add one drop of mineral oil and PCR under the following conditions: 30 cycles of 94°C for 30 s, 41°C for 2 min, 72°C for 30 s; hold at 72°C for 10 min, then 4°C.

3.5. Differential Display Gel Electrophoresis

1. Mix the following in 500 mL (light solution): 75 mL of 40% acrylamide, 50 mL of 5X TBE, 230 g of ultrapure urea.
2. Mix the following in 200 mL (heavy solution): 30 mL of 40% acrylamide, 100 mL of 5X TBE, 92 g of ultrapure urea, 20 g of sucrose, 10 mg of bromophenol blue.
3. Siliconize one glass plate and assemble gel-pouring unit.
4. Catalyze 10 mL of the heavy solution with 10 µL of 25% ammonium persulfate, and immediately inject between glass plates at the bottom of gel.
5. On polymerization, catalyze 10 mL of the bottom solution and 35 mL of the top solution with 10 and 35 µL, respectively, of 25% ammonium persulfate.
6. Draw 9 mL of the top solution followed by 9 mL of the bottom solution into a 25-mL pipet, slightly mix with air bubbles, and pour between glass plates. Fill the space with the remainder of the top solution.

7. Let the gel polymerize and preferably leave overnight covered with TBE-drenched tissues and Saran wrap.
8. Prerun the gel for 1 h to warm up (60 W constant power).
9. Run 3 μL of each sample on a 6% acrylamide sequencing gel, 60 W constant power (850 V, 69 mA) for 3 h.
10. Dry the gel at 80°C for 3 h on Whatman 3M paper.
11. Expose the dried gel to Kodak X-Omat AR-5 film overnight.

3.6. Phosphorylation of DNA Markers (Phosphoexchange Reaction)

1. Mix the following: 5 μL of DNA marker with 5′ terminal phosphates (e.g.,123-bp ladder) (5 μg), 5 μL of 10X exchange reaction buffer, 3 μL of 5 mM adenosine 5′-diphosphate, 5 μL of α-^{32}P-ATP (specific activity 3000 Ci/mmol) (5–10 mCi), 30 μL of double deionized H$_2$O, 2 μL of T4 polynucleotide kinase (10 U/μL), for a total volume of 50 μL.
2. Incubate at 37°C for 30 min.
3. Add 2 μL of 0.5 M EDTA, 8.0, and 20 μL of TE.
4. Purify by 30,000 molecular weight cutoff spin column.
5. Store at –20°C; use 5–10 × 10^5 cpm/lane.

3.7. Identification and Isolation of Differentially Displayed Gene Products

In lanes of approximately equal overall intensity, carefully screen for bands of the same size of higher or lower intensity consistently associated with the treatment under study (*see* **Note 6**). These bands are subsequently processed as follows:

1. Precisely align the autoradiogram and the dried gel, and pierce the corners of a band in a sample in which the band is overexpressed.
2. Remove the autoradiogram, and cut the band out with a clean scalpel. Place in a microfuge tube.
3. Add 100 μL of sterile water and soak at room temperature for 10 min. Then boil for 15 min.
4. Remove paper by centrifugation.
5. Add 50 μg of glycogen in 5 μL, 1/10 vol of 3 M NaOAc, and 2 vol of ethanol; maintain on dry ice for 30 min.
6. Centrifuge at 14,000g for 10 min.
7. Wash the pellet in 85% EtOH.
8. Dissolve the pellet in H$_2$O. Use half for one round of reamplification.
9. Use for reamplification under identical conditions, without the radiolabeled nucleotide.
10. Run the product on a low-melt agarose gel, 1.5% in TAE buffer.
11. Cut the band from the gel in minimal volume under long-wave or low-intensity UV light.

3.8. Preparation of Bluescript (pBSsk+) T-Vector for PCR Cloning

1. Mix the following: 5 µL of Qiagen purified plasmid pBSsk+ (1 µg/µL), 11 µL of H_2O, 2 µL of 10X React 2 (Gibco), 2 µL of *Eco*RV (Gibco), for a total volume of 20 µL.
2. Digest for 1 h at 37°C.
3. Incubate with the following: 3 µL of 10X PCR buffer (500 m*M* KCl, 10 m*M* Tris-HCl, pH 8.0, 25 m*M* $MgCl_2$), 6 µL of 10 m*M* dTTP (final 2 m*M*), 1 µL of *Taq* DNA polymerase (5 U/µL (Gibco) (use 1 U/µg of plasmid), for a total volume of 30 µL.
4. Incubate for 2 h at 70°C.
5. Add 220 µL TE, pH 8.0, and mix.
6. Add 250 µL of Tris-saturated phenol and extract the aqueous (upper) phase.
7. Precipitate with 1/10 vol of NaOAc, pH 5.2, and 2.5 vol of EtOH overnight at –20°C.
8. Resuspend in 20 µL of H_2O and measure the optical density.
9. Dilute to 50 ng/µL and store at –20°C (*see* **Note 7**).

3.9. Cloning and Amplification of Fragments

1. Melt fragments in agarose at 70°C for 10 min.
2. Prewarm microfuge tubes at 37°C.
3. Combine 9 µL of melted agarose and 1 µL of T-vector.
4. Add 4 µL of 5X ligase buffer.
5. Add 1 µL of ligase.
6. Mix quickly with a pipet tip.
7. Keep at room temperature overnight.
8. Add 3 µL of dimethyl sulfoxide to 200 µL of competent XL1-Blue (~3 × 10^8 bacteria).
9. Combine with ligated plasmid.
10. Keep on ice for 30 min.
11. Keep at 42°C for 90 s.
12. After 2 min at 4°C, add 1 mL of LB without ampicillin, and gently shake at 37°C for 2 h.
13. Plate on LB agar plates containing 60 µg/mL of ampicillin, 10 µg/mL of tetracycline, 40 µg/mL 5-bromo-4-chloro-3-indolyl-β-D-galactoside, and 0.5 *M* isopropylthio-β-D-galactoside.
14. Incubate at 37°C overnight.
15. Transfer white colonies to LB with ampicillin and tetracycline.
16. Grow shaking at 37°C overnight.
17. Prepare glycerol stock and reisolate plasmid, e.g., with a Promega miniprep kit.
18. Use the plasmid for sequence analysis (M13 primers) and to prepare more of the fragment of interest for Northern analysis by restriction enzyme digestion followed by gel electrophoresis and reisolation of the fragment.

3.10. Preparation of cDNA Probe for Northern Analysis

1. Mix the following: 23 μL of 100 ng of template DNA fragment in H_2O, 15 μL Random Prime Buffer Mix (Gibco), 2 μL of dCTP, 2 μL of dTTP, 2 μL dGTP, 5 μL of α-^{32}P-dATP (10 μCi/μL), 1 μL of Klenow enzyme, for a total volume of 50 μL.
2. Heat denature DNA for 5 min at 95°C, and cool on ice to prevent renaturation.
3. Anneal random primers and transcribe at 37°C for 1 h.
4. Store at –20°C until use.
5. Prior to use, boil for 3 min.
6. Cool on ice to prevent renaturation.

3.11. 1.2% Gel for Northern Analysis

1. Add 0.36 g of agarose to 18 mL of water.
2. Boil and cool.
3. Add 6 mL of 5X MESA running buffer.
4. Add 5.4 mL of formaldehyde.
5. Mix and pour, and leave for 1 h at room temperature.

3.12. Northern Blotting

1. Combine the following: 4.5 μL of DEPC water + RNA (25 μg), 2 μL of 5X MESA running buffer, 3.5 μL of formaldehyde, 10 μL of formamide, for a total volume of 20 μL.
2. Heat denature RNA samples at 55°C for 15 min.
3. Add 2 μL of sterile Northern loading dye.
4. Run in 1X MESA running buffer (4–6 V/cm; constant voltage) for 3.5 h.
5. Transfer by capillary diffusion to Nytran or other charged membrane in 10X SSC, and mark the membrane for 28 and 18S as markers or use RNA markers.
6. Prehybridize the membrane with hybridization solution.
7. Add labeled probe and hybridize for 16 h at 42°C.
8. Extensively wash the blot with 1X SSC and 0.1% SDS at room temperature for 20 min and wash three times in 0.2X SSC and 0.1% SDS at 68°C. Check for loss of radioactivity. Further removal of background can be done after exposure.
9. Dry and expose to Kodak X-Omat AR-5 film with a reflection screen at –80°C for 16–72 h, depending on the intensity of the signal (*see* **Note 8**).
10. Repeat hybridization of the blot, probing with a standard for loading such as β-actin or glyceraldehyde-3-phosphate dehydrogenase.

3.13. Sequencing of Differentially Expressed Fragments

1. Prepare 6% gradient polyacrylamide gradient sequencing gel as described for differential display.
2. Following polymerization, cover with tissues drenched in TBE and Saran wrap overnight.

3. The next day combine 2–3 µg of purified plasmid DNA with 1/10 vol of 2 *M* NaOH and 2 m*M* EDTA.
4. Incubate for 30 min at 37°C.
5. Precipitate in the presence of 1/10 vol of 3 *M* NaOAc (pH 5.2) and 2–4 vol of ethanol at –70°C for 15 min.
6. Spin at 14,000*g* at 4°C for 15 min.
7. Wash the pellet with 70% ethanol, air-dry, and suspend in 8 µL of H_2O.
8. Add 1 µL of 10X Klenow buffer and 1 µL of (5 ng/µL) M13 primer.
9. Incubate at 37°C for 15 min to anneal, and then place on ice.
10. Add 5 U of Klenow fragment per tube.
11. Add 4 µL of ^{32}P-dATP (10 µCi/µL, 800 Ci/mmol).
12. Add 3 µL of each Klenow nucleotide mix to four separate tubes.
13. Add 3 µL of annealed primer/radiolabel mix to each tube and incubate at 37°C for 15 min.
14. Add 1 µL of chase solution and incubate at 37°C for 15 min.
15. Add 5 µL of stop solution; the reaction can be stored overnight at –70°C.
16. Load 2.5 µL/slot after heating at 70°C for 3 min to denature.
17. Mix and keep refrigerated until loading.
18. Prerun the sequencing gel for 45 min.
19. Heat the samples at 80°C for 2 min, and load the gel immediately as GATC (2.5 µL/lane).
20. Run at 60 W (constant power) for 2 to 3 h. (In a 6% gel, the bromophenol blue comigrates with a 26 nucleotide DNA fragment, and xylene cyanol with a 106 nucleotide DNA fragment.)
21. Soak the gel in 5% acetic acid with 15% methanol for 10 min to remove urea.
22. Blot the gel onto 3MM Whatman paper and dry at 80°C for 3 h.
23. Cover with Saran wrap and expose to Kodak X-Omat AR-5 film overnight at room temperature.
24. The sequence should be read by two people individually. If loaded as prescribed, the complementary strand can be read by flipping the autoradiogram, assuming the same nucleotide order and reading from the bottom.

3.14. Database Search

1. Enter the sequence from a file on disk (or manually) into the appropriate window of the Basic Local Alignment Search Tool (BLAST) program available through the NCBI/NIH Web site in sequence analysis under topics related to molecular biology of the scientific resources section.
2. Set the database to search either to (nr) for nonredundant GenBank, EMBL, DDBJ, and PDB databases or to the human or mouse EST databases.
3. Enter the search command and inspect the results (queries are queued). For homology to be considered significant, the expect value (E-value) should be well below 1, because this describes the number of hits to be found by chance alone for the given database size. The value of E decreases exponentially with increasing scores (S-values).

4. If significant homology is found for a range of sequences with unrelated functions or localizations, this is likely to be caused by the presence of repetitive sequences such as ALU. In such cases, select a search for homology to the ALU database and subsequently delete the repetitive part of the sequence. The revised sequence can be used to perform a new search.

5. Additional information can be acquired directly from the search results, by clicking on the code assigned to the homologous sequence. A longer stretch of the sequence, information regarding potential function of the expressed gene, and the availability of the homologous clone can be found. In case of an unknown sequence, *see* **Note 9**.

4. Notes

1. The method used for RNA isolation is not critical; other potential methods of isolation include standard RNAzol, Tri-Reagent, and Qiagen RNA spin column methodology, as indicated by the manufacturer. The RNA is best stored until use before DNase treatment.

2. A problem frequently encountered specifically when amplifying RNA isolated from pigment cells is that melanin is coisolated with nucleic acids and interferes with subsequent PCR amplifications. A published method to avoid such inhibition consists of adding bovine serum albumin to the amplification reaction in amounts of 0.6 mg/mL *(26)*. Nonconstitutive high melanin content in cultured cells can be avoided by culturing cells in media containing low tyrosine concentrations *(27)*.

3. The availability of kits to perform differential display has greatly facilitated analysis of differential gene expression. Apart from GenHunter, founded by differential display pioneer Peng Liang, kits are presently available from Clontech, GenPak, Stratagene, Bio101, and Genomyx, with slight variations in strategy. GenHunter and Operon will provide primer combinations suitable for differential display. In fact, kits are available to cover most steps in this procedure, from primer combinations through plasmid isolation to sequencing procedures.

4. Although just 1 primer combination can suffice to find a differentially expressed gene, more are required to analyze differential expression of all messages found in the cell. In combination with the two-anchor primers used, approx 25 upstream primers are required to represent >95% of all mRNA species present in the cell, assuming 15% of 100,000 genes to be expressed *(6)*.

5. The radiolabel described here for differential display is ^{32}P. ^{35}S can also be used and provides increased band resolution; however, an accompanying increase in contaminatation can occur *(28)*. Another alternative is ^{33}P, which is more expensive but provides resolution equivalent to ^{35}S without the increased contamination problems.

6. In every application of the technique, a substantial number of fragments that are reamplified from the display gels were not confirmed as differentially expressed. This can be attributed to several factors. Northern blotting, traditionally used to confirm differential expression, is too insensitive to detect small yet potentially

significant differences of <30% in levels of expression. Also, the absolute content of the original message may be too little to confirm by traditional Northern blotting. The finding that such unconfirmed messages frequently represent DNA fragments not previously identified attests to their infrequency yet certainly does not invalidate their involvement in a process under study. However, it is also possible that a band represents more than one fragment, and a reamplified band that is subsequently cloned may not represent the differentially expressed species.

7. Cloning vectors for PCR fragments (T-vectors) are also commercially available, but, in our experience, these kits have not worked nearly as well as the self-prepared version according to Marchuk et al. *(29)*.

8. A difficulty in weeding out false positive fragments has been reported by several researchers *(30–33)*. To prevent false positive bands, it is important to compare more than two samples in the original display. Also, repeating the reverse transcriptase-PCR reaction is essential. In addition, reversed methods have recently been introduced to validate mRNA fragments obtained by differential display. Such methods involve blotting of the fragment of interest onto a membrane and probing it with the samples in which differential expression was observed. In this respect, we have introduced reverse dot blotting as a simple and sensitive technique to confirm differential expression. This method involves blotting the fragment onto two separate membranes suitable for Southern blotting in exponentially increasing amounts of 5 pg to 5 ng per dot following heat denaturation. Twenty nanograms of RNA representing the samples of interest (but preferably from a separate source) is reverse transcribed and PCR amplified following the exact protocol used for differential display, in the presence of radiolabeled dNTP. We have used 0.25 µL (2.5 µCi) of ^{32}P-dCTP in a 20-µL PCR reaction. Incorporation is checked on a differential display gel using 3 µL of the radiolabeled product, which also provides an extra control for differential expression. Subsequently, the labeled samples are run over a Bio-Rad BioSpin 30 column to remove unincorporated nucleotides, and the flow-through is used to hybridize to the separate membranes following heat denaturation. The 1X hybridization buffer containing 0.5% SDS to which the membranes have been exposed for 2 h is not replaced. Hybridization is performed at 42°C for 16 h. The blots are subsequently washed in 0.1% SDS in 2X SSPE for 15 min at room temperature. The wash buffer is replaced, and the blots are washed for 30 min at 42°C. The blots are exposed at –80°C for 72 h to Kodak X-Omat AR5 film. If the blotted fragment is truly differentially expressed, the extent of hybridization will differ between the two samples compared *(13)*. Methods using only reverse-transcribed RNA (reverse Northern) are also available but may not be sensitive enough to detect the fragment of interest.

9. In the event that a differentially expressed cDNA fragment has not been previously described as defined by a BLAST search, a cDNA library may be screened to further characterize the gene of interest. Some libraries are commercially available through Research Genetics, including a human and a mouse melanocyte

library as well as a human melanoma cDNA library. Because of the high sensitivity of the technique and the small sample required, it is to be expected that the differential display will continue to reveal novel and existing genes associated with pigmentary abnormalities.

References

1. Welch, D. R. and Goldberg, S. F. (1997) Molecular mechanisms controlling human melanoma progression and metastasis. *Pathobiology* **65,** 311–330.
2. Nordlund, J. J (1997) The epidemiology and genetics of vitiligo. *Clin. Dermatol.* **15,** 875–878.
3. Liang, P. and Pardee, A. B. (1992) Display of eukaryotic messenger RNA by means of the polymerase chain reaction. *Science* **257,** 967–970.
4. Liang, P., Averboukh, L., Keyomarsi, K., and Pardee, A. B. (1994) Distribution and cloning of eukaryotic mRNAs by means of differential display: refinements and optimization. *Nucleic Acids Res.* **21,** 3269–3275.
5. Mou, L., Miller, H., Li, J., Wang, E., and Chalifour, L. (1994) Improvements to the differential display method for gene analysis. *Biochem. Biophys. Res. Commun.* **199,** 564–569.
6. Bauer, D., Muller, H., Reich, J., Riedel, H., Ahrenkiel, V., Warthoe, P., and Strauss, M. (1993) Identification of differentially expressed mRNA species by an improved display technique (DDRT-PCR). *Nucleic Acids Res.* **21,** 4272–4280.
7. Lipman, D. J. (1997) Making (anti)sense of non-coding sequence conservation. *Nucleic Acids Res.* **25,** 3580–3583.
8. Kwon, B. S., Halaban, R., Kim, G. S., Usack, L., Pomerantz, S., and Haq, A. K. (1987) A melanocyte-specific complementary DNA clone whose expression is inducible by melanotropin and isobutylmethyl xanthine. *Mol. Biol. Med.* **4,** 339–355.
9. Dakour, J., Jimbow, K., Vinayagamoorthy, T., Luo, D., and Chen, H. (1993) Characterization of melanosome-associated proteins by establishment of monoclonal antibodies and immunoscreening of a melanoma cDNA library through an anti-melanosome antibody. *Melanoma Res.* **3,** 331–336.
10. Frohmann, M. A. (1994) On beyond classic RACE (Rapid Amplification of cDNA Ends). *PCR Meth. Appl.* **4,** 40–48.
11. Jiang, H., Lin, J. J., Su, Z. Z., Goldstein, N. I., and Fisher, P. B. (1995) Subtraction hybridization identifies a novel melanoma differentiation associated gene, *mda-7*, modulated during human melanoma differentiation, growth and progression. *Oncogene* **11,** 2477–2486.
12. Schena, M., Shalon, D., Davis, R. W., and Brown, P. O. (1995) Quantitative monitoring of gene expression patterns with a complementary DNA microaaray. *Science* **270,** 467–470.
13. Le Poole, I. C., Yang, F., Brown, T. L., Cornelius, J., Babcock, G. F., Das, P. K., and Boissy, R. E. Altered gene expression in melanocytes exposed to 4-tertiary butyl phenol (4-TBP): upregulation of the A2b adenosine receptor. *J. Invest. Dermatol.* **113,** 725–731.

14. Bennett, D. C., Cooper, P. J., and Hart, I. R. (1987) A line of non-tumorigenic mouse melanocytes syngeneic with the B16 melanoma and requiring a tumor promotor for growth. *Int. J. Cancer* **39,** 414–418.
15. Maiorana, A., Cavallari, V., Maiorana, M. C., Fano, R. A., Scimone, S., Fante, R., and Garbisa, S. (1992) Metastatic capacity and differentiation in murine melanoma cell lines: a morphometric study. *Pathol. Res. Pract.* **188,** 657–662.
16. Ishiguro, T., Nakajima, M., Naito, M., Muto, T., and Tsuruo, T. (1996) Identification of genes differentially expressed in B16 murine melanoma sublines with different metastatic potentials. *Cancer Res.* **55,** 6237–6243.
17. van Groningen, J. J. M., Bloemers, H. P. J., and Swart, G. W. M. (1995) Identification of melanoma inhibitory activity and other differentially expressed messenger RNAs in human melanoma cell line with different metastatic capacity by messenger RNA differential display. *Cancer Res.* **55,** 4109–4115.
18. Gómez, L. A., Strasberg Rieber, M., and Rieber, M. (1996) PCR-mediated differential display and cloning of a melanocyte gene decreased in malignant melanoma and up-regulated with sensitization to DNA damage. *DNA Cell Biol.* **15,** 423–427.
19. Hashimoto, Y., Shindo-Okada, N., Tani, M., Takeuchi, K., Toma, H., and Yokota, J. (1996) Identification of genes differentially expressed in association with metastatic potential of K-1735 murine melanoma by messenger RNA differential display. *Cancer Res.* **56,** 5266–5271.
20. Francia, G., Mitchell, S. D., Moss, S. E., Hanby, A. M., Marshall, J. F., and Hart, I. R. (1996) Identification by differential display of annexin-VI, a gene differentially expressed during melanoma progression. *Cancer Res.* **56,** 3855–3858.
21. Hildebrandt, T., Freiherr, J., Klostermann, S., Kaul, S., Zendman, A. J. W., van Muijen, G. N. P., and Weidle, U. H. (1999) Identification of URIM, a novel gene up-regulated in metastasis. *Anticancer Res.* **19,** 525–530.
22. Duncan, L. M., Deeds, J., Hunter, J., Shao, J., Holmgren, L. M., Woolf, E. A., Tepper, R. I., and Shyjan, A. W. (1998) Down-regulation of the novel gene *melastatin* correlates with potential for melanoma metastasis. *Cancer Res.* **58,** 1515–1520.
23. van Groningen, J. J. M., Egmond, M. R., Bloemers, H. P. J., and Swart, G. W. M. (1997) *nmd,* A novel gene differentially expressed in human melanoma cell lines, encodes a new and atypical member of the family of lipases. *FEBS Lett.* **404,** 82–86.
24. Vogt, T. M. M., Welsh, J., Stolz, W., Kullman, F., Jung, B., Landthaler, M., and McCleland, M. (1997) RNA fingerprinting displays UVB-specific disruption of transcriptional control in human melanocytes. *Cancer Res.* **57,** 3554–3561.
25. Furumura, M., Sakai, C., Potterf, S. B., Vieira, W. D., Barsh, G. S., and Hearing, V. J. (1998) Characterization of genes modulated during pheomelanogenesis using differential display. *Proc Natl Acad Sci USA* **95,** 7374–7378.
26. Giambernardi, T. A., Rodeck, U., and Klebe, R. J. (1998) Bovine serum albumin reverses inhibition of RT-PCR by melanin. *BioTechniques* **25,** 564–566.

27. Smit, N. P. M., Van der Meulen, H., Koerten, H. K., Kolb, R. M., Lentjes, E. G., and Pavel, S. (1997) Melanogenesis in cultured melanocytes can be substantially influenced by L-tyrosine and L-cysteine. *J. Invest. Dermatol.* **109,** 796–800.

28. Trentmann, S. M., Van der Knaap, E., and Kende, H. (1995) Alternatives to ^{35}S as a label for the differential display of eukaryotic messenger RNA. *Science* **267,** 1186.

29. Marchuk, D., Drumm, M. , Saulino, A., and Collins, F. S. (1991) Construction of T-Vectors, a rapid and general system for direct cloning of unmodified PCR products. *Nucleic Acids Res.* **19,** 1154.

30. Callard, D., Lescure, B., and Mazzolini, L. (1994) A method for the elimination of false positives generated by the mRNA differential display technique. *BioTechniques* **16,** 1100–1103.

31. Wadha, R., Duncan, E., Kaul, S. C., and Reddel, R. R. (1996) An effective elimination of false positives isolated from differential display of mRNAs. *Mol. Biotechnol.* **6,** 213–217.

32. Luce, M. J. and Burrows, P. D. (1998) Minimizing false positives in differential display. *BioTechniques* **24,** 766–768, 770.

33. Miele, G., MacRae, L., McBride, D., Manson, J., and Clinton, M. (1998) Elimination of false positives generated through PCR re-amplification of differential display cDNA. *BioTechniques* **25,** 138–144.

10

Fluorescence *In Situ* Hybridization as a Tool in Molecular Diagnostics of Melanoma

Lionel J. Coignet

1. Introduction

Structural and numerical chromosomal abnormalities have been observed in all types of malignancies. These events are associated with neoplastic pathogenesis and progression *(1)*. For a long time, conventional cytogenetics analysis was the prevalent approach in assessing chromosomal rearrangements. Many data were collected initially from hematologic malignancies because of ease of analysis, despite the fact that they represent only 10% of all malignancies *(2)*. Cytogenetic data on solid tumors were hampered by the technical difficulties in obtaining dividing malignant cells. During the last two decades, these problems were solved and data have been quickly acquired. Karyotyping of malignant melanoma cell lines reveals more than 95% of the cases presenting aneuploidy (numerical chromosome abnormalities: near triploidy) *(3)*, and all the cell lines present structural abnormalities (balanced and unbalanced translocations, inversions and deletions) (*see*, e.g., German Collection of Microorganisms and Cell Cultures [Dr. H. Drexler] at <http://www.dsmz.de> *(4,5)*. Cytogenetic analysis of malignant melanoma cells allowed the identification of nonrandom karyotypic changes involving chromosomes 1, 6, and 7 and, to some extent, chromosomes 9 and 10.

In recent years, fluorescence *in situ* hybridization (FISH) was developed as a new molecular cytogenetic approach to overcome the culture difficulties regarding solid tumors. The so-called interphase cytogenetics allows the study of multitargets/multichromosome copy in nondividing cells. With this approach, all cells are studied, and the bias always introduced by the in vitro cell culture is thus eliminated. Some recent reports have presented data using

From: *Methods in Molecular Medicine, Vol. 61: Melanoma: Methods and Protocols*
Edited by: B. J. Nickoloff © Humana Press Inc., Totowa, NJ

from 1 to 13 chromosome-specific probes *(5–11)*. Smaller locus-specific probes can also be used to detect loss, gain, or disruption of specific regions of the genome *(6,11–14)*.

A variation of FISH called comparative genomic hybridization (CGH) *(15,16)* allows the scanning of the whole genome for changes in DNA copy number by using DNA probes for total genomic tumor DNA. CGH bypasses the need for intact tumor cells and allows analysis using a small amount of tumor DNA. With degenerated oligonucleotides (degenerate oligonucleotide-primed polymerase chain reaction [DOP-PCR]) *(17)*, it is even possible to amplify the whole DNA complement from a few malignant cells and then compare the variation in DNA copy number within a single tumor. The most recent advance in molecular cytogenetics consists of spectral karyotyping *(18)* in which each chromosome is "painted" with a different and specific color.

The operational principles of the FISH technique are as follows.

1.1. Samples

The FISH techniques can be used with various target samples. Whatever the nature of the sample, DNA hybridization can be performed.

1.1.1. Tissue Section

Classically, tissue sections are embedded in paraffin and fixed in formalin. These sections can be used for FISH. They will be processed once positioned on slides and will require quenching and permeabilization pretreatments.

1.1.2. Single Cell Suspensions

Single cell suspensions are relatively easy to isolate by mechanical or enzymatic disaggregation of fresh solid tumors. Removal of cytoplasm and nuclear proteins can be achieved by alcohol/acetic acid fixation prior to spotting the cells on glass slides and pretreating them with enzymatic digestion (pepsin).

1.1.3. Metaphase Spreads from Tumor and/or Cultured Cell Lines

Metaphase spreads are obtained using conventional cytogenetic techniques, using synchronization and colcemid to arrest cells at the metaphase of the cell cycle.

1.2. Probes Used for FISH

1.2.1. Centromere-Specific Probes

Centrome-specific probes are used to assess chromosome aneuploidy (copy number) in a sample. They hybridize specifically to a given centromere. The number of signals detected reflects the number of chromosomes present in the cells. They are usually commercially available either labeled with haptens (biotin or digoxigenin) or directly labeled (several fluorochromes available).

1.2.2. Painting Probes

Painting probes allow one to "paint" specifically a whole chromosome or a whole chromosome arm. It is possible to visualize gross chromosomal breakage. These probes must be preferentially used on a chromosome metaphase spread to give their full efficiency. Use on interphase cells is not recommended.

1.2.3, Nonrepetitive Clones

Nonrepetitive clones includes genomic probes such as cosmids, phage artificial chromosome/bacterial artificial chromosome (BAC/PAC), and yeast artificial chromosome (YAC). Depending on their respective insert size, they can be used for different purposes. These clones are often used for mapping of break points, for specific rearrangement screening.

1.2.4. Probes for Spectral Karyotyping

As mentioned earlier, spectral karyotyping or multicolor FISH allows one to paint each separate chromosome pair with one specific color. Whole chromosome-specific probes are mixed together after being separately labeled using different combinations of five differential labels or fluorochromes. Because each chromosome is painted with a unique color, it is then possible to visualize and characterize a translocation event present in a metaphase spread, circumventing the recognition problem of marker chromosomes when morphology is of poor quality, as is often the case in solid tumor.

1.3. Whole Genomic DNA

CGH, a new development in FISH, allows the scanning of the entire genome for changes in DNA sequence copy number by generating DNA probes from total genomic tumor DNA. The CGH approach bypasses the need for intact and/or dividing tumor cells and permits analysis with a relatively small amount of tumor DNA.

1.3.1 Isolation of Genomic DNA from Large Amount of Malignant Tissue/Cell Lines

The isolation from a large amount of tumor cells/cell lines is performed using classic phenol/chloroform techniques.

1.3.2. Isolation of Genomic DNA from Small amount of Cells

Quite often, malignant tissue is not present in large quantities to allow a large-scale genomic DNA extraction. Also, in a tumor, malignant cells are infiltrated in normal cells. The best approach is to dissect malignant cells from tissue sections obtained from routine pathology examination. Using micromethods, it is possible to obtain a small quantity of DNA. To perform CGH with a sufficient quantity of DNA, a DOP-PCR technique can be used to generate sufficient material.

1.3.3. Degenerate Oligonucleotide Polymerase Chain Reaction

DOP-PCR is based on the amplification of the whole genome DNA that is present in one tube, using degenerated oligonucleotides. This way, the whole genomic DNA can be amplified because degenerated oligoprimers can be anchored randomly throughout the DNA that is present and thus be used ultimately for CGH experiments.

1.4. Fluorescence In Situ Hybridization

FISH is now a well-known, established technique that allows the hybridization of a known DNA segment to a target. Different strategies can be used with the FISH principle and variations consist in the choice of probe and target support. Next, we summarize a limited number of protocols that can be adapted to all situations.

1.4.1. Comparative Genomic Hybridization (CGH)

One of the FISH variations consists of using whole genomic tumor DNA as a probe. Whole genomic tumor DNA is extracted and labeled in one color (usually green). Whole normal genomic DNA is extracted in parallel and differentially labeled (usually red). Both DNAs are mixed in a 1:1 ratio and simultaneously hybridized onto normal chromosome metaphase spreads. At each hybridization site, a competition phenomenon takes place between the tumor and the normal DNA. If identical copy numbers of DNA are present in both the tumor and normal DNA, an equal amount of each DNA will hybridize to the given sequence. The resulting color ratio will be an average ratio and will produce a merge color from the two original ones (usually yellow). If there is amplification in the tumor DNA, the tumor DNA will "win" the competition against the normal DNA. The resulting color ratio then will be shifted in favor of the tumor DNA and produce a color predominantly from tumor origin (usually green). Inversely, if there is a deletion in the tumor DNA, the color ratio will be shifted and produce a color from normal DNA (usually red). Using software that is able to analyze color ratio between tumor and normal DNA, it is then possible to visualize the amplification/deletion status from a given tumor DNA.

1.4.2. Spectral Karyotyping—Multicolor FISH

This new advanced FISH technology, multicolor FISH, has been developed recently to obtain a molecular cytogenetic karyotype. As mentioned earlier, each chromosome is painted with one specific color. Therefore, it is possible to identify any part of chromosome that is translocated to another chromosome. This will allow the identification, in a single experiment, of marker chromosomes that remain quite often unidentified and uncharacterized. The important limitation of this particular approach is the production and obtention of malignant metaphases from the tumor.

2. Materials
2.1. Probe Labeling

1. 10X Nick translation buffer (0.5 *M* Tris-HCl, pH 7.8; 50 m*M* MgCl$_2$; 0.5 mg of bovine serum albumin (BSA)/mL.
2. Nucleotide mix (0.5 m*M* dATP, dCTP, dGTP; 0.1 m*M* dTTP) (Roche, Indianapolis, IN).
3. 0.1 *M* DL-dithiothreitol (DTT) (Sigma, St. Louis, MO).
4. DNase I (1 mg) (Roche) dissolved in 20 m*M* Tris-HCl, 50 m*M* NaCl, 1 m*M* DTT, 0.1 mg/mL BSA, 50% glycerol (v/v), pH 7.6.
5. DNA polymerase I (10 U/µL)(Roche).
6. Yeast tRNA (10 mg/mL) (Sigma).
7. Sonicated herring sperm DNA (10 mg/mL) (Sigma).
8. Hapten or fluorochrome (e.g., biotin, digoxigenin, fluorescein isothiocyanate [FITC], Texas Red, rhodamine, dUTP).
9. Cot1 DNA (Life Technologies, Rockville, MD).
10. 3 *M* sodium acetate, pH 5.5.
11. 100% Ethanol (−20°C).
12. Hybridization solution: 50% deionized formamide; 2X saline sodium citrate [SSC]; 50 m*M* sodium phosphate, pH 7.0; 10% dextran sulfate.
13. Water bath in a cold room/refrigerator.
14. Refrigerated centrifuge.

2.2. Slide Pretreatments

1. RNase A (100 µg/mL in 2X SSC) (Roche).
2. 2X SSC.
3. Pepsin (Sigma).
4. Ethanol series (70, 90, and 100%).
5. Glass jar containing 10 slides.
6. Moist chamber.
7. Water bath.

2.3. Hybridization

1. Hybridization solution: 50% deionized formamide, 2X SSC, 50 m*M* sodium phosphate, pH 7.0; 10% dextran sulfate.
2. Probe stock solutions.
3. Denaturation solution 70% deionized formamide, 2X SSC, 50 m*M* sodium phosphate, pH 7.0.

4. 37°C Water bath.
5. Moist chamber (with 50% formamide, 2X SSC).
6. Heating block set for 70 °C.
7. 37°C Dry incubator.

2.4. Posthybridization Washes

1. 1X SSC solution.
2. 0.1X SSC solution.
3. TNT: 0.1 M Tris-HCl, 0.15 M NaCl, 0.05% Tween-20.
4. Ethanol series (70, 90, and 100%).
5. Water bath 45 and 60 °C.
6. Glass jar.

2.5. Immunologic Detection

1. TNB: 0.1 M Tris-HCl, 0.15 M NaCl, 0.5% Boehringer blocking reagent (Roche).
2. Sheep antidigoxigenin (Fab fragment)-TRITC conjugated (Roche).
3. Streptavidin-FITC conjugated (Vector, Burlingame, CA).
4. TNT.
5. Vectashield-DAPI (Vector).
6. Ethanol series (70, 90, and 100%).
7. 37°C Dry incubator.
8. Glass jar.
9. Moist chamber (water).

3. Methods
3.1. Tissue Section

The classic deparaffinization protocols can be used: xylene, rehydration (100–95% ethanol), and then water. Immerse the slides in 1% H_2O_2 in 100% methanol for 30 min. Wash in two changes of 100% methanol for 5 min each and air-dry the slides. Then incubate in pepsin solution (4 mg of pepsin/mL in 0.2 M Cl) for 5–60 min at 37°C; thirty minutes is standard. Pepsin time is to be determined for each tissue studied. Pepsin in combination with HCl is recommended although proteinase K can also be used for proteolytic digestion. After pepsin treatment, wash the slides in phosphate-buffered saline, dehydrate through ethanol series (70, 90, and 100% ethanol), and air-dry.

3.2. Single Cell Suspension

Collect tumors in RPMI-1640 medium (Life Technologies, Rockville, MD) with 10–20% fetal calf serum (Life Technologies), 50 mg/mL of penicillin, and streptomycin. Mechanically disaggregate tissues by scraping and cutting in a Petri dish and filtering. Fix the cell suspension obtained with either ethanol or methanol : acetic acid (3 : 1). The latter seems more appropriate because the acetic acid participates actively in the removal of cytoplasm and nuclear proteins. Store cell suspensions at –20°C until use.

3.3. Obtention of Metaphases from Tumors and/or Cell Lines

Cell lines allow one to obtain good morphology metaphases rather easily. For tumor material, after mechanical disaggregation, set cells in culture for 3–9 d. Harvesting and fixation have been described elsewhere *(19)*.

3.4. Probes Used for FISH

Centromere-specific, whole-chromosome, and multicolor FISH are now commercially available from numerous companies. Company specifications must be followed to obtain the best efficiency in hybridization. The non-repetitive probes are prepared and extracted using classic cosmid, PAC, and YAC extraction techniques.

3.5. Whole DNA Extraction

Genomic DNA is extracted using conventional phenol/chloroform techniques. If DNA is extracted from paraffin-embedded tissue sections, 20–60 sections must be collected. Dissolve paraffin in 1 mL of xylene for 10 min. Remove xylene by washing twice with 100% ethanol and allow sections to dry. Then digest sections in 400 µL of 50 mM Tris-HCl, pH 8.5, 1 mM EDTA, 0.5% Tween-20, and 200 mg/mL of proteinase K at 55°C for 3 d. **Caution:** Fresh proteinase K must be added every 24 h. Then extract DNA using standard phenol/chloroform procedure. In case of microdissection from tissue section and microextraction of the tumor DNA, volumes must be adjusted.

To obtain sufficient material to perform the CGH, DOP-PCR can be used prior to CGH. DOP-PCR employs oligonucleotides of partially degenerated sequence. This degeneracy, together with a PCR protocol utilizing a low initial annealing temperature, ensures priming from multiple, evenly dispensed sites within a given DNA or whole genome.

3.6. Fluorescence In Situ Hybridization (20–22)

3.6.1. Probe Labeling

Commercially available probes are usually labeled and can be used directly in the hybridization procedure. For the nonrepetitive probes (cosmid, PAC, and YACs), a nick-translation labeling procedure is usually applied. Commercial kits are available and will produce similar results as the one described in **Subheading 2.1.**

In the following protocol, it is assumed that the DNA probe concentration is 1 µg/µL; if not, the volume of water will have to be adjusted. Mix all of the following together: 26 µL of water, 5 µL of 10X nick translation buffer, 5 µL of DTT, 4 µL of nucleotide mix, 2 µL of labeling dUTP molecule, 1 µL of DNA probe, 2 µL of DNA polymerase I (10 U/µL), and 5 µL of DNase I (1:1000 from the 1 mg/mL stock solution). The final volume should be 50 µL. Place the labeling mixture in a 15°C water bath for 2 h. After the incubation, add 5 µL of sonicated herring sperm DNA, 5 µL of yeast tRNA, and the required amount of Cot-1 DNA (50- to 200-fold excess—to be assessed for each probe). Precipitate labeled DNA by adding 0.1 vol of 3 M sodium acetate (pH 5.5) and 2.5X vol of 100% ethanol (–20°C). Place the solution at –20°C for 30 min, spin down for 30 min at +4°C, and resuspend the pellet in hybridization solution. Probes can be stored at –20°C. For CGH, better results are achieved when longer DNA fragments are generated during labeling. It is thus advised to reduce the amount of DNase I in the labeling mixture to 2 µL.

3.6.2. Slide Pretreatments

As mentioned earlier, tissue sections are pretreated with pepsin solution. For the other types of target DNA, it is also recommended to pretreat the sample preparations in order to obtain an optimal permeability for the probes and possibly for the antibody in case of hapten labeling.

Apply 100–120:1 of RNase A solution on the slide and incubate for 1 h at 37°C in a moist chamber humidified with water. Wash the slides in 2X SSC. Place the slides for 10 min (standard) in a 10 mg of pepsin/100 mL of 0.01 M HCl solution in a 37°C water bath. Wash the slides in 2X SSC and dehydrate through an ethanol series.

If the loss of cells after the pepsin treatment appears to be too important, either the length of the pepsin treatment can be shortened or a postfixation step can be added by placing the slides for 10 min in a 1% acid-free formaldehyde, 1X PBS, 50 mM MgCl$_2$ solution at room temperature. Then formaldehyde is removed by washing in 1X PBS and slides are dehydrated.

3.6.3. Hybridization

The protocol differs whether a centromere-specific probe or other probes are used.

3.6.3.1. Centromere-Specific Probes

Centromere-specific probes consist usually of short sequences corresponding to highly repetitive satellite DNA, specific for (almost) each centromere. They do not need a preincubation with unlabeled competitive Cot-1 DNA. Apply the probe (2–5 ng/µL) to the target area. Denature the slide and the

DNA probe simultaneously for 2 to 3 min at 70 °C. Hybridize overnight at 37°C in a moist chamber.

3.6.3.2. OTHER PROBES

Whole chromosome painting probes and spectral karyotyping probes, even though they are commercially available already labeled, need a competition preanneling step, to allow the Cot-1 to suppress repetitive sequences. Depending on the nature of the probe, a working solution is prepared to reach the requested concentration (5 ng/μL of cosmid, 10 ng/μL of PAC/BAC, 20 ng/μL of YAC; for commercially available probes, follow manufacturer's instructions). Denature the DNA by placing it for 5 min in boiling water. Place the DNA for 1 min on ice, spin down briefly, and preanneal by placing the DNA for 1–2 h in a 37°C water bath. During the preannealing of the DNA probe, apply denaturation solution to the target DNA. Place the slide on a heating block set at 70°C for 2 to 3 min. Wash off the denaturation solution once with 2X SSC and then dehydrate the slides through ethanol series. After preannealing, place the probe on the target DNA and allow to hybridize overnight at 37°C in a moist chamber.

3.6.4. Posthybridization Washes

All the washing solutions need to be prewarmed at 45°C and 60°C, respectively, before use.

Wash the slides three times for 5 min in 1X SSC at 45°C. Then wash the slides in high-stringency washes (0.1X SSC) at 60°C. Wash the slides for 5 min in TNT solution. Directly labeled (FITC, TRITC, Texas Red) probes do not need immunologic detection. Then directly dehydrate the slides in ethanol series and air-dry.

3.6.5. Immunologic Detection

The hapten-labeled probes (biotin, digoxigenin) need to be detected using fluorochrome-conjugated antibodies. The protocol given here is for the detection of two different probes labeled with biotin and digoxigenin, respectively, with a single-layer detection procedure. For smaller probes, a three-layer detection procedure might be necessary. However, the use of small probes on paraffin-embedded tissue section is rather difficult. The antibodies mentioned here can be substituted by others, giving similar results.

After washing in TNT, incubate slides for 30 min with the sheep antidigoxigenin-TRITC antibody (2 μg/μL) and streptavidin-FITC (2.5 μg/μL) in TNB solution at 37°C in a moist chamber. Then wash slides three times for

5 min in TNT and dehydrate through ethanol series. Mount the slides in Vectashield with 4,6-diamidino-2-phenylindole·2HCl. Chromosomes and nuclei will be counterstained in blue.

3.7. Comparative Genomic Hybridization

Tumor and normal DNA are usually directly labeled with fluorochromes. Because the red/green ratio will be used to estimate the amplification/deletion status of the tumor DNA, the use of fluorochrome-labeled DNA avoids variability owing to the use of immunologic detection. The different ratios are calculated and interpreted using specific software packages, now available through several companies. In our laboratory, the Perspective Scientific Instrument (PSI) system has been chosen.

3.8. Multicolor FISH/Spectral Karyotyping

The 26 color probes are also directly labeled. Similar to CGH, the analysis is possible through specific software packages commercially available. As mentioned, we chose to use the PSI system. For both applications, this system meets our needs in good FISH capture and analysis software coupled with an excellent karyotyping package.

4. General Conclusion and Future Insight of FISH in Molecular Cytogenetics of Melanoma

FISH is a very important tool to study the molecular events that may arise in malignant melanoma. Indeed, the applications are numerous, because even if some clues on the importance of some chromosomes have been demonstrated, the central and original event is still unknown. It is hoped that the FISH approaches described in this chapter will help in this search, since cytogenetic techniques have improved in recent years. Undoubtedly, the development of techniques such as CGH and especially multicolor FISH will provide many data that will be used further in more targeted FISH with sequence-specific probes. Once the event is characterized at the chromosome level, the insight to the molecular and genetic level will follow. This will certainly help us in improving our understanding of the pathogenesis of malignant melanoma.

References

1. Vogelstein, B, et al. (1993) *Trends Genet.* **9,** 138–141.
2. Rabbitts, T. H., et al. (1994) *Nature* **372,** 143–149.
3. Trent, J. M., et al. (1989) *Cancer Res.* **49,** 420–423.
4. Thompson, C. T. (1994) *Pathology* **2,** 401–412.
5. Parmiter, A. H., et al. (1993) *J. Invest. Dermatol.* **100,** 254–585.
6. Dopp, E., et al. (1997) *Cancer Lett.* **120,** 457–463.

7. Barks, J. H., et al. (1997) *Genes Chrom. Cancer* **19,** 278–285.
8. Balazs, M., et al. (1999) *Cancer Genet. Cytogenet.* **109,** 114–118.
9. Matsuta, M., et al. (1997) *J. Cutan. Pathol.* **24,** 201–251.
10. Poetsch, M., et al. (1998) *Lab. Invest.* **78,** 883–887.
11. Poetsch, M., et al. (1998) *Cancer Genet. Cytogenet.* **104,** 146–152.
12. Nelson, M. A., et al. (1999) *Cancer Genet. Cytogenet.* **108,** 91–99.
13. Zhang, J., et al. (1999) *Cancer Genet. Cytogenet.* **111,** 119–123.
14. Robertson, G. P., et al. (1999) *Oncogene* **18,** 3173–3180.
15. Kallioniemi, A., et al. (1992) *Science* **258,** 818–821.
16. Glazvini, S., et al. (1996) *Cancer Genet. Cytogenet.* **90,** 95–101.
17. Telenius, H., et al. (1992) *Genomics* **13,** 718–725.
18. Speicher, M. R., et al. (1996) *Nat. Genet.* **12,** 368–375.
19. Prescher, G., et al. (1995) *Cancer Genet. Cytogenet.* **80,** 40–46.
20. Coignet, L., et al. (1996) *Blood* **87,** 1512–1519.
21. Coignet, L. J., et al. (1996) *Leukemia* **10,** 1065–1071.
22. Coignet, L. J., et al. (1999) *Gene Chrom. Cancer* **25,** 222–229.

III

TREATMENT

11

Antigen-Pulsed Dendritic Cell Approach to Melanoma

Frank O. Nestle, Adrian Tun-Kyi, and Michel F. Gilliet

1. Introduction

Dendritic cells (DCs) are potent antigen-presenting cells (*1*) with wide tissue distribution. They are classified based primarily on their localization: as Langerhans cells when present in the epidermis and as dermal DCs when found in the dermis. DCs exhibit several common features: an irregular shape with elongated dendritic processes, a distinctive cell-surface phenotype, low buoyant density, active motility, and the ability to stimulate vigorous proliferation of unprimed T-cells. DCs are able to ingest, process, and present antigen in the context of major histocompatibility complex (MHC) molecules. However, because of their high expression of MHC class I and II, as well as costimulatory molecules and adhesion molecules, DCs have the ability to induce primary T-cell-dependent immune responses in vivo and in vitro. This outstanding feature gives DCs a central role in controlling adaptive T-cell-based immunity.

For years the low frequency of DCs throughout the human body (e.g., <0.2% of human mononuclear cells are mature blood DCs) has been a major obstacle to the development of immunotherapeutic strategies based on the ex vivo antigen loading of DCs.

Recently, several laboratories have developed new culture methods for the generation of high numbers of human DCs from blood, bone marrow, or CD34+ stem cells. The first report on the generation of DCs from peripheral human blood was described by Caux et al. (*2*) in 1992. This approach, based on the isolation and culture of proliferating CD34+ cells, is less practical for small samples of blood, in which the frequency of CD34+ cells is very low (0.1%). A major breakthrough was the description of a method to generate blood-derived

From: *Methods in Molecular Medicine, Vol. 61: Melanoma: Methods and Protocols*
Edited by: B. J. Nickoloff © Humana Press Inc., Totowa, NJ

DCs from monocytes by culture with granulocyte macrophage colony-stimulating factor (GM-CSF) and interleukin-4 (IL-4) *(3,4)*. This allowed the design of novel immunotherapeutic strategies using ex vivo–generated DCs as adjuvants *(5,6)*. Although reaching a good level of maturation at d 7, these culture conditions involved xenologous sera such as fetal calf serum (FCS), which may be suboptimal in clinical applications. FCS-free autologous conditions necessitate an additional maturation step for the generation of mature DCs. In this two-step culture system, peripheral blood mononuclear cells (PBMCs) are first differentiated in autologous plasma-supplemented medium with the addition of GM-CSF and IL-4 for 7 d and then stimulated for an additional 3 d with monocyte-conditioned medium *(7,8)*. This completely autologous culture system may have the disadvantage of an unpredictable DC quality owing to the variation in the content of maturation-inducing cytokines in the conditioned medium. An improved method came with the identification of IL-1, IL-6, and tumor necrosis factor-α (TNF-α) as substitutes for the monocyte-conditioned medium *(9,10)*. Prostaglandin E_2 (PGE$_2$) was found to further enhance the yield and the quality of DCs generated *(9)*.

The in vitro maturation of blood-derived DCs has many similarities to the in vivo physiologic maturation of Langerhans cells upon antigen uptake and migration to the T-cell areas of lymphoid organs. Like skin-resident Langerhans cells, immature blood-derived dendritic cells have an efficient antigen uptake and processing machinery with highly recirculating MHC complexes *(11)*. Mature BDC, with their strong T-cell stimulatory capacity, correspond qualitatively to Langerhans cells after migration into the lymph node. Profound insight into their maturation pathway (**Fig. 1**) makes BDC optimal tools for immunotherapy based on DCs as adjuvants. Full protein antigens may be preferentially delivered at the immature stage, when the processing machinery is highly activated. Further in vitro culture will generate mature DCs, which are less able to capture new proteins but are better at stimulating resting CD4 and CD8, therefore representing optimal candidates for immunization. An additional maturation to "superactivated DCs" takes place in vivo after DC vaccination: interaction with CD40L on T-cells will license DCs to fully activate cytotoxic T-cells without bystander T-cell help *(12–14)* (**Fig. 2**).

The use of DCs as adjuvants for antigen-based immunointervention strategies in melanoma will open new ways for the treatment of this deadly disease *(15)*.

2. Materials
2.1. Culture Medium

DC cultures are grown in X-VIVO 15 supplemented with 1% heat-inactivated autologous plasma.

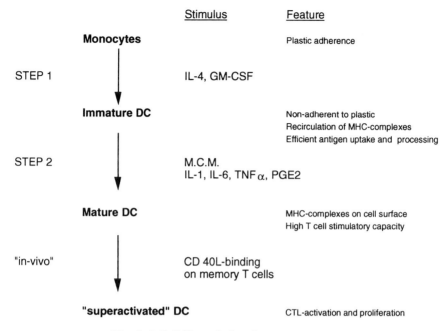

Fig. 1. DC differentiation from monocytes.

1. Centrifuge 10 mL of heparinized autologous whole blood for 10 min at 1300g.
2. Collect the clear cell-free supernatant (plasma) and transfer into a 15-mL tube. Keep the cellular components for PBMC isolation.
3. Heat inactivate in a 56°C water bath for 1 h.
4. Centrifuge and collect the supernatant (heat-inactivated plasma).
5. Prepare complete culture medium (CM): 96% X-VIVO 15 (03-418Q; Bio-Whittaker), 1% heat-inactivated autologous plasma, 2% 200 mM L-glutamin (K0282; Seromed, Berlin, Germany), 1% penicillin/streptomycin (10,000 IU/mL) (15140-114; Gibco, Basel, Switzerland).
6. Filtrate through a 0.2-μm filter and store at 4°C.

2.2. Reagents

1. Phosphate-buffered saline (PBS).
2. EDTA (E-5134; Sigma, Buchs, Switzerland).
3. Bovine serum albumin (BSA) (A-7906; Sigma).
4. Formaldehyde solution (47608; Fluka, Buchs, Switzerland).
5. Ficoll-Paque (17-0840-02; Pharmacia Biotech, Dübendorf, Switzerland).
6. Tissue culture flasks (75 cm^2) with 0.2-μm vented plug seal cap (3111; Falcon, B&D, Meylan, France).

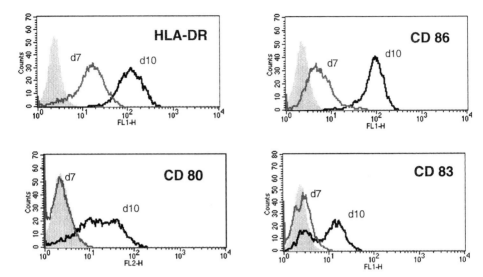

Fig. 2. Flow cytometry analysis of immature (d 7) and mature (d 10) monocyte-derived DCs.

7. Recombinant human cytokines: GM-CSF (Leukomax, Sandoz, Bern, Switzerland), IL-4 (204-IL-005; R&D, Wiesbaden-Nordenstadt, Germany), IL-1β (201-LB-005; R&D), IL-6 (206-IL-001; R&D), TNF-α (210-TA-010; R&D).
8. FACS buffer: PBS, 1% BSA, 5 mM EDTA, 0.01% NaN$_3$. Store at 4°C.
9. FACS fixative solution: FACS buffer, 0.5% formaldehyde. Solution is light sensitive; store at 4°C and do not expose to light for prolonged periods.
10. Mouse antihuman monoclonal antibody: CD 83 FITC (4210; Immunotech, Marseille, France), CD 80 PE (340294; B&D), CD 86 FITC (33404; Pharmingen, Hamburg, Germany), HLA-DR FITC (7363; B&D).
11. Isotype controls: IgG$_{2b}$ FITC (284-040; Ancell, Bayport, MN), IgG$_1$ PE (9043; B&D), IgG$_1$ FITC (9041; B&D), IgG$_{2a}$ FITC (9010; B&D).
12. Polytron (Kinematica AG, Switzerland).
13. Millex-GP (SLGPR25CS; Millipore, Switzerland).
14. Bio-Rad Protein Assay (500-0006; Bio-Rad, Switzerland).

3. Methods

3.1. Step 1: Generation of Immature DCs

1. Collect 80 mL of heparinized peripheral blood from patients or healthy donors.
2. Separate into four 50-mL tubes and dilute 1:1 in PBS (20 mL of blood + 20 mL of PBS).
3. Underlay carefully the 40-mL diluted blood sample with 10 mL of Ficoll-Paque and centrifuge for 20 min at 666g.

4. Isolate PBMCs by gently aspirating the interface between the plasma and the Ficoll-Paque with a 10-mL pipet. Transfer to a clean centrifuge tube, wash twice with at least 3 vol of PBS, and resuspend in 15 mL of CM.
5. Incubate for 2 h at 37°C and 5% CO_2 in a 75-cm^2 culture flask (adherence step).
6. Discard nonadherent cells and wash the flask surface twice with PBS (at room temperature) to eliminate residual lymphocytes and thrombocytes.
7. Incubate adherent cells (monocytes) overnight at 37°C, 5% CO_2 with 15 mL of CM (without cytokines).
8. At d 2, substitute CM with 15 mL of fresh medium supplemented with 800 U/mL of GM-CSF and 1000 U/mL of IL-4.
9. Incubate for another 6 d at 37°C and 5% CO_2.
10. At d 7 rinse off nonadherent cells (immature DCs) and wash once with PBS.

3.2. Step 2: Generation of Mature DCs

1. Transfer the d 7 immature DCs to new 75-cm^2 culture flask with 15 mL of CM supplemented with 800 U/mL of GM-CSF and 1000 U/mL of IL-4. Use either monocyte-conditioned medium (protocol 1) or proinflammatory cytokines (protocol 2) as maturation stimuli:
   a. Protocol 1 (modified from Bender/Romani *[7,8]*): Add 20% monocyte-conditioned medium, generated as described in **Subheading 3.3.**
   b. Protocol 2 (modified from Jonuleit *[9]*): Add 10 ng/mL of IL-1β, 1000 U/ml of IL-6, and 10 ng/mL of TNF-α. Add 1 μg/mL of PGE_2.
2. Incubate at 37°C and 5% CO_2 for 3 d (until d 10) and rinse off the nonadherent mature DCs. Wash once with PBS.
3. Count the cells, determine viability, and perform quality control.

3.3. Generation of Monocyte-Conditioned Medium

1. Apply 10 mL of 10 mg/mL of human γ-globulin solution to a bacteriologic 10-mL dish and swirl the plate until the entire surface is coated. Leave for 1 min and then aspirate back the fluid.
2. Leave the coated plates at room temperature for 30 min.
3. Just before use, gently wash the plates with cold PBS twice: add PBS slowly to the side of the plate and let it run down onto the surface. Swirl the plate to cover and "rinse" the surface. Aspirate off between washes and before the addition of cells.
4. Draw 50 mL of peripheral blood, isolate PBMCs (approx 50×10^6) by Ficoll centrifugation as described in **Subheading 3.1.** and resuspend in 10 mL of CM. Add cells to coated plates and incubate at 37°C and 5% CO_2 for 30 min.
5. Vigorously rinse off the nonadherent cells.
6. Add 10 mL of CM on adherent cells (monocytes adhering to IgG-coated plates via Fc-receptor) and incubate at 37°C and 5% CO_2 for 24 h.
7. Isolate the cell-free supernatant and store at 4°C for a maximum of 1 wk or at –20°C for longer periods.

3.4. Quality control

Phenotypic changes are monitored by light microscopy and flow cytometric analysis of surface marker expression: CD83 as DC maturation markers and CD80, CD86, and HLA-DR as functional relevant markers.

1. Put 10^5 DCs into eight FACS tubes. Keep the cells at 4°C on ice.
2. Wash twice with FACS buffer (keep the solution at 4°C).
3. Add antibodies (anti-CD83, -CD80, -CD86, -HLA-DR and respective isotype controls) diluted in 100 μL of FACS buffer and incubate for 30 min at 4°C in the dark.
4. Wash twice with FACS buffer. Do not expose stained cells to light for prolonged periods, to avoid bleaching of the fluorescent dye.
5. Fix cells by adding 400 μL of FACS fixative solution and keep at 4°C until flow cytometric analysis (should be done within 3 d for optimal results).

3.5. Tumor Lysate

1. Excise pigmented tumor material, and disperse the tumor material with a mixer after the addition of 1 mL of PBS.
2. Centrifuge the homogenate for 5 min at 666g.
3. Put the supernatant into a new tube and submit it to three freeze-thaw cycles.
4. Pass the solution through a 0.2-μm filter.
5. Irradiate the lysate using a gamma irradiation unit (12,000 rad).
6. Measure the protein concentration using the Bio-Rad protein assay according to the manufacturer's guidelines.
7. Adjust the protein concentration to 10 μg/μL with sterile PBS.
8. Make 10-μL aliquots and store at –80°C.

4. Notes

1. Culture conditions involving FCS-supplemented media produce fairly mature DCs within 7 d, which are much more potent than "immature" cells generated under non-FCS conditions, but may be inappropriate for human applications owing to the presence of xenologous proteins. The use of autologous plasma requires an additional maturation step after the classic 7-d culture period in order to generate mature DCs with potent T-cell stimulatory capacity.
2. Heat inactivation of plasma is an essential procedure to prevent complement activation.
3. The addition of 5 mM EDTA to wash solution (PBS) may enhance the PBMC yield by avoiding clumping of cells.
4. Alternatively, to plastic adherence, T- and B-cells may be eliminated by immunomagnetic depletion with CD19 and CD3 Dynabeads. This procedure, aiming at the purity of the monocyte preparation, may not be suitable for subsequent in vivo use of generated DCs. We therefore prefer a simple 2-h adherence step that gives us routinely a recovered DC population of >80%.
5. Adherent cells are cultured at approx $0.5 \times x10^6$ cells/mL, which allows an easy 7-d culture period without the need of medium and cytokine replacement. The

convenience of the procedure and its safety regarding possible contamination steps by avoiding repetitive handling of cells make this protocol suitable for clinical applications. Increasing the cell density to 1×10^6 cells/mL by culturing the cells in six-well plates (3×10^6 cells in 3 mL/well) slightly increases the yield of mature CD83-positive DCs but necessitates a CM replacement every other day and bears the risk of contaminations.

6. Mature DCs should be isolated between d 9 and d 10.
7. Mature DCs ($4.0 [\pm 2.4] \times 10^6$) can be generated from 80 mL of peripheral blood ($n = 29$). As role of thumb: 1×10^6 PBMCs/mL of blood is obtained after Ficoll centrifugation, 10% of PBMCs is plastic-adherent monocytes, and half can be isolated as mature DCs at d 10 of culture.
8. Monocyte-conditioned medium was described as the stimulus for the generation of mature DCs in an FCS-free culture system *(7,8)*. A major advantage of this cocktail is that it does not contain any foreign serum and can be obtained from autologous human blood. However, the considerable and unpredictable variations of the quality of monocyte-conditioned medium represent a hazard for the generation of standardized mature DCs. The identification of the growth factors mediating the monocyte-conditioned medium effect *(9,10)* allows the substitution of monocyte-conditioned medium with a well-defined cytokine cocktail (IL-1β, IL-6, TNF-α) for the generation of uniformly mature DCs.
4. PGE$_2$ enhances the maturation, homogeneity, and quality of DCs when used as described *(9)*. It is, however, important to keep in mind that the effects of PGE$_2$ on DC maturation are strictly dependent on culture conditions and the presence of additional activation signals such as IL-1 and TNF-α. Some investigators have shown that in FCS-containing conditions, the addition of PGE$_2$ in the absence of proinflammatory cytokines inhibits the maturation of DC precursors. Furthermore, the addition of PGE$_2$ before d 5 of culture completely inhibits the maturation of DCs and results in differentiation of macrophage-like cells *(16)*.
9. The protocol described in **Subheading 3.** may be used for vaccination therapies in a single center approach and does not correspond in every aspect to good manufacturing practice criteria depending on different countries.
10. Homogenization should be performed on ice.
11. Centrifugation is performed to remove nondispersed tissue.
12. Freeze-thaw cycles, filtration, and irradiation are performed in order to make sure that the lysate is free of viable tumor cells.

References

1. Banchereau, J. and Steinman, R. M. (1998) Dendritic cells and the control of immunity. *Nature* **392,** 245–252.
2. Caux, C., Dezutter Dambuyant, C., Schmitt, D., and Banchereau, J. (1992) GM-CSF and TNF-alpha cooperate in the generation of dendritic Langerhans cells. *Nature* **360,** 258–261.
3. Sallusto, F. and Lanzavecchia, A. (1994) Efficient presentation of soluble antigen by cultured human dendritic cells is maintained by granulocyte/macrophage

colony-stimulating factor plus interleukin 4 and downregulated by tumor necrosis factor alpha. *J. Exp. Med.* **179,** 1109–1118.

4. Romani, N., Gruner, S., Brang, D., Kampgen, E., Lenz, A., Trockenbacher, B., Konwalinka, G., Fritsch, P. O., Steinman, R. M., and Schuler, G. (1994) Proliferating dendritic cell progenitors in human blood. *J. Exp. Med.* **180,** 83–93.

5. Hsu, F. J., Benike, C., Fagnoni, F., Liles, T. M., Czerwinski, D., Taidi, B., Engleman, E. G., and Levy, R. (1996) Vaccination of patients with B-cell lymphoma using autologous antigen-pulsed dendritic cells. *Nat. Med.* **2,** 52–58.

6. Nestle, F. O., Alijagic, S., Gilliet, M., Sun, Y., Grabbe, S., Dummer, R., Burg, G., and Schadendorf, D. (1998) Vaccination of melanoma patients with peptide- or tumor lysate-pulsed dendritic cells. *Nat. Med.* **4,** 328–332 (see comments).

7. Bender, A., Sapp, M., Schuler, G., Steinman, R. M., and Bhardwaj, N. (1996) Improved methods for the generation of dendritic cells from nonproliferating progenitors in human blood. *J. Immunol. Methods* **196,** 121–135.

8. Romani, N., Reider, D., Heuer, M., Ebner, S., Kampgen, E., Eibl, B., Niederwieser, D., and Schuler, G. (1996) Generation of mature dendritic cells from human blood: an improved method with special regard to clinical applicability. *J. Immunol. Methods* **196,** 137–151.

9. Jonuleit, H., Kuhn, U., Muller, G., Steinbrink, K., Paragnik, L., Schmitt, E., Knop, J., and Enk, A. H. (1997) Pro-inflammatory cytokines and prostaglandins induce maturation of potent immunostimulatory dendritic cells under fetal calf serum-free conditions. *Eur. J. Immunol.* **27,** 3135–3142.

10. Reddy, A., Sapp, M., Feldman, M., Subklewe, M., and Bhardwaj, N. (1997) A monocyte conditioned medium is more effective than defined cytokines in mediating the terminal maturation of human dendritic cells. *Blood* **90,** 3640–3646.

11. Sallusto, F., Cella, M., Danieli, C., and Lanzavecchia, A. (1995) Dendritic cells use macropinocytosis and the mannose receptor to concentrate macromolecules in the major histocompatibility complex class II compartment: downregulation by cytokines and bacterial products. *J. Exp. Med.* **182,** 389–400 *(see comments).*

12. Ridge, J. P., Di Rosa, F., and Matzinger, P. (1998) A conditioned dendritic cell can be a temporal bridge between a CD4+ T-helper and a T-killer cell. *Nature* **393,** 474–478 (see comments).

13. Bennett, S. R., Carbone, F. R., Karamalis, F., Flavell, R. A., Miller, J. F., and Heath, W. R. (1998) Help for cytotoxic-T-cell responses is mediated by CD40 signalling. *Nature* **393,**478–480 (see comments).

14. Schoenberger, S. P., Toes, R. E., van der Voort, E. I., Offringa, R., and Melief, C. J. (1998) T-cell help for cytotoxic T lymphocytes is mediated by CD40-CD40L interactions. *Nature* **393,** 480–483 (see comments).

15. Nestle, F. O., Burg, G., and Dummer, R. (1999) New perspectives on immunobiology and immunotherapy of melanoma. *Immunol. Today* **20,** 5–7.

16. Kalinski, P., Hilkens, C. M., Snijders, A., Snijdewint, F. G., and Kapsenberg, M. L. (1997) Dendritic cells, obtained from peripheral blood precursors in the presence of PGE2, promote Th2 responses. *Adv. Exp. Med. Biol.* **417,** 363–367.

12

Gene Therapy in Melanoma

Giorgio Parmiani, Flavio Arienti, Cecilia Melani, Filiberto Belli, Gianfrancesco Gallino, and Arabella Mazzocchi

1. Introduction: Different Approaches to Cancer Gene Therapy

The identification of genes involved in different biologic functions and in the pathogenesis of diseases has paved the way to the possibility of either interfering with the role of such genes or replacing them in somatic cells in case of loss, which may occur in some genetic diseases or cancer. Such progress has been accomplished thanks to advances in molecular biology and applied technology that allow the transport and insertion of genes into recipient cells by viral or physical vectors as well as the inhibition of gene transcription by antisense oligonucleotides. Methods have also been devised to transfer genes not only in vitro but also in vivo, although this latter approach is still limited owing to poor selectivity and targeting of most vectors when given systemically. Viral and physical vectors have been employed; each of these vectors has distinct advantages and disadvantages, and, therefore, the appropriate vector should be selected according to the therapeutic system involved (*1*). Retroviral vectors have been used largely for their ability to selectively transfect proliferating cells, a feature that can be advantageous in case one wishes to target only proliferating tumor cells. Owing to the heterogeneous proliferation rate in different parts of a tumor, however, it could be desirable, under some circumstances, to be able to target even the fraction of nonproliferating tumor cells. This can now be obtained by the use of lentivirus (*2*) or by switching to the use of adenoviruses that can target both dividing and quiescent cells but also induce unwanted inflammmatory reactions from the host.

Among the many different genetic changes occurring in cancer cells, activation of oncogenes or inactivation of tumor suppressor genes plays an important

From: *Methods in Molecular Medicine, Vol. 61: Melanoma: Methods and Protocols*
Edited by: B. J. Nickoloff © Humana Press Inc., Totowa, NJ

role in the development of human cancer. Therefore, gene therapy theoretically can make use of two opposite strategies: disruption of oncogene transcription by antisense oligonucleotides (in the case of oncogenes) and replacement of tumor suppressor genes that have been lost in cancer cells. Both these strategies have been found to meet with some success in several human tumors when experiments were carried out ex vivo with in vitro growing cell lines, whereas the in vivo application was more problematic owing to the limited ability to convey either oligos or therapeutic genes into single cells of a tumor mass growing in distant organs. In addition, as in the case of melanoma, knowledge of the genes involved in the process of carcinogenesis and progression may not be sufficient to identify the precise target of this direct type of gene therapy.

Another strategy is that of the suicide genes, or genetic prodrug activation. In such a case, tumor cells need to be transfected with genes encoding proteins (usually enzymes) of prokaryotes that are absent or weakly or inefficiently expressed by mammalian cells and allow the transfected cells to metabolize a prodrug into a cytotoxic compound. The administration of the prodrug to cancer-bearing individuals results to the destruction not only of tumor cells that had received the gene, but also of surrounding cells owing to the so-called bystanding phenomenon that is probably mediated by a release of the activated drug from gene-transfected cells. Even with this strategy, however, the in vivo targeting of cancer cells with the given gene that confers the ability to metabolize the drug remains difficult. This limitation can be bypassed at least partially by intralesional injections with the vector bearing the appropriate gene as may occur in brain tumors that can be precisely targeted by the stereotaxic technique.

Another strategy is to use indirect approaches in the control of tumor growth. Two main approaches can be envisaged: one is immunologic and the other is based on the attempt to block neoangiogenesis by the growing tumor. The immunologic approach is aimed at constructing more efficient reagents to be used in the immunotherapy of cancer *(3)*. This approach is applicable to those human neoplasms that are well characterized from the immunologic standpoint such as melanoma, whereas it appears less suitable for tumors (e.g., lung cancer) for which the knowledge of factors necessary for setting up a specific immunologic therapy is scanty. In fact, to devise a sound immunotherapy protocol, one needs to know the genes that encode tumor-specific antigens, along with those that may confer either a better immunogenicity to a vaccine or a precise recognizing function to antitumor immune cells. Such genes can then be transfected into normal or tumor cells and exploited in an attempt to increase the efficiency of imunologically based cancer therapy. The exciting recent developments in basic and applied immunology are providing new information that can be exploited in constructing reagents for a more effective tumor immuntherapy. In such a context, gene manipulation represents a crucial technology.

The antiangiogenetic approach is still in its early use, but several studies with animal models or in vitro have shown the possibility of transferring into tumor cells genes that can inhibit the function of those genes (e.g., vascular endothelial growth factor [VEGF]) that are known to promote tumor neoangiogenesis and whose disruption or blocking will result in tumor regression or cytostasis *(4)*. Even in such an exciting approach, however, limitations lie in the selection and targeting of metastatic lesions in the body.

Thus, a variety of strategies is available that need to be modulated according to the different tumors and different clinical conditions to be treated. These strategies include approaches that make use of different vector systems, different genes, and even combinations of different approaches.

After a period of overoptimism, gene therapy of tumors has now entered into a more realistic time in which preclinical and clinical studies are aimed at testing scientifically sound hypotheses without emphasizing possible and immediate widespread clinical applications.

2. Melanoma: The Disease and Its Immunobiologic Features

Melanoma is a skin tumor that affects a relatively limited number of individuals in the Western world. However, when not cured by early surgical intervention, metastatic disease is often fatal. Moreover, possibly owing to an increased acute exposure to ultraviolet light for recreational reasons, the rate of incidence and mortality of melanoma has risen rapidly during the last 10 yr in the Western world, with the incidence in the United States jumping from fewer than 3 in 100,000 individuals to more than 12 in 100,000 today. A similar trend is present in Western European countries. Many efforts, therefore, have been made worldwide to understand better the biology of this dreadful disease, which still remains practically incurable after the appearance of visceral metastases. Skin melanoma can progress through several histologically and biologically defined steps from precursor nevi to dysplastic nevi to *in situ* primary tumor to vertical growth phase primary melanoma with metastatic competence to distant metastasis *(5)*. Transition from one step to another is usually accompanied by biologic and genetic changes, some of which have been identified and molecularly characterized. However, information about which genes are involved in neoplastic transformation of melanocytes in humans and by which mechanism remains scanty, despite the work of several groups of investigators.

Even immunologic changes during progression, however, are less well understood both in terms of expression of antigens recognized by immune cells and of alterations in the ability of the patient's immune system to be activated by such antigens. In general, two opposite trends can be found during the progression of melanoma from the primary, nonmetastatic horizontal growth phase through metastases: a trend in the reduction of expression of T-cell-defined antigens of the differentiation type (e.g., tyrosinase, Melan-A/MART-1, gp100, tyrosine-related protein-1 [TRP-1], TRP-2) possibly owing to immunoselection *(6)*, and a tendency to a more frequent expression, at least at the mRNA level, of other, apparently less immunogenic antigens such as the melanoma antigen (MAGE) and B-antigen (BAGE) families *(7)*.

In any event, the large number of antigenic epitopes recognized by T-cells that is now available renders the analysis of the role of each of them in stimulating or inhibiting the immune response rather difficult. Note, however, that recent work of different research groups has indicated that nearly 50% of patients with metastatic melanoma have a high frequency of melanoma antigen-specific memory cytotoxic T-lymphocyte (CTL) precursors in their blood *(8)*. Such effectors should therefore be easily activated by different immunologic maneuvers, including vaccination and administration of cytokine or adoptive immunotherapy.

3. Gene Therapy of Melanoma

3.1. Immunologic Approaches

The immunologic gene therapy of cancer can be divided into two main approaches: genetic modification of neoplastic or normal cells to construct vaccines, and insertion of genes into lymphocytes to be used in adoptive immunotherapy. These two approaches are discussed next.

3.1.1. Vaccination with Gene-Modified Normal or Tumor Cells

Many animal studies have shown that cytokine gene-transduced neoplastic cells of different histology can elicit tumor growth inhibition that is frequently followed by a systemic antitumor immunity, although the underlying mechanisms are slightly different according to the type of cytokine released by tumor cells *(9)*. Vaccines derived from these gene-modified cells were shown to induce regression of established murine neoplasms, although in a fraction of cases *(10)*. Based on this rationale, several pilot or phase I/II clinical trials have been initiated using either autologous or allogeneic cytokine gene-transduced tumor cells (*see* **Table 1**). To avoid the need to obtain a tumor line from each patient, a goal that is often difficult to achieve, normal cells also have been used as recipients of cytokine genes; such cells were then admixed with fresh tumor cells and injected into the patients. **Table 2** lists clinical protocols that are either initiated or at least approved by regulatory bodies and that involve the use of gene-transduced normal cells. However, only a limited number of reports

Table 1
Clinical Protocols of Vaccination with Gene-Modified Melanoma Cells

Transduced melanoma cells	Transduced gene (cytokine)	Vector	Transduction approach	Administration	Phase	Responsible investigator[a]
Autologous	GM-CSF	Adenovirus	Ex vivo	id and sc	I	Suzuki, T., Kansas City, KS
Autologous	GM-CSF	Adenovirus	Ex vivo	sc	I	*Dranoff, G., Boston, MA*
Autologous	GM-CSF	Vaccinia virus	In vivo	Intratumoral	I/II	*Mastrangelo, M. J., Philadelphia, PA*
Autologous	GM-CSF	Gold particle	Ex vivo	id	I/IB	Mahvi, D. M., Madison, WI
Autologous	GM-CSF	Retrovirus	Ex vivo	id	I	Chang, A. E., Ann Arbor, MI
Autologous	IL-2	Retrovirus	Ex vivo	sc	I	Economou, J. S., Los Angeles, CA
Autologous	IL-2	Adenovirus	Ex vivo	id and sc	I	*Stingl, G., Vienna*
Autologous	IL-2	Adenovirus	In vivo	Intratumoral	I	*Stewart, A. K., Toronto*
Autologous	IL-2	Retrovirus	Ex vivo	id and sc	I/II	Rosenberg, S. A., Bethesda, MD
Autologous	IL-2	Plasmid	In vivo	Intratumoral	I/II	*Hersh, E. M., Tucson, AZ*
Autologous	IL-2	Retrovirus	Ex vivo	sc	I	*Palmer, K., London*
Autologous	IL-7	Plasmid	Ex vivo	sc	I/II	Schmidt-Wolf, I. G. H., Berlin
Autologous	IL-7	Plasmid	Ex vivo	sc	I	*Schadendorf, D., Berlin*
Autologous	TNF	Retrovirus	Ex vivo	id and sc	I/II	Rosenberg, S. A., Bethesda, MD
Autologous	IL-12	Canarypox virus	In vivo	Intratumoral	IB	Conry, R. M., Birmingham, AL
Autologous	IL-12	Plasmid	Ex vivo	sc	I	*Schadendorf, D., Heidelberg*
Autologous	IFN-γ	Retrovirus	In vivo	Intratumoral	I	*Nemunaitis, J., Dallas, TX*
Autologous	IFN-γ	Retrovirus	Ex vivo	sc	I	*Nemunaitis, J., Dallas, TX*
Autologous	IFN-γ	Retrovirus	In vitro	sc	I	*Siegler, H. F., Durham, NC*
Autologous	IFN-γ	Adenovirus	In vivo	Intratumoral	I	Rosenblatt, J. D., Rochester, NY
Allogeneic	IL-2	Retrovirus	In vitro	sc	Pilot	Gansbacher, B., New York, NY
Allogeneic	IL-2	Retrovirus	In vitro	im	I	Das Gupta, T. K., Chicago
Allogeneic	IL-2	Retrovirus	In vitro	sc	I/II	Osanto, S., The Netherlands
Allogeneic	IL-2	Retrovirus	In vitro	sc	I/II	*Parmiani, G., Milan*
Allogeneic	IL-4	Retrovirus	In vitro	sc	I/II	*Parmiani, G., Milan*
Allogeneic	IL-7	Retrovirus	In vitro	sc	I	Economou, J. S., Los Angeles, CA

(continued)

Table 1 (continued)

Transduced	Transduced gene	Vector	approach	Administration	Phase	Responsible investigator[a]
Costimulating molecule						
Autologous	B7.1	Adenovirus	In vivo	Intratumoral	I	Schuchter, L., Philadelphia, PA
Allogeneic	B7	Plasmid	In vitro	sc	I	Sznol, M., Bethesda
Allogeneic HLA molecule						
Autologous	HLA-B7	Plasmid	In vivo	Intratumoral	I	*Nabel, G. J., Ann Arbor, MI*
Autologous	HLA-B7	Plasmid	In vivo	Intratumoral	II	Dreicer, R., Denver, CO
Autologous	HLA-B7	Plasmid	In vivo	Intratumoral	III randomized	Thomson, J. A., New York
Autologous	HLA-B7	Plasmid	In vivo	Intratumoral	III randomized	Park, C. H., Seoul
Autologous	HLA-B7	Plasmid	In vivo	Intratumoral	II	Park, C. H., Seoul
Autologous	HLA-B7	Plasmid	In vivo	Intratumoral	I	Gonzales, R., Denver, CO
Autologous	HLA-B7	Plasmid	In vivo	Intratumoral	I	*Stopeck, A. T., Tucson, AZ*
Autologous	HLA-B7+ β2 microglobulin	Plasmid	In vivo	Intratumoral	I	Hersh, E. M., Tucson, AZ
Autologous	HLA-B7+ β2 microglobulin	Plasmid	Ex vivo	sc	I	Fox, B. A., Portland, OR
Autologous	HLA-B13 or murine H-2K^k	Plasmid	In vivo	Intratumoral	I	*Hui, K. M., Singapore*
Combination of genes						
Autologous	HLA-B7 and IL-2	Plasmid	In vivo	Intratumoral	I	Gonzales, R., Denver, CO
Autologous	B7.1 with or without IL-12	Canarypox	In vivo	Intratumoral	IB	Conry, R. M., Birmingham
Autologous	IL-2 and Staphylococcus enterotoxin B	Plasmid	In vivo	Intratumoral	I	Walsh, P., Denver, CO
Other						
Autologous	HSV-1-thymidine kinase	Adenovirus	In vivo	Intratumoral	I	Morris, J. C., Bethesda, MD

[a] Italics indicate clinical trials whose results have been published (see Table 3). id, intradermally; sc, subcutaneously; im, intramuscularly.

Table 2
Clinical Protocols of Vaccination with Gene-Modified Normal Cells

Transduced cell	Gene transduced	Vector	Transduction	Administration	Phase	Principal investigator[a]
Autologous CD8+ TIL	TNF	Retrovirus	Ex vivo	iv	I/II	Rosenberg, S. A., Bethesda, MD
Xenogeneic fibroblast	*IL-2*	Plasmid	In vitro	Intra tumoral	I/II	*Rochlitz, C., Basel*
Autologous fibroblast	*IL-4*	Retrovirus	Ex vivo	id	Pilot	Lotze, M. T., Pittsburgh, PA
Autologous fibroblast	IL-12	Adenovirus	Ex vivo	Peritumoral	II	Lotze, M. T., Pittsburgh, PA
Autologous dendritic	MART-1	Adenovirus	Ex vivo	id or iv	I	Economou, J. S., Los Angeles, CA
Autologous dendritic	MART-1 and *gp100*	Adenovirus	Ex vivo	sc	I/II	Haluska, F., Boston, MA
Autologous skin	*gp100* and/or GM-CSF	DNA-coated gold beads	In vivo	id	I	Albertini, M. R., Madison, WI
Autologous	*gp100*	Plasmid	In vivo	id or im	II	Rosenberg, S. A., Bethesda, MA
Autologous	MART-1	Plasmid	In vivo	im	I	Conry, R. M., Birmingham, AL
Autologous	MART-1 or *gp100*	Adenovirus	In vivo	sc or im	I	*Rosenberg, S. A., Bethesda, MD*
Autologous	MART-1	Fowlpox virus	In vivo		I	Rosenberg, S. A., Bethesda, MD
Autologous	*gp100*	Fowlpox virus	In vivo	iv or im	I	Rosenberg, S. A.–Bethesda, MD
Autologous	Tyrosinase	Fowlpox virus and vaccinia virus	In vivo	im	II randomized	Topalian, S. L., Bethesda, MD
Autologous	*MART-1*	Vaccinia virus			I	Rosenberg, S. A., Bethesda, MD
Autologous hematopoietic progenitor	Mutant-MGMT-G156A[b]	Retrovirus	Ex vivo	iv	I	Gerson, S. L., Ohio
Allogenic fibroblasts	IL-2	Plasmid	Ex vivo	sc + id	I	Veelken, H., Freiburg
Xenogeneic fibroblasts	IL-2	Plasmid	In vitro	Intratumoral	I/II	Rochlitz, C., Basel

[a]Italics indicate clinical trials whose results have been published (see Table 3).
[b]*G156A* is a mutant form of MGMT [O(6)-methylguanine DNA methyltransferase] gene. This gene codes a DNA repair protein that protects cells against nitrosourea cytotoxicity: id, intradermally; sc, subcutaneously; im, intramuscularly; iv, intravenous.

describing the results of these studies in melanoma patients have been published (**Table 3**). The most relevant end point of these trials was the induction or increase in tumor-specific T-cell responses, but toxicity and clinical activity were also considered.

In the case of melanoma patients, vaccines have been constructed ex vivo with both autologous and allogeneic melanoma cells (*see* **Table 1**). Autologous vaccines offer the advantage that only tumor antigens can be recognized by the host's immune system, whereas allogeneic lines can generate anti-allogeneic human leukocyte antigen (HLA) or even anti–minor histocompatibility antigen responses that, however, do not seem to impair recognition of tumor antigens. However, the choice of autologous cell lines carries several disadvantages such as the need to resect a tumor mass of a certain size in order to be able to generate the line to be transduced, the variability in gene transfer from culture to culture, the labor intensity and economic cost of preparing the necessary amount of vaccine and performing the required safety assays before injection into patients, and the need to characterize the line for expression of melanoma antigens and other molecules as well. These problems can be avoided by using allogeneic melanoma lines that can be selected for the high expression of melanoma antigens, expanded, gene transduced, stabilized, used for safety assays, and irradiated in enough quantity to be administered in patients when needed. However, the majority of early planned protocols was based on autologous cell vaccines (**Table 1**) although only a few of these studies were completed owing to the long time required for enrollment of patients from whom the autologous melanoma lines could be established *(12,17,19,28)*.

Altogether, the results of protocols of vaccination with cytokine gene-transduced cells were similar whether autologous or allogeneic vaccines were used inasmuch as clinical responses were weak (**Table 3**) and T-cell-specific immune reactions, when appropriately assessed, were obtained in a minority (20–30%) of patients. It is also evident that, given the fact that cytokine gene transduction was carried out ex vivo, no major difference was found in immunogenic terms between cell lines transduced with retroviral and adenoviral vectors.

A limited number of studies were conducted by a direct intratumoral injection of the cytokine gene by using adenoviral or retroviral vectors or a plasmid (*see* **Table 1**). Although by this approach only local clinical responses may be expected, only in one study *(17)* were such responses reported in 4 of 17 patients treated.

In addition to cytokines, other genes have been transduced into tumor cells with the purpose of increasing their stimulatory activity, such as *B7*, a gene encoding a costimulatory molecule that may deliver the second signal to activate naïve T-lymphocytes *(29)*. In vitro studies demonstrated that melanoma

Summary of Clinical Responses Observed in Melanoma Patients Treated According with Gene Therapy Trials

Transduced cell	Transduced gene	Phase	Number of patients	Clinical responses					References
				PRO	SD	MR	PR	CR	
Autologous melanoma	IL-2	I	15	15[a]					11
Autologous melanoma	IL-2	I	12	8	4				12
Autologous melanoma	IL-2	I	14	9	4	1			13
Autologous melanoma	IL-2	I/II	16		3		1		14
Autologous melanoma	IL-7	I	8	2	4	2			15
Autologous melanoma	IL-12	I	6	3	3				16
Autologous melanoma	IFN-γ	I	17[b]	8	5		2[g]	2[g]	17
Autologous melanoma	IFN-γ	I	12[c]	not evaluable since tumors were removed after 8 d					18
Autologous melanoma	GM-CSF	I/II	29	24	3	1	1	0	19
Autologous melanoma	GM-CSF	I/II	7	2		3	1	1	20
Allogeneic melanoma	IL-2	I/II	12	7	2	3			21
Allogeneic melanoma	IL-4	I/II	12	9	1	2			22
Autologous melanoma	HLA-B7	I	5	4		1[d]			23
Autologous melanoma	HLA-B7	I	14	5	4	7	0	1	24
Autologous melanoma	HLA-B13 or H-2K^K	I	2	2					25
Autologous skin or muscle	MART-1 or gp100	I	36[e]/18[f]				2[e]/0[f]	3[e]/1[f]	26
Xenogenic fibroblast	IL-2	I/II	1		1				27
Autologous melanoma	HSV-1 thymidine kinase	I/II	8[b]	8					28

[a] Including five local responses.

[b] In this protocol transduction was performed in vivo (intratumor administration).

[c] In this protocol transduction was performed ex vivo (sc administration).

[d] Complete response of treated cutaneous nodule and of some untreated distant metastases.

[e] Patients receiving adenovirus MART-1.

[f] Patients receiving adenovirus gp100.

[g] Local response only.

PRO, progression of disease; SD, stable disease; MR, mixed response; PR, partial response; CR, complete response.

cells transduced with *B7.1* show an increased immunogenicity for autologous and allogeneic patients' T-cells *(30)*. Animal models indicate that tumors expressing *B7* can elicit a strong immunity when transplanted in syngeneic mice *(31)*. As shown in **Table 1**, at least three clinical studies (responsible investigators are L. Schuchter, M. Sznol and R. M. Conry, respectively) have been initiated with vaccines expressing B7 or B7 plus IL-2, but results are not yet available.

Another approach of immunologic gene therapy that has been applied in melanoma patients is the in vivo intratumoral injection of plasmid coding for the allogeneic HLA-B7 (Allovectin-7; Vical, San Diego, CA) with the intent of inducing an immune/inflammatory reaction at the tumor site that will activate recognition and destruction of melanoma cells. Such a study reported the generation of T-cell-specific cytotoxicity against the autologous melanoma in treated patients *(23)*. Based on this rationale, some clinical protocols have been proposed; two such studies have resulted in published reports (**Table 3**). One of the studies recorded seven minor responses in the injected metastases (≥25% reduction) and one complete response out of 17 treated melanoma patients *(24)*; toxicities related to the injections or biopsies included pain, hemorrage, pneumothorax, and hypotension.

Because tumor cells to be used as recipients of genes are often available in a limited number and are unable to grow in vitro, normal fibroblasts that can be easily obtained from the normal skin have been used. On cytokine gene transduction, fibroblasts have been admixed with fresh tumor cells (to provide antigens) and injected into patients. There are no convincing preclinical data, however, suggesting that this approach is superior to provision of the exogenous cytokine (e.g., interleukin-4[IL-4] or IL-12) to tumor cells, and the preliminary results of these clinical studies are rather disappointing. Allogeneic, long-term, cultured human fibroblasts transduced with the IL-2 gene were also used to vaccinate melanoma patients after admixing with fresh autologous tumor cells *(32)*. Melanoma-specific cytotoxic T-cells could be isolated from the tumor infiltrate after vaccination, but only in a few patients.

A variant form of this approach is the intratumoral injection of xenogeneic (monkey) fibroblasts transduced with the IL-2 gene to cause an inflammatory reaction that may result into tumor shrinkage; however, this occurred in only a limited number of cases *(27)*.

It should be emphasized that gene therapy of cancer is aimed at controlling metastatic disease, and, therefore, approaches that envisage the injection of genes into tumor nodules, although important to prove a principle, will hardly be used in the clinic, where the large majority of patients require treatment of visceral lesions usually not accessible without invasive techniques. Thus, the problem of in vivo targeting remains a major issue of gene therapy, particularly in metastatic melanoma because cutaneous, lymph node, and even lung lesions can be approached easily by surgery.

A new development in cancer vaccination lies in the use of dendritic cells (DCs), the most potent antigen-presenting cells (APCs) that can now be obtained from patients' blood in such a quantity that allows their clinical use *(33)*. **Table 2** lists examples of clinical studies in which autologous DCs have been transfected with genes coding for one or more T-cell-defined melanoma antigens and then injected into melanoma patients to elicit a melanoma-specific immune response. In vitro studies have shown that these DCs can elicit primary T-cell responses from peripheral blood lymphocytes (PBLs) of melanoma patients *(34)*. As shown in **Table 2**, different vectors can be used in clinical protocols along with different routes of administration. However, no published data are available from these studies.

Altogether, the studies of vaccination with autologous or allogeneic gene-transduced neoplastic or normal cells suggest that only in a limited number of cases a specific, T-cell-defined antimelanoma response can be elicited and that clinical consequences of such a response are modest. However, important information has also been collected from several of these studies that, together with the new findings of animal models, now allows optimization of this approach in order to obtain more convincing clinical responses. More specifically, one should construct vaccines whose cells express high density of known, immunogenic melanoma antigens and release a cytokine that can provide a microenvironment that favors the recruitment of DCs and their maturation to enable the antigens to be taken into draining lymph nodes where immunization of T-cells may occur. Whether or not expression of class I and II major histocompatibility complex and of costimulatory molecules is important is debatable (*see* **ref. *3***). In fact, although cross-priming is recognized as the most important mechanism of antigen presentation to naïve T-cells, when patients are already primed against melanoma antigens *(8)*, a direct APC function might be carried out by tumor cells themselves and help generate an efficient T-cell response. Indeed, memory T-cells can be reactivated even in the absence of costimulatory molecules. Recent observations indicate also that the mechanism by which tumor cells die (in the case of gene-modified vaccines, this occurs by radiaton) and release their antigens can be crucial for the immunogencity of tumors that appears to be increased when heat-shock proteins are involved *(35)*.

3.1.2. Adoptive Immunotherapy with Gene-Modified Lymphocytes

Available technology allows the transfer of genes into lymphocytes. Thus, it is possible to confer to such cells an antitumor activity superior to that they may have acquired spontaneously in vivo or after in vitro stimulation. In fact, previous studies showed that, despite the injection of high amounts of lymphokine-activated killer cells or of tumor-infiltrating lymphocytes (TILs) into melanoma patients, the clinical response rate was relatively low for the former without a clear advantage over the administration of high doses of IL-2 alone *(36)*, whereas TIL provided a 34% response rate but at the expense of costly and labor-intensive procedures *(37)*. Note, however, that the majority of lymphocytes transferred into patients in these early studies were not tumor specific and probably ineffective.

It was therefore decided to use retroviral vectors to transduce TILs first with marker genes (e.g., that coding for neomycin resistance) to evaluate their in vivo long-term tissue distribution by polymerase chain reaction (PCR) analysis of tissue biopsies. The results of these studies indicate that TILs can survive up to 260 d in the circulation although no preferential tumor localization could be demonstrated *(38)*.

More recent approaches to adoptive immunotherapy involve genetic manipulation of lymphocytes to overcome previous drawbacks in their use. To bypass the need to generate and expand tumor-specific T-cells from each patient even in case T-cell-defined antigens are not known, a procedure that may be successful in <50% of individuals, one can use chimeric receptors containing the V regions of antibodies directed to tumor antigens, joined to the C regions of the T-cell receptor (TCR) *(39)*. Such an approach allows retargeting of tumor cells expressing antigens frequently recognized by antibodies (e.g., gangliosides in melanoma) and was shown to be effective in animal models of ovarian carcinoma *(40)*. However, no clinical studies in melanoma patients have been initiated, and, therefore, the effectiveness of this approach remains to be determined.

To overcome the difficulty of generating large numbers of tumor-specific T-cells from TILs, an alternative strategy is that of genetically modifying patients' PBLs. This can be obtained by the transfer of genes coding for the TCR of melanoma-specific antigens that will confer the ability to recognize such antigens on the autologous tumor cells *(41)*.

Thanks to new information on the molecular nature of melanoma antigens recognized by T-cells and the availability of new technology, it is now possible to select and expand in vitro autologous T-cell populations enriched for their ability to recognize specific melanoma antigens (e.g., Melan-A/MART-1, gp100) by using either anti-TCRV antibodies or tetramers *(42,43)*. These populations also can be modified further to express genes that may confer selective tissue-targeting properties (homing receptors) or additional killing activity (e.g., tumor necrosis factor-α). Again, these reagents are being prepared and validated in several laboratories, but clinical trials have yet to be designed to test the antitumor activity of such genetically modified T-lymphocytes.

3.2 Genetic Prodrug Activation Therapy

3.2.1. Rationale

One of the aims of the gene therapy approach is to create an artificial difference between normal and tumor cells in terms of susceptibility or resistance to cytotoxic drugs in order to improve the selectivity of the therapeutic intervention. The possibility of modifying tumor cells in order to make them more sensitive to an otherwise nontoxic agent is known as suicide gene therapy or genetic prodrug activation therapy. This approach involves the insertion of a gene encoding an enzyme, usually viral or bacterial, that modifies a nontoxic compound, the prodrug, into an active metabolite interfering with DNA synthesis, or transforms the prodrug into a more powerful cytotoxic agent able to kill the genetically modified cells.

The thymidine kinase encoded by the herpes simplex virus type 1 (HSV1-TK) is the best known example of the former class of enzymes and the most commonly used. It catalyzes the phosphorylation of nucleoside analogs that are poor substrates of the cellular endogenous thymidine kinase, including the guanosine analogs ganciclovir (GCV) and acyclovir (ACV). Once triphosphorylated by HSV1-TK, GCV or ACV become substrates of the DNA polymerase and are incorporated into newly synthesized DNA, resulting in DNA chain termination and the death of proliferating cells. The cytosine deaminase encoded by bacteria and fungi is an example of the latter class of enzymes: it catalyzes the deamination of cytosine to uracil and is able to transform the nontoxic prodrug 5-fluorocytosine into the cytotoxic agent 5-fluorouracil. In addition to these systems, several other enzymatic activities have been described that can be used as suicide genes, such as the *Escherichia coli* xanthine guanine phosphoribosyl transferase or the nitroreductase, and many others are under development *(44)*.

3.2.2. Mechanisms of Antitumor Effects

The positive outcome of the suicide gene therapy relies on successful in vivo targeting of tumor cells with the suicide gene, and the choice of vector for gene transfer is therefore crucial. However, experimental models demonstrated that at least two other components are involved in the destruction of tumor by the activated prodrug: the so-called bystander effect and the inflammatory/immunologic response activated *in situ* by tumor cell destruction.

The bystander effect refers to the observation that the activated prodrug has killed not only the transduced but also nontransduced tumor cells that are in close contact. This phenomenon relies either on the passive diffusion of the activated metabolite from the genetically modified cells to neighboring counterparts, as occurs for 5-fluorouracil, or on an active process of transferring of the toxic drug through gap junctions, as is the case for GCV. Moreover, apoptotic vesicles released by dying transduced cells and phagocytosed by nearby cells have also been considered possible vehicles of activated metabolites *(45)*. An immunologic component is also involved in the amplification of both the suicide and the bystander effect in vivo. Studies in experimental models have shown active mononuclear cell infiltration of regressing tumors in immunocompetent hosts with release of cytokines *in situ* and generation of a protective immune response *(46,47)*.

Many characteristics of this gene therapy approach make it suitable for the treatment of melanoma patients. In fact, certain localizations of melanoma lesions (skin, subcutaneous tissue, lymph nodes) make them easily accessible to surgical maneuvers and favor their direct transduction via injection of gene therapy vectors. Otherwise, when melanoma lesions are difficult to reach, as in the case of visceral or cerebral metastasis, the possibility of using tumor-specific promoters, such as the tyrosinase or the tyrosinase-related protein-1 promoter, may allow the selective expression of the suicide gene into melanoma cells, preventing toxicity in nearby normal tissues *(48,49)*. Moreover, the possibility of amplifying the therapeutic response through the bystander effect will permit significant killing of tumor cells also in the presence of low gene transduction efficiency (as low as 10%) *(45)*. Finally, the activation of local inflammation with immune cell infiltration provides an opportunity to break local tolerance to melanoma antigens and activate a systemic immune response. Therefore, the murine melanoma model B16 has been widely used to test the efficacy and study the mechanisms underlying the suicide gene therapy in view of its use in clinical trials.

Although nonviral vectors have been used to transduce suicide genes into B16 melanoma cells in vivo, such as cationic liposomes *(49)* and attenuated strains of *Salmonella (50)*, viral vectors are still the most efficient system to transduce melanoma cells both in vitro and in vivo. In fact, adenoviral vectors can target both dividing and quiescent cells, resulting in efficient but transient gene expression. An improvement to the gene transduction was recently obtained with the use of replication competent adenoviral vectors also capable of exerting an oncolytic effect and spreading the suicide gene to many more replicating tumor cells, as demonstrated in a xenograft model of human melanoma *(51)*. Although potentially hazardous, the use of infective adenoviruses may offer a further advantage owing to their strong immunogenicity, a characteristic that also can be employed to potentiate antitumor immune response.

Intratumoral injection of replication defective adenoviral vectors efficiently transduced HSV1-TK into sc B16 melanoma, resulting in a significant reduction in tumor growth on ip treatment with GCV *(51)*. The observation that transduced tumor growth was impaired also in the absence of GCV treatment in immunocompetent hosts but not in athymic mice suggested an immune response to viral antigens and prompted the investigators to design a combined immunotherapy protocol to amplify this response. The combination of in vivo tumor transduction with suicide gene and cytokines, such as IL-2 or granulocyte macrophage colony-stimulating factor (GM-CSF), via adenoviral vectors improved the therapeutic response to GCV and induced tumor cell–specific CTL activity *(52)*.

The mechanisms by which tumor cells are killed in vivo may be important in activating specific immune responses by providing an inflammatory stimulus that helps convert an otherwise tolerogenic presentation of tumor antigens into a stimulatory signal. The expression of suicide genes has been used to induce the death of tumor cells used as live vaccine, so that an immunostimulatory environment is created at the site where tumor antigens are released and presented. To this aim, polycistronic retroviral vectors have been used to transduce B16 melanoma cells with HSV1-TK and immunostimulatory cytokines, such as GM-CSF or IL-2. Vaccination with these melanoma cells followed by GCV treatment generated a long-term immune protection to challenge with parental B16, especially when GM-CSF was associated to the HSV1-TK. On the other hand, in a therapeutic setting, the release of IL-2 before GCV killing of vaccine cells resulted in a significant slowing of contralateral B16 established tumors *(53)*. In fact, further studies have demonstrated that the mechanisms of cell death can control the immunogenicity of tumor cells. Although an alternative pathway of cell death may depend on the cell line considered, the treatment of B16 expressing HSV1-TK with GCV induces more tumor cell necrosis than apoptosis. This process is responsible for the induction and release of heat-shock proteins whose uptake by APCs preludes the re-presentation of tumor antigens and immunization against them *(35)*.

3.2.3. Clinical Studies

A phase I/II clinical trial has been performed to establish the tolerance of intratumoral injection of retroviral packaging cells in order to transduce HSV1-TK into melanoma lesions and evaluate the effect of the subsequent administration of GCV *(28)* (*see* **Table 3**). The treatment was well tolerated and unwanted retroviral dissemination was not found. Histologic modification of the treated tumors that included necrosis but not lymphocytic infiltration was evident in two of eight patients; signs of distant bystander effect were detected in one patient. Although reductions in tumor volume on GCV treatment were recorded, the efficacy was limited. This was probably owing to inefficient gene transduction (<1% of tumor cells), as demonstrated by the poor detection of the HSV1-TK gene in tumor biopsies by PCR, a result expected in view of the xenogeneic nature of the packaging cells injected. However, the histologic signs of response to GCV, the safety of the treatment, and the absence of toxic side effects warrant further development of this gene therapy approach that will take advantage of new gene transfer vectors available and combination with other immunotherapy approaches.

4. Conclusion

Several strategies are being applied in the gene therapy of human melanoma but none of them appears successful at present. However, the wealth of information that has been collected through both preclinical investigations and appropriate clinical trials will certainly be used to improve our understanding of the mechanism of the diverse approaches of gene therapy in patients bearing metastatic melanoma. Although, as in other types of cancer, in vivo delivery and targeting remain the major unresolved issues of gene therapy, the immunologic approach should be able to improve its efficacy both in the vaccination and in the adoptive immunotherapy with gene-modified lymphocytes. We do believe, therefore, that gene therapy of melanoma deserves to be studied further through a synergistic effort that should include investigators from different disciplines to improve its clinical impact for a disease that remains without effective cures when recurring in distant organs.

References

1. Caplen, N. J. (1998) Gene therapy: different strategies for different applications. *Mol. Med. Today* **5,** 374,375.
2. Verma, I. M. and Somia, N. (1997) Gene therapy: Promises, problems and prospects. *Nature* **389,** 239–242.
3. Parmiani, G. (1998) Editorial. Immunological approach to gene therapy of human cancer: improvements through the understanding of mechanism(s). *Gene Ther.* **5,** 863,864.
4. Nguyen, J. T., Wu, P., Clouse, M. E., Hlatky, L., and Terwillinger, F. (1998) Adeno-associated virus-mediated delivery of antiangiogenic factors as an antitumor strategy. *Cancer Res.* **58,** 5673–5677.
5. Meier, F., Satyamoorthy, K., Nesbit, M., Hsu, M.-Y., Schittek, B., Garbe, C., and Herlyn, M. (1998) Molecular events in melanoma development and progression. *Front. Biosci.* **3,** 1005–1010.
6. Jäger, E., Ringhoff, M., Karbach, J., Arand, M., Oesch, F., and Knuth, A. (1996) Inverse relationship of melanocyte differentiation antigen expression in melanoma

tissues and CD8+cytotoxic T cell response: evidence for immunoselection of antigen-loss variants in vivo. *Int. J. Cancer* **66,** 470–476.

7. Brasseur, F., Rimoldi, D., Liénard, D., et al. (1995) Expression of MAGE genes in primary and metastatic cutaneous melanoma. *Int. J. Cancer* **63,** 375–380.

8. Anichini, A., Molla, A., Mortarini, R., Tragni, G., Bersani, I., Di Nicola, M., Gianni, A. M., Pilotti, S., Dunbar, R., Cerundolo, V., and Parmiani, G. (1999) An expanded peripheral T cell population to a CTL-defined melanocyte-specific antigen in metastatic melanoma patients impact on generation of peptide-specific CTL, but does not overcome tumor escape from immune surveillance in metastatic lesions. *J. Exp. Med.* **190,** 651–667.

9. Musiani, P., Modesti, A., Giovarelli, M., Cavallo, F., Colombo, M. P., Lollini, P. L., and Forni, G. (1997) Cytokines, tumour-cell death and immunogenicity: a question of choice. *Immunol. Today* **18,** 32–36.

10. Parmiani, G., Colombo, M. P., Melani, C., and Arienti, F. (1997) Cytokine gene transduction in the immunotherapy of cancer. *Adv. Pharmacol.* **40,** 259–307.

11. Stewart, A. K., Lassam, N. J., Quirt, I. C., et al. (1999) Adenovector-mediated gene delivery of interleukin-2 in metastatic breast cancer and melanoma: results of a phase 1 clinical trial. *Gene Ther.* **6,** 350–363.

12. Palmer, K., Moore, J., Everard, M., et al. (1999) Gene therapy with autologous, interleukin 2-secreting tumor cells in patients with malignant melanoma. *Hum. Gene Ther.* **10,** 1261–1268.

13. Schreiber, S., Kampgen, E., Wagner, E., et al. (1999) Immunotherapy of metastatic malignant melanoma by a vaccine consisting of autologous interleukin 2-transfected cancer cells: outcome of a phase I study. *Hum. Gene Ther.* **10,** 983–993.

14. Galanis, E., Hersh, E. M., Stopeck, A. T., et al. (1999) Immunotherapy of advanced malignancy by direct gene transfer of an interleukin-2 DNA/DMRIE/DOPE lipid complex: phase I/II experience. *J. Clin. Oncol.* **17,** 3313–3323.

15. Moller, P., Sun, Y., Dorbic, T., Alijagic, S., Makki, A., Jurgovsky, K., Schroff, M., Henz, B. M., Wittig, B., and Schadendorf, D. (1998) Vaccination with IL-7 gene-modified autologous melanoma cells can enhance the anti-melanoma lytic activity in peripheral blood of patients with a good clinical performance status: a clinical phase I study. *Br. J. Cancer* **77,** 1907–1916.

16. Sun, Y., Jurgovsky, K., Moller, P., Alijagic, S., Dorbic, T., Georgieva, J., Wittig, B., and Schadendorf, D. (1998) Vaccination with IL-12 gene-modified autologous melanoma cells: preclinical results and a first clinical phase I study. *Gene Ther.* **5,** 481–490.

17. Nemunaitis, J., Fong, T., Robbins, J. M., Edelman, G., Edwards, W., Paulson, R. S., Bruce, J., Ognoskie, N., Wynne, D., Pike, M., Kowal, K., Merritt, J., and Ando, D. (1999) Phase I trial of interferon-gamma (IFN-γ) retroviral vector administered intratumorally to patients with metastatic melanoma. *Cancer Gene Ther.* **6,** 322–330.

18. Nemunaitis, J., Bohart, C., Fong, T., Burrows, F., Bruce, J., Peters, G., Ognoskie, N., Meyer, W., Wynne, D., Kerr, R., Pippen, J., Oldham, F., and Ando, D. (1998) Phase I trial of interferon-gamma retroviral vector administered intratumorally

with multiple courses in patients with metastatic melanoma. *Hum. Gene Ther.* **10,** 1289–1298.

19. Soiffer, R., Lynch, T., Mihm, M., et al. (1998) Vaccination with irradiated autologous melanoma cells engineered to secrete human granulocyte-macrophage colony-stimulating factor generates potent antitumor immunity in patients with metastatic melanoma. *Proc. Natl. Acad. Sci. USA* **95,** 13,141–13,146.

20. Mastrangelo, M. J., Maguire, H. C. Jr., Eisenlohr, L. C., Laughlin, C. E., Monken, C. E., McCue, P. A., Kovatich, A. J., and Lattime, E. C. (1999) Intratumoral recombinant GM-CSF-encoding virus as gene therapy in patients with cutaneous melanoma. *Cancer Gene Ther.* **6,** 409–422.

21. Belli, F., Arienti, F., Cascinelli, N., and Parmiani, G. (1997) Active immunization of metastatic melanoma patients with interleukin-2-transduced allogeneic melanoma cells: evaluation of efficacy and tolerability. *Cancer Immunol. Immunother.* **44,** 197–203.

22. Arienti, F., Belli, F., Cascinelli, N., Napolitano, F., Sulé-Suso, J., Mazzocchi, A., Gallino, G. F., Cattelan, A., Sanantonio, C., Rivoltini, L., Melani, C., Colombo, M. P., Cascinelli, N., Maio, M., and Parmiani, G. (1999) Vaccination of melanoma patients with IL-4 gene-transduced allogeneic melanoma cells. *Hum. Gene Ther.*, **10,** 2907–2916.

23. Nabel, G. J., Nabel, E. G., Yang, Z.-Y., Fox, B. A., Plautz, G. E., Gao, X., Huang, L., Shu, S., Gordon, D., and Chang, A. E. (1993) Direct gene transfer with DNA-liposome complexes in melanoma:expression, biologic activity, and lack of toxicity in humans. *Proc. Natl. Acad. Sci. USA* **90,** 11,307–11,311.

24. Stopeck, A. T., Hersh, E. M., Akporiaye, E. T., Harris, D. T., Grogan, T., Unger, E., Warnecke, J., Schluter, S. F., and Stahl, S. (1997) Phase I study of direct gene transfer of an allogeneic histocompatibility antigen, HLA-B7, in patients with metastatic melanoma. *J. Clin. Oncol.* **15,** 341–349.

25. Hui, K. M., Ang, P. T., Huang, L., and Tay, S. K. (1997) Phase I study of immunotherapy of cutaneous metastases of human carcinoma using allogeneic and xenogeneic MHC DNA-liposome complexes. *Gene Ther.* **4,** 783–790.

26. Rosenberg, S. A., Zhai, Y., Yang, J. C., Schwartzentruber, D. J., Hwu, P., Marincola, F. M., Topalian, S. L., Restifo, N. P., Seipp, C. A., Einhorn, J. H., Roberts, B., and White, D. E. (1998) Immunizing patients with metastatic melanoma using recombinant adenoviruses encoding MART-1 or gp100 melanoma antigens. *J. Natl. Cancer Inst. USA* **90,** 1894–1900.

27. Rochlitz, C., Jantscheff, P., Bongartz, G., Dietrich, P. Y., Quinquerez, A. L., Schatz, C., Mehtali, M., Courtney, M., Tartour, E., Dorval, T., Fridman, W. H., and Herrmann, R. (1999) Gene therapy study of cytokine-transfected xenogeneic cells (Vero-interleukin-2) in patients with metastatic solid tumors. *Cancer Gene Ther.* **6,** 271–281.

28. Klatzmann, D., Cherin, P., Bensimon, G., Boyer, O., Coutellier, A., Charlotte, F., Boccaccio, C., Salzmann, J. L., and Herson, S. (1998) A phase I/II dose-escalation study of herpes simplex virus type 1 thymidine kinase "suicide" gene therapy for metastatic melanoma. *Hum. Gene Ther.* **9,** 2585–2594.

29. Liu, Y. and Linsey, P. S. (1992) Costimulation of T cell growth. *Curr. Op. Immunol.* **4**, 265–270.

30. Sulé-Suso, J., Arienti, F., Melani, C., Colombo, M. P., and Parmiani, G. (1995) A B7-1 transfected human melanoma line stimulates proliferation and cytotoxicity of autologous and allogeneic lymphocytes. *Eur. J. Immunol.* **25**, 2737–2742.

31. Towsend, S. E. and Allison, J. P. (1993) Tumor rejection after direct costimulation of CD28+ T cells by B7-transfected melanoma cells. *Science* **259**, 368–370.

32. Veelken, H., Mackensen, A., Lahn, M., et al. (1997) A phase I clinical study of autologos tumor cells plus interleukin-2-gene-transfected allogeneic fibroblasts as a vaccine in patients with cancer. *Int. J. Cancer* **70**, 269–277.

33. Siena, S., Di Nicola, M., Bregni, M., Mortarini, R., Anichini, A., Lombardi, L., Ravagnani, F., Parmiani, G., and Gianni, A. M. (1995) Massive ex-vivo generation of functional dendritic cells from mobilized CD34+ blood progenitors for anticancer therapy. *Exp. Hematol.* **23**, 1463–1471.

34. Tuting, T., Wilson, C., Martin, D. M., Kasamon, Y. L., Rowles, J., Ma, D. I., Slingluff, C. L. Jr., Wagner, S. N., van der Bruggen, P., Baar, J., Lotze, M. T., and Storkus, W. J. (1998) Autologous human monocyte-derived dendritic cells genetically modified to expressed melanoma antigens elicit primary cytotoxic T cell responses *in vitro*: enhancement by co-transfection of genes encoding the Th1-biasing cytokines IL-12 and IFN-α. *J. Immunol.* **160**, 1139–1147.

35. Melcher, A., Todryk, S., Hardwick, N., Ford, M., Jacobson, M., and Vile, R. G. (1998) Tumor immunogenicity is determined by the mechanism of cell death via induction of heat shock protein expression. *Nat. Med.* **4**, 581–587.

36. Parkinson, D. R., Abrams, J. S., Wiernik, P. H., Rayner, A. A., Margolin, K. A., Van Echo, D. A., Sznol, M., Dutcher, J. P., Aronson, F. R., Doroshow, J. H., Atkins, M. B., and Hawkins, M. J. (1990) Interleukin-2 therapy in patients with metastatic malignant melanoma: a phase II study. *J. Clin. Oncol.* **8**, 1650–1656.

37. Rosenberg, S. A., Yannelli, J. R., Yang, J. C., Topalian, S. L., Schwartzentruber, D. J., Weber, J. S., Parkinson, D. R., Seipp, C. A., Einhorn, J. H., and White, D. E. (1994) Treatment of patients with metastatic melanoma with tumor-infiltrating lymphocytes. *J. Natl. Cancer Inst. USA* **86**, 1159–1166.

38. Merrouche, Y., Negrier, S., Bain, C., Combaret, V., Mercatello, A., Coronel, B., Moskovitchenko, J.-F., Tolstoshev, P., Moen, R., Philip, T., and Favrot, M. C. (1995) Clinical application of retroviral gene transfer in oncology: results of a French study with tumor-infiltrating lymphocytes transduced with the gene of resistance to neomycin. *J. Clin. Oncol.* **13**, 410–418.

39. Eshhar, Z., Waks, T., Gross, G., and Schindler, D. (1993) Specific activation and targeting of cytotoxic lymphocytes through chimeric single chains consisting of antibody binding domain and the gamma or zeta subunit of the immunoglobulin and T-cell receptors. *Proc. Natl. Acad. Sci. USA* **90**, 720–724.

40. Hwu, P., Yang, J. C., Cowherd, R., Treisman, J., Shafer, G. E., Eshhar, Z., and Rosenberg, S. A. (1995) In vivo antitumor activity of T cells redirected with chimeric antibody/T-cell receptor genes. *Cancer Res.* **55**, 3369–3373.

41. Clay, T. M., Custer, M. C., Sachs, J., Hwu, P., Rosenberg, S. A., and Nishimura, M. I. (1999) Efficient transfer of a tumor antigen-reactive TCR to human peripheral blood lymphocytes confers anti-tumor reactivity. *J. Immunol.* **163,** 507–513.

42. Maccalli, C., Farina, C., Sensi, M., Parmiani, G., and Anichini, A. (1997) TCR β-chain variable region-driven selection and massive expansion of HLA-class I-restricted antitumor CTL lines from HLA-A*0201+ melanoma patients. *J. Immunol.* **158,** 5902–5913.

43. Valmori, D., Pittet, M. J., Rimoldi, D., Liénard, D., Dunbar, R., Cerundolo, V., Lejeune, F., Cerottini, J.-C., and Romero, P. (1999) An antigen-targeted approach to adoptive transfer therapy of cancer. *Cancer Res.* **59,** 2167–2173.

44. Encell, L. P., Landis, D. M., and Loeb, L. A. (1999) Improving enzymes for cancer gene therapy. *Nat. Biotechnol.* **17,** 143–147.

45. Pope, I. M., Poston, G. J., and Kinsella, A. R. (1997) The role of the bystander effect in suicide gene therapy. *Eur. J. Cancer* **33,** 1005–1016.

46. Vile, R. G., Castleden, S., Marshall, J., Camplejohn, R., Upton, C., and Chong, H. (1997) Generation of an anti-tumour immune response in a non-immunogenic tumour: HSVtk killing in vivo stimulates a mononuclear cell infiltrate and a Th1-like profile of intratumoural cytokine expression. *Int. J. Cancer* **71,** 267–274.

47. Consalvo, M., Mullen, C. A., Modesti, A., Musiani, P., Allione, A., Cavallo, F., Giovarelli, M., and Forni, G. (1995) 5-fluorocytosine-induced eradication of murine adenocarcinomas engineered to express the cytosine deaminase suicide gene requires host immune competence and leaves an efficient memory. *J. Immunol.* **154,** 5302–5312.

48. Hart, I. R. (1996) Tissue specific promoters in targeting systemically delivered gene therapy. *Semin. Oncol.* **23,** 154–158.

49. Szala, S., Missol, E., Sochanik, A., and Strozyk, M. (1996) The use of cationic liposomes DC-CHOL/DOPE and DDAB/DOPE for direct transfer of Escherichia coli cytosine deaminase gene into growing melanoma tumors. *Gene Ther.* **3,** 1026–1031.

50. Pawelek, J. M., Low, K. B., and Bermudes, D. (1997) Tumor-targeted *Salmonella* as a novel anticancer vector. *Cancer Res.* **57,** 4537–4544.

51. Wildner, O. M., Morris, J. C., Vahanian, N. N., Ford, H. Jr., Ramsey, W. J., and Blaese, R. M. (1999) Adenoviral vectors capable of replication improve the efficacy of HSVtk/GCV suicide gene therapy of cancer. *Gene Ther.* **6,** 57–62.

52. Bonnekoh, B., Greenhalgh, D. A., Chen, S. H., Block, A., Rich, S. S., Krieg, T., Woo, S. L., and Roop, D. R. (1998) Ex vivo and in vivo adenovirus-mediated gene therapy strategies induce a systemic anti-tumor immune defence in the B16 melanoma model. *J. Invest. Dermatol.* **110,** 867–871.

53. Castleden, S. A., Chong, H., Garcia-Ribas, I., Melcher, A. A., Hutchinson, G., Roberts, B., Hart, I. R., and Vile, R. G. (1997) A family of bicistronic vectors to enhance both local and systemic antitumor effects of HSVtk or cytokine expression in a murine melanoma model. *Hum. Gene Ther.* **20,** 2087–2102.

13

Use of Gene Gun for Genetic Immunotherapy

In Vitro and In Vivo Methods

Alfred E. Chang, Keishi Tanigawa, Joel G. Turner, Edwin C. Chang, and Hua Yu

1. Introduction

A major thrust in the application of gene transfer technology for cancer therapy has been the modulation of the immune response. There has been a veritable explosion of information regarding the components of the immune response that are required to generate a meaningful cellular response to tumor-associated antigens (TAAs) capable of eliciting rejection of established tumor. Many of the preclinical and clinical immunogenetic studies have focused on melanoma. Historically, melanoma has been an immunoresponsive tumor for which several melanoma TAAs have been identified.

1.1. Immunogenetic Strategies

A variety of different immunogenetic strategies have been explored in preclinical animal models and, in some instances, in phase I clinical trials. The schematic diagram depicted in **Fig. 1** gives an overview of these approaches. Several different target cells have been used to transfect genes encoding immunoregulatory or immunostimulatory molecules and proteins. These target cells include tumor cells, fibroblasts, antigen-presenting cells (APCs) such as dendritic cells (DCs), and lymphoid cells or their progenitor lineage of stem cells. The immunostimulatory molecules include cytokines, costimulatory molecules, major histocompatibility complex (MHC) molecules, adhesion molecules, TAAs, and components of T-cell receptors. The underlying goal of these strategies is to develop more effective T-cell responses to tumor antigen.

From: *Methods in Molecular Medicine, Vol. 61: Melanoma: Methods and Protocols*
Edited by: B. J. Nickoloff © Humana Press Inc., Totowa, NJ

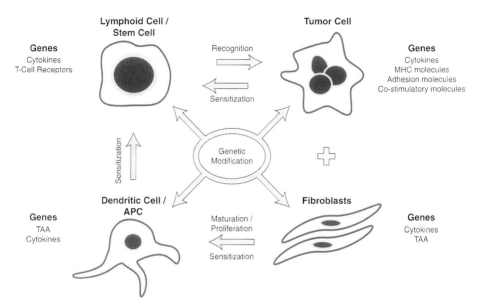

Fig. 1. Schematic diagram of various gene transfer approaches for modulating the immune response to tumors.

One such approach would be to genetically modify lymphoid cells or stem cells ex vivo for subsequent adoptive transfer in vivo. This subject is reviewed in detail elsewhere *(1)*. Briefly, investigators have examined ways to augment tumor-reactive T-cells to kill tumor cells more efficiently, prolong the in vitro or in vivo life span of such cells, or improve their ability to localize preferentially to sites of tumor on adoptive transfer. The use of stem cells genetically altered to express T-cell receptor genes targeted to specific TAAs has the potential to provide patients with a self-replicating source of memory T-cells.

In contrast to these approaches, the vast majority of immunogenetic therapeutic strategies employ the "vaccine" approach. Vaccination in this context spans a broad definition. Basically, it involves introducing an immunologic reagent into the host that incorporates the presence of TAAs to induce an active immunologic response against epitopes of the TAAs. As opposed to the adoptive transfer of an immunologically competent tumor-reactive lymphoid cell, which is known as passive immunotherapy, the use of a vaccine requires an intact host immune system to respond to the vaccine and is known as active immunotherapy. Different forms of genetically engineered tumor vaccines are reviewed in the next section.

1.2. Gene-Based Tumor Vaccines

One of the reasons that gene-based vaccines are of interest is the assumption that the host immune system to amplify the biologic effect of the transgenic protein that is expressed by the vaccine. Hence, the efficiency and level of expression of the therapeutic gene is not as restrictive as gene therapies that are designed to replace defective oncogenes/tumor suppressor genes, incorporate "suicide" genes, or target cellular signaling pathways. The end point of any tumor vaccine strategy is to induce a host immune response to TAAs that will result in the regression of established tumor, or prevent the growth of micrometastatic disease in the adjuvant setting. To date, tumor vaccines have been tested only in patients with diagnosed tumors, either after resection of a primary tumor or in the advanced disease setting. In these clinical studies, tumor response and time to progression are evaluated as potential end points. In addition, immunologic end points can be measured to monitor the biologic effects of the therapy. Several different immunologic tools are reviewed in this book that are helpful in monitoring the effects of vaccine therapies. Tumor-induced immunosuppression is a potential barrier in the induction of immune responses to vaccine therapies. In the future, preventive vaccines may be devised to immunize noncancer-bearing individuals identified to have a high risk of developing certain malignancies based on the presence of cancer susceptibility genes.

1.2.1. Noncellular DNA Vaccines

DNA encoding TAAs has been investigated as a method to stimulate an immune response by in vivo gene transfer methods. Examples of human TAAs evaluated in this context include CEA-derived antigens for colorectal cancer, prostate-associated antigen (i.e., prostate-specific antigen [PSA], prostate membrane surface antigen for prostate cancer, and papilloma virus–associated antigens (i.e., E6, E7) for cervical cancer. The form of gene delivery has varied according to the preference of the investigator. Viral vectors utilizing the vaccinia virus or other pox viruses have been used for immunization to CEA and PSA epitopes in clinical trials (2,3). Intradermal inoculation of viral vectors can potentially transfect an array of dermal cells along with inflammatory cells attracted by the viral vector. Gene gun utilization has been performed in preclinical animal models for E6 antigen and is discussed further in **Subheading 3.4.** Skin bombardment of DNA by gene gun delivery presumably transfects keratinocytes and dermal constituents such as Langerhans cells. Naked DNA, when injected into myoblasts, can efficiently express the transgenic protein (4).

An indirect method of vaccinating the tumor-bearing host has been the in vivo transfection of a tumor with a foreign MHC gene. In syngeneic animal models, Plautz et al. *(5)* reported the regression of established sc tumors by the intratumoral inoculation of an allogeneic MHC class I gene using DNA complexed with liposomes. They found that the tumor expressed the alloantigen and induced a cellular response not only to the alloantigen but also to parental tumor antigens. Presumably, the allogeneic response engendered a local tumor milieu conducive to the upregulation of tumor antigen sensitization. These observations led to clinical studies to evaluate the toxicity, immunologic responses, and antitumor responses of intratumoral inoculation of melanoma nodules with an allogeneic MHC class I gene complexed with liposomes *(6)*. Transgene expression by tumor cells was observed in the majority of patients treated. This was associated with an influx of tumor-infiltrating lymphocytes. In a small subgroup of patients, tumor regression of the injected nodules was observed.

1.2.2. Genetically Modified Tumor Cell Vaccines

The use of tumor cells (either whole or lysates) plus the admixture of an immune adjuvant has been the traditional approach to generate cellular responses to TAAs. The tumor cells (either autologous or allogeneic) provide the source of antigens and the adjuvant elicits a local microenvironment conducive to antigen processing and presentation to host lymphoid cells. The availability of molecular tools to introduce genes into cells has provided alternate means of providing the adjuvant. There have been numerous reports involving animal models in which tumor cells are genetically altered with immunostimulatory genes ex vivo and then reintroduced to normal, syngeneic hosts in which the transduced tumor cells fail to grow. On subsequent challenge with parental tumor cells, these animals are found to be immune and reject the challenge inoculum.

The list of immunostimulatory genes is extensive, with cytokines being the more common adjuvants examined. Several review articles summarize this topic *(7,8)*. In comparative studies of genetically modified tumor cell vaccines, granulocyte macrophage colony-stimulating factor (GM-CSF) appears to be one of the more potent cytokines in promoting T-cell responses to tumor antigen *(9,10)*. The utility of GM-CSF as an adjuvant is postulated to be owing to its role in causing an infiltration of DCs into the site of vaccination, thereby promoting antigen processing and presentation. Other cytokines appear to have different mechanisms of action. Restifo et al. *(11)* reported that tumor cells transduced to secrete interferon-γ result in enhanced MHC expression as well as increased ability of the tumor cell to present antigen to lymphoid cells, making these genetically altered tumor cells "nonprofessional" APCs. Besides cytokines, numerous immunomodulatory genes have been introduced into tumor cells to enhance immunogenicity. These include costimulatory molecules (i.e., B7.1), MHC molecules, adhesion molecules, and foreign proteins. Many of these models have helped increase our understanding regarding the mechanisms involved in the induction of antitumor immunity.

1.2.3. Genetically Altered Fibroblasts as Vaccines

A major impediment in generating tumor cells transduced with immunostimulatory genes for clinical therapy is the difficulty in establishing stable cultures from human tumors. Human melanoma tumor cultures are relatively easy to establish compared with, e.g., breast and colorectal cancer tumors. An alternative for clinical application is to establish fibroblast cultures from individual patients using skin biopsies. Fibroblasts are readily able to grow in culture and can be transfected with immunostimulatory genes. In animal studies, fibroblasts transduced to secrete interleukin-12 (IL-12) have been inoculated at sites of established tumor with resultant tumor regression *(12)*. More commonly, genetically altered fibroblasts that secrete cytokines have been admixed with tumor cells and utilized as effective vaccines *(13,14)*. Systemic immunity against a challenge of parental tumor cells can be established in this manner. Allogeneic fibroblasts have been used in a similar manner with effective adjuvant effect. We have noted that syngeneic transduced fibroblasts appear to be superior to allogeneic fibroblasts in the paracrine delivery of adjuvant cytokines *(15)*.

1.2.4. Genetically Altered DCs as Vaccines

DCs are considered to be the most potent APCs in the immune response. These cells process antigens and present them to lymphoid cells in association with MHC molecules. DCs play a central role in the induction of antigen-specific B- and T-cells. Several animal studies have demonstrated that the in vitro "pulsing" of DCs with tumor antigen in the form of whole tumor cells, tumor lysates, or tumor peptides generates DCs capable of priming naïve T-cells *(16–18)*. The id or iv inoculation of DCs has been reported to result in the regression of established murine tumors *(19)*. In clinical studies, investigators have reported that the iv or intranodal inoculation of antigen-pulsed DCs has resulted in regressions of metastatic tumors in patients *(20,21)*.

Methods to enhance the therapeutic efficacy of DCs include gene modification. Liposomal transfection, retroviral gene transfer, and the gene gun have been used to modify DCs successfully. Genes encoding tumor antigens have been transferred successfully into DCs to enhance their ability to sensitize lymphoid cells *(22–25)*. Reeves et al. *(25)* retrovirally transduced human DC with the melanoma TAA, MART-1. These DCs were able to elicit antigen-specific cytotoxic T-lymphocytes (CTLs) and stimulate greater levels of cytokine release by MART-1-specific TIL. In an in vivo murine model, Ribas et al. *(26)* demonstrated the superior induction of immunity with MART-1-transduced murine DCs compared with that of tumor cells expressing MART-1 as a vaccine.

1.3. Gene Gun Technology

The gene gun offers a useful method to introduce DNA or RNA into cells without the need of viral vectors. In 1987, Klein et al. *(27)* were the first to report using a "particle gun" to accelerate RNA or DNA attached to tungsten microprojectiles into intact epidermal cells of an onion. The microprojectiles were 4 µm and could be applied to a 1-cm^2 area where about 90% of the cells were found to contain the particles. Expression of the RNA or DNA was observed, and this method was proposed as an easy and rapid way of introducing nucleic acids into plant cells. In 1992, the first application of the gene gun to immunize animals to foreign protein was reported by Tang et al *(28)*. In this study, mice were bombarded in the skin with gold microprojectiles coated with plasmids encoding human growth hormone or human α1-antitrypsin. Antibodies to both foreign proteins could be detected, which was boosted by a subsequent treatment with the gene gun. Furthermore, direct injection of the plasmid into the skin was not effective in eliciting an antibody response. Tang et al. *(28)* proposed that this technique may provide a tool for manipulating the immune response.

The technology of "biolistics" has improved over time and its application in a wide range of biologic systems has been reported *(29)*. It is not only applicable to transfecting skin in vivo but also visceral organs such as the pancreas and liver. Microscopic gold particles ranging from approx <1 to 3 µm are typically utilized as microprojectiles. Using submicrogram quantities of DNA, thousands to tens of thousands of DNA copies can be delivered into cells in vivo. Single or multiple gene constructs can be delivered simultaneously in appropriate molar ratios. It takes only 5 s to complete a single transfection. Sequential application to the same targeted tissue in vivo can be employed to give multiple doses of genetic material. In addition to in vivo applications, the gene gun technology is useful to transfection of tissue explants, cell clumps, organoids, or other cultured cells such as tumor cells. Cells do not need to be actively proliferating for particle-mediated gene gun delivery. Cells of the myeloid lineage (i.e., T-cells, stem cells, macrophages), which are notoriously difficult to transfect by viral vectors, can be transfected with the gene gun for transient gene expression *(30–32)*. Gene expression lasts for a relatively short period ranging from 7 to 10 d. For immunologic modulation, this often is all that is required.

The mechanisms involved in the induction of both humoral and cellular T-cell responses by genetic immunization of the skin with the gene gun has been examined experimentally. When DNA vaccines are administered by gene gun bombardment of the skin, the majority of the plasmid is taken up by keratinocytes as well as APCs. The relative contribution of these two cell populations in the development of primary and memory immunity has been examined. Among the APCs in the epidermis, there are resident Langerhans cells as well as migratory cells from the bone marrow. From several studies, it appears that DCs (both Langerhans cells and bone marrow–derived DCs) that are transfected at the site of gene gun administration play a key role in the induction of immunity. These transfected cells rapidly migrate to the draining lymph nodes where cross-presentation of antigen to CD8+ T-cells occurs *(33)*. These migratory transfected DCs alone are responsible for immunologic memory *(34)*. The role of the nonmigratory transfected keratinocytes that express antigen is minimal, as demonstrated by grafting of skin vaccine sites to naïve recipients (24 h after gene gun treatment when migratory cells have left the skin site *(35)*.

2. Materials

 1. Ultrapure nitrogen gas.
 2. Helium gas (bone dry).
 3. 0.05 *M* Spermidine (Sigma, St. Louis, MO).
 4. 1 *M* CaCl$_2$ (Sigma).
 5. Absolute ethanol (anhydrous).
 6. Isopropanol (anhydrous) (Sigma).
 7. Polyvinylpyrrolidone (PVP) (Sigma).
 8. Tefzel tubing (id, 0.93 in.; od, 1/8 in.) (McMaster-Carr, Elmhurst, IL).
 9. Gold particles (1–3 µm) (Bio-Rad, Hercules, CA, or Aldrich, Milwaukee, WI).
10. Microcentrifuge tubes (1.5 mL), 5- to 10-mL capped tubes, and 10-cc syringe.
11. Culture media appropriate to the cells being transfected.
12. Sterile 50-mL conical tubes.
13. Sterile 35-mm tissue culture dishes.
14. Sterile pipets (5 mL); 20-, 200-, and 1000-µL pipettors with sterilized tips.
15. Large orifice universal pipet tips (200 µL).
16. Gene gun.
17. Tubing prep station (tube turner) and tubing cutter (Bio-Rad).
18. Vortex mixer.
19. Ultrasonic water bath.
20. Analytical balance.
21. Microcentrifuge.

3. Methods
3.1. Preparation of Gene Gun Cartridges

In this method, plasmid DNA is attached to gold particles and coated onto the inner wall of Tefzel tubing. The following steps describe a generalized method that will work for most protocols, but it is recommended that the transfection efficiency be optimized, varying sizes of gold particles, loading rates, and DNA/gold particle ratios (*see* **Note 1**).

1. Before starting, insert a length of Tefzel tubing into the tube turner apparatus. The tubing should be approx 3 in. longer than the tube turner. Purge the tubing for 1 h with 1.0 liter per minute (LPM) of nitrogen.
2. Weigh out 25 mg of gold (1- to 3-μm particle size) into a 1.5-mL microfuge tube, add 100 μL of 0.05 M spermidine, and sonicate briefly (5–10 s) in a ultrasonic water bath. After sonication, add 75 μg of DNA (3 μg of DNA/mg of gold) and vortex briefly. The spermidine/DNA mix should be no greater than 200 μL; if necessary, concentrate the DNA prior to making the prep.
3. Dropwise add 100 μL of 1 M $CaCl_2$ to the DNA/spermidine while vortexing, and allow the mixture to precipitate for 10 min. Flick the tube to get any residual gold particles off the sides and allow to precipitate an additional 10 min.
4. Centrifuge briefly and remove the clear liquid supernatant. Wash the DNA/gold pellet twice with 1 mL of absolute ethanol (anhydrous), and then wash once with 1 mL of isopropanol (anhydrous). With each wash vortex the mixture and centrifuge briefly to pellet the DNA/gold.
5. After washing, bring up the DNA/gold in 3.5 mL of isopropanol and place in a 5- to 10-mL capped tube. For in vivo transfections, the isopropanol should contain 0.1 mg/mL of PVP.
6. Briefly (5–10 s) sonicate the gold/DNA isopropanol slurry and mix well by shaking. Attach a 10-mL syringe to the purged length of tefzel tubing, and draw up the mixture into the tubing. Place in the tube turner and let settle for 5 min.
7. Remove the isopropanol by drawing very slowly with the syringe. Switch on the tube turning apparatus to 10 rpm and immediately turn on nitrogen gas to 1.5 LPM. Purge with nitrogen for 8 min while turning.
8. Using a razor or a Bio-Rad tubing cutter, slice the tubing into 0.5-in. cartridges. Store the cartridge tubes in an airtight vial at -20C°C, preferably desiccated. There are commercially available desiccant pellets that can be placed in the vials (United Desiccants, Belen, NM). Alternatively, purge the vial with nitrogen gas before sealing.

3.2. In Vitro and Ex Vivo Transfection of Cultured Cells

Proper assembly of the gene gun to the helium and electrical service may vary; therefore, refer to the manual supplied by the manufacturer. To optimize the helium pressures used to transfect the cells, transfect different samples in a stepwise fashion starting at 100 psi and increasing in increments of 50–400 psi. Generally, 200–300 psi is best for cell transfections. Green fluorescent protein, luciferase, or β-galactosidase plasmids are excellent reporter genes for optimizing the specific transfection protocol. In addition, it is important to try different particle loading rates (between 0.25 and 0.5 mg of gold/cartridge) and DNA to gold ratios (between 0.5 and 5 μg of DNA/mg of gold).

1. Make a suspension of the cells to be transfected of between 50 and 250 million cells per milliliter of culture media and store on ice. The actual number of cells transfected at these concentrations is between 1×10^6 and 5×10^6 cells in a 20-µL vol.
2. For ex vivo vaccine, irradiate the cells before transfection (3500–10,000 rad), depending on cell types and applications.
3. Transfections should be performed in a sterile tissue culture hood. It is helpful to clamp the gene gun to a large ring stand with the barrel pointing down. Using a large orifice pipet tip, plate a 20-µL vol of cell suspension in a 1.5-cm circle on the center of a 35-mm culture dish. It is useful to draw a 1.5-cm circle with a marker on the hood surface as a guide (a dime is about the right size). Hold the 35-mm culture dish firmly against the gene gun barrel with the cells centered and press the discharge button (200–300 psi).
4. For ex vivo vaccination, add 1 mL of media with a 5-mL pipet, gently suspend the cells in the media by tapping the dish, and collect the cell suspension into a 50-mL sterile conical tube. Wash the plate with a second 1-mL vol of culture media and collect in the 50-mL tube. Before vaccine injection, wash the cells twice with sterile phosphate-buffered saline.

3.3. In Vivo Transfection

Optimize the helium pressures used to transfect tissues. Transfect different samples in a stepwise fashion starting at 200 psi and increasing in increments of 50–500 psi. Generally, between 300 and 500 psi is the best range for in vivo transfections. Like ex vivo transfection, plasmids encoding green fluorescent protein, luciferase, or β-galactosidase are excellent for optimizing transfection efficiencies. Different particle loading rates and DNA to gold ratios described for ex vivo transfection should also be used to optimize in vivo transfection efficiency.

1. For skin transfections, remove hair from the area of transfection with electric clippers. DNA penetration of living tissues via gene gun is limited to the first 10 cell layers depending on the tissue being transfected and helium pressure.
2. Hold the tip of the gene gun firmly against the skin and discharge the gun (300–500 psi). Wearing ear and eye protection is recommended when higher pressures are used. (The gene gun is adaptable for transfection of internal organs or tissues.)

3.4. Examples
3.4.1. Example of In Vivo Cytokine Gene Treatment
of Established sc Tumor with Gene Gun Technology (from **ref. 36**)

GM-CSF plasmid was bombarded onto skin overlying implanted sc tumor nodules in mice. Prior to performing these experiments, the conditions of DNA delivery to normal skin were optimized. Gold particles of 0.6-, 1.0-, and

1.6-μm particles were superior. In subsequent studies, the amount of DNA (1.0–2.0 μg/mL) and pressure (200–500 psi) used to project the DNA/gold particles was evaluated (**Table 1**). Transgeneic GM-CSF protein was measured 24 h after particle bombardment by enzyme-linked immunosorbent assay (ELISA) with proteins extracted from minced specimens. As shown in **Table 1**, optimal skin transfection was observed with 1.6-μm particles, coated with 2.0 μg/mL of DNA, and projected at 300 psi. This demonstrates that optimizing the conditions of transfection for each experimental model is necessary to achieve maximal gene expression.

Subsequent in vivo transfection of growing sc tumors revealed diminished growth compared with controls, but no complete regressions of tumor. Transfection appeared to be confined to the skin overlying the tumor. Significant induction of tumor-reactive T-cells in the tumor-draining lymph nodes was observed, and the GM-CSF was found to enhance this sensitization.

3.4.2. Example of In Vivo TAA Gene Transfection of Skin Combined with Cytokine Gene for Tumor Immunization (from **ref. 37**)

As reviewed in **Subheading 1.**, genetic immunization with genes encoding TAAs is being examined for potential clinical applications. In animal models, the gene gun has been used to induce immunity to human TAAs. In this example, the E6 oncoprotein of human papillomavirus was used as a TAA for genetic immunization. Papillomaviruses are involved in the cellular transformation leading to the growth of certain cervical cancers. In addition, the cytokine gene for murine IL-12 was utilized in cotransfection studies. IL-12 has been reported to be a potent immune adjuvant in the setting of antitumor vaccines.

A plasmid encoding for E6 and human factor IX (hFIX) was constructed and called pvRE6hFIX *(37)*. hFIX was included as a marker protein that could be assayed by ELISA. Vaccination using the gene gun with pvRE6hFIX with or without mIL-12 gene was performed twice to the abdominal skin of mice spaced 1 or 2 wk apart. Approximately 1 wk after the last vaccination, splenocytes were harvested for assessment of functional antitumor reactivity, and mice were challenged with syngeneic Renca tumor transfected to express E6-E7 protein. As shown in **Fig. 2**, vaccination with E6hFIX plasmid resulted in CTLs in the spleen that were specific for E6-E7-expressing tumor cells (**Fig. 2A,B**). Cotransfection with mIL-12 gene enhanced the CTL generation (**Fig. 2C**). **Figure 3** shows challenge with E6-E7-expressing tumor cells (**Fig. 3A**) and parental tumor cells (**Fig. 3B**). Vaccination with E6hFIX or IL-12 resulted in protection of a small percentage of animals that were free of tumor. By contrast, cotransfection with E6hFIX and IL-12 genes resulted in significant antitumor immunity that appeared synergistic. The antitumor response was

Table 1
GM-CSF Transgenic Protein Expression
by Skin After Gene Gun Application

Gold particle size (μ)	DNA (μg/mL)	GM-CSF expression with varying psi[a]			
		200	300	400	500
1.0	1.0	3.3 (2.4)	41.3 (5.8)	20.3 (9.6)	13.8 (3.1)
	2.0	10.3 (9.5)	31.0 (2.4)	17.2 (0.5)	20.3 (3.2)
	3.0	1.5 (0.3)	14.8 (7.5)	15.2 (0.4)	13.4 (3.3)
1.6	1.0	8.5 (0)	28.3 (3.5)	53.7 (20.4)	63.6 (0.1)
	2.0	10.1 (3.1)	<u>74.7 (8.8)</u>	29.9 (3.4)	28.6 (6.4)
	3.0	7.0 (0.4)	29.0 (10.0)	17.8 (3.8)	42.7 (20.0)

[a]Skin was excised 24 h after gene gun application and GM-CSF production assayed as described in **Subheading 3.** Values represent mean nanograms/milliliter (SD) from triplicate skin samples. psi, pounds per square inch of gold particle pressure. The maximal GM-CSF expression is underlined.

owing to induction of E6 immunity because parental tumor challenge resulted in tumor growth in the majority of animals receiving the genetic immunizations.

These studies illustrate the relative ease of performing in vivo transfections of two genes at the same time. They also demonstrate how two different immunostimulatory genes (i.e., TAA and cytokine) can interact to enhance antitumor immunity.

3.4.3. Example of In Vitro Cytokine Gene Transfection of Tumor Cells Utilizing the Gene Gun

As reviewed in **Subheading 1.**, another approach to developing vaccines for cancer therapy is to genetically modify tumor cells ex vivo with immunostimulatory genes. These cells can then be used as vaccines to induce host immunity. We present here an example of genetically modifying tumor cells to secrete GM-CSF with the use of the gene gun. The D5 murine melanoma is an established tumor cell line that has been characterized by our laboratory as poorly immunogenic *(10)*. Utilizing the methods described herein, the D5 cells were transfected at different conditions with a plasmid encoding for murine GM-CSF *(36)*. After transfection, the cells were plated into 2-mL wells and culture supernatants harvested 24 h later for GM-CSF quantification. As shown in **Fig. 4**, the conditions of transfection dramatically influenced the expression of transgenic protein. Optimal conditions were obtained with 1-μm particles at a DNA loading rate of 2 μg of DNA/mg of gold. Bombardment of particles at 200 psi was better than at 100 psi. The level of gene expression was excellent

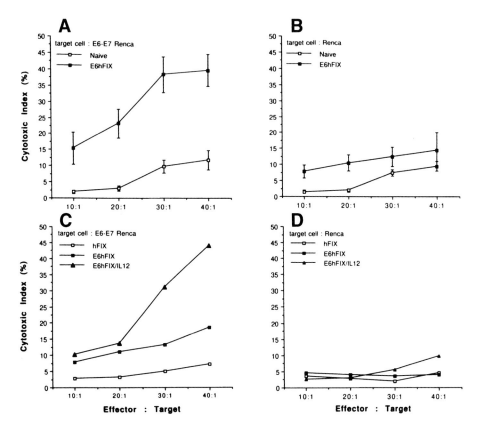

Fig. 2. Vaccination with pVRE6hFIX DNA results in E6-specific CTLs, and the E6 CTL is potentiated by cotransfection with the IL-12 cDNA vector. Splenocytes were prepared from mice after two immunizations. [51]Cr release assays were performed after in vitro restimulation with irradiated E6-E7 Renca cells for 5 d. The target cells used for the assays were E6-E7 Renca (**A,C**) and Renca (**B,D**).

under these conditions with GM-CSF production in the range of 60,000 pg/ (mL·24 h). The duration of transgenic GM-CSF was documented to be present for at least 4 d after the transfected cells were irradiated (**Fig. 5**).

4. Notes

1. The presence of moisture is a major problem when producing gene gun cartridges. It is extremely important when making gene gun cartridges that both the ethanol and isopropanol be anhydrous. Another source of moisture is the nitrogen gas used to dry the tubes. Always use ultrapure (bone-dry) nitrogen gas. If the tubing is not coated uniformly, the presence of moisture is the most likely cause. It is not unusual to get imperfectly coated tubing. Whereas clumping or uncoated sections of tubing is unacceptable, some streaking and banding usually cause little harm.

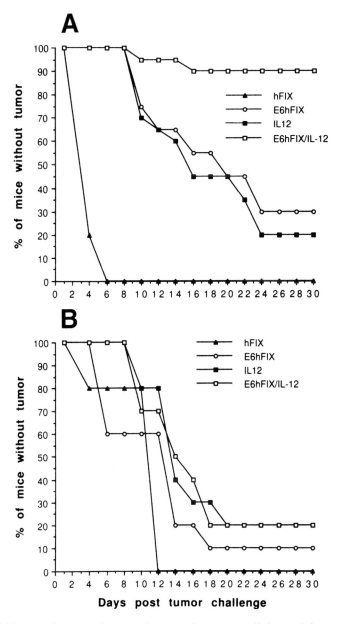

Fig. 3. Skin transfection with an E6 expression vector elicits an E6-specific antitumor immune response that is greatly enhanced by cotransfection of the IL-12 cDNA vector. A total of 2×10^5 of either (A) E6-E7 Renca cells or (B) parental Renca cells (E6-negative) were inoculated subcutaneously. Data are expressed as the percentage of tumor-free animals.

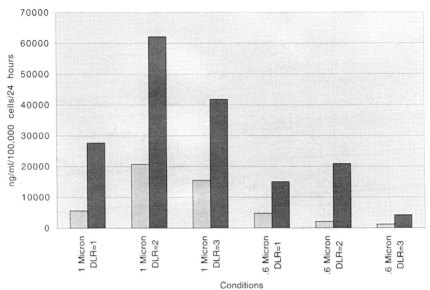

Fig. 4. In vitro gene transfection of D5 melanoma cells with GM-CSF cDNA. Transfection conditions, which were varied, included bombardment pressure (psi), particle size (0.6 vs 1.0 μm), and DNA loading rate (μg DNA/mg gold).

2. Smaller sizes of gold particles give more uniform tubing but less penetration of DNA/gold into cells and tissues.
3. Irradiation (5000 rad) of the Tefzel tube prior to coating with gold/DNA can produce markedly better cartridges. Irradiation applies a charge to the inner wall of the tube and results in more even coating.
4. Most of the materials needed to make gene gun cartridges can be obtained from Bio-Rad, including an optimization kit.

References

1. Chang, A. E. and Salas, A. P. (1999) Applications of gene transfer in the adoptive immunotherapy of cancer, in *Gene Therapy of Cancer* (E. C. Lattime and S. L. Gerson, eds.), Academic Press, San Diego, CA, pp. 349–358.
2. Marshall, J. L., Hawkins, M. J., Tsang, K. Y., Richmond, E., Pedicano, J. E., Zhu, M. Z., and Schlom, J. (1999) Phase I study in cancer patients of a replication-defective avipox recombinant vaccine that expresses human carcinoembryonic antigen. *J. Clin. Oncol.* **17(1),** 332–337.
3. Sanda, M. G., Smith, D. C., Charles, L. G., Hwang, C., Pienta, K. J., Schlom, J., Milenic, D., Panicali, D., and Montie, J. E. (1999) Recombinant vaccinia-PSA

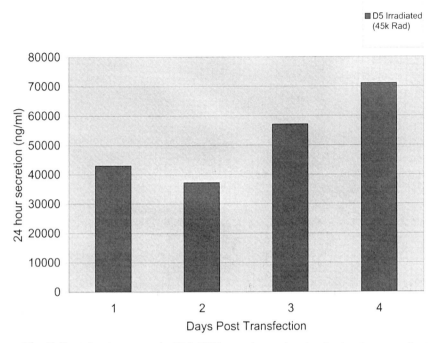

Fig. 5. Sustained transgenic GM-CSF protein production by in vitro transfected D5 melanoma cells. After transfection, D5 cells were irradiated with 45,000 cGy (rad) and cultured in 2-mL wells. Culture supernatants were replaced daily and assayed for GM-CSF. The slowly rising levels of protein production are owing to persistent proliferation of the irradiated tumor cells.

(PROSTVAC) can induce a prostate-specific immune response in androgen-modulated human prostate cancer. *Urology* **53(2),** 260–266.

4. Wolff, J. A., Malone, R. W., Williams, P., Chong, W., Acsadi, G., Jani, A., and Felgner, P.L. (1990) Direct gene transfer into mouse muscle in vivo. *Science* **247(4949 Pt. 1),** 1465–1468.

5. Plautz, G. E., Yang, Z., Wu., B, Gao, X., Huang, L., and Nabel, G. J. (1993) Immunotherapy of malignancy by in vivo gene transfer into tumors. *Proc. Natl. Acad. Sci. USA* **90,** 4645–4649.

6. Nabel, G. J., Gordon, D., Bishop, D. K., Nickoloff, B. J., Yang, Z., Aruga, A., Cameron, M. J., Nabel, E. G., and Chang, A. E. (1996) Immune response in human melanoma after transfer of an allogeneic class I major histocompatibility complex gene with DNA-liposome complexes. *Proc. Natl. Acad. Sci. USA* **93,** 15,388–15,393.

7. Miller, A. R., McBride, W. H., Hunt, K., and Economou, J. S. (1994) Cytokine-mediated gene therapy for cancer. *Ann. Surg. Oncol.* **1(5),** 436–450.

8. Péron, J. M., Shurin, M. R., and Lotze, M. T. (1999) Cytokine gene therapy of cancer, in *Gene Therapy of Cancer* (E. C. Lattime and S. L. Gerson, eds.), Academic Press, San Diego, CA, pp. 359–371.

9. Dranoff, G., Jaffee, E., Lazenby, A., Golumbek, P., Levitsky, H., Brose, K., Jackson, V., Hamada, H., Pardoll, D., and Mulligan, R. C. (1993) Vaccination with irradiated tumor cells engineered to secrete murine granulocyte-macrophage colony-stimulating factor stimulates potent, specific, and long-lasting anti-tumor immunity. *Proc. Natl. Acad. Sci. USA* **90**, 3539–3543.

10. Arca, M. J., Krauss, J. C., Aruga, A., Cameron, M. J., Shu, S., and Chang, A. E. Therapeutic efficacy of T cells derived from lymph nodes draining a poorly immunogenic tumor transduced to secrete granulocyte-macrophage colony-stimulating factor. *Cancer Gene Ther.* **1996, 3(1),** 39–47.

11. Restifo, N. P., Spiess, P. J., Karp, S. E., Mulé, J. J., and Rosenberg, S. A. (1992) A nonimmunogenic sarcoma transduced with the cDNA for interferon γ elicits CD8+ T cells against the wild-type tumor: correlation with antigen presentation capability. *J. Exp. Med.* **175**, 1423–1431.

12. Zitvogel, L., Tahara, H., Robbins, P. D., Storkus, W. J., Clarke, M. R., Nalesnik, M. A., and Lotze, M. T. (1995) Cancer immunotherapy of established tumors with IL-12: effective delivery by genetically engineered fibroblasts. *J. Immunol.* **155**, 1393–1403.

13. Shawler, D. L., Dorigo, O., Gjerset, R. A., Royston, I., Sobol, R. E., and Fakhrai, H. (1995) Comparison of gene therapy with interleukin-2 gene fibroblasts and tumor cells in the murine CT-26 model of colorectal carcinoma. *J. Immunother.* **17(4)**, 201–208.

14. Tahara, H., Zeh, H. J. III, Storkus, W. J., Papp, I., Watkins, S. C., Gubler, Y., Wolf, S. F., Robbins, P. D., and Lotze, M. T. (1994) Fibroblasts genetically engineered to secrete interleukin-12 can suppress tumor growth and induce antitumor immunity to a murine melanoma in vivo. *Cancer Res.* **54**, 182–189.

15. Aruga, A., Aruga, E., and Chang, A. E. (1997) Reduced efficacy of allogeneic versus syngeneic fibroblasts modified to secrete cytokines as a tumor vaccine adjuvant. *Cancer Res.* **57**, 3230–3237.

16. Zitvogel, L., Mayordoma, J. I., Tjandrawan, T., DeLeo, A. B., Clarke, M. R., Lotze, M. T., and Storku, W. J. (1996) Therapy of murine tumors with tumor peptide-pulsed dendritic cells: dependence on T cells, B7 costimulation, and T helper cell 1-associated cytokines. *J. Exp. Med.* **183**, 87–97.

17. Nair, S. K., Boczkowski, D., Snyder, D., and Gilboa, E. (1997) Antigen-presenting cells pulsed with unfractionated tumor-derived peptides are potent tumor vaccines. *Eur. J. Immunol.* **27**, 589–597.

18. Fields, R. C., Shimizu, K., and Mulé, J. J. (1998) Murine dendritic cells pulsed with whole tumor lysates mediate potent antitumor immune responses in vitro and in vivo. *Proc. Natl. Acad. Sci. USA* **95(16)**, 9482–9487.

19. Shimizu, K., Fields, R. C., Giedlin, M., and Mulé, J. J. (1999) Systemic administration of interleukin 2 enhances the therapeutic efficacy of dendritic cell-based tumor vaccines. *Proc. Natl. Acad. Sci. USA* **96**, 2268–2273.

20. Hsu, F. J., Benike, C., Fagnont, F., Liles, T. M., Czerwinski, D., Taidi, B., Engleman, E. G., and Levy, R. (1996) Vaccination of patients with B-cell lymphoma using autologous antigen-pulsed dendritic cells. *Nat. Med.* **2(1)**, 52–58.
21. Nestle, F. O., Alijagic, S., Gilliet, M., Sun, Y., Grabbe, S., Dummer, R., Burg, G., and Schadendorf, D. (1998) Vaccination of melanoma patients with peptide- or tumor lysate-pulsed dendritic cells. *Nat. Med.* **4(3)**, 328–332.
22. Boczkowski, D, Nair, S. K., Snyder, D, and Gilboa, E. (1996) Dendritic cells pulsed with RNA are potent antigen-presenting cells in vitro and in vivo. *J. Exp. Med.* **184**, 465–472.
23. Butterfield, L. H., Jilani, S. M., Chakraborty, N. G., Bui, L. A., Ribas, A., Dissette, V. B., Lau, R., Camradt, S. C., Glaspy, J. A., McBride, W. H., Muhkherji, B., and Economou, J. S. (1998) Generation of melanoma-specific cytotoxic T lymphocytes by dendritic cells transduced with a MART-1 adenovirus. *J. Immunol.* **161**, 5607–5613.
24. Henderson, R. A., Nimgaonkar, M. T., Watkins, S. C., Robbins, P. D., Ball, E. D., and Finn, O. J. (1996) Human dendritic cells genetically engineered to express high levels of the human epithelial tumor antigen mucin (MUC-1). *Cancer Res.* **56**, 3763–3770.
25. Reeves, M. E., Royal, R. E., Lam, J. S., Rosenberg, S. A., and Hwu, P. (1996) Retroviral transduction of human dendritic cells with a tumor-associated antigen gene. *Cancer Res.* **56**, 5672–5677.
26. Ribas, A., Butterfield, L. H., McBride, W. H., Jilani, S. M., Bui, L. A., Vommer, C. M., Lau, R., Dissette, V. B., Hu, B., Chen, A. Y., Glaspy, J. A., and Economou, J. S. (1997) Genetic immunization for the melanoma antigen MART-1/Melan-A using recombinant adenovirus-transduced murine dendritic cells. *Cancer Res.* **57(14)**, 2865–2869.
27. Klein, T. M., Wolf, E. D., Wu, R., and Sanford, J. C. (1987) High-velocity microprojectiles for delivering nucleic acids into living cells. *Nature* **327**, 70–73.
28. Tang, D., DeVit, M., and Johnston, S. A. (1992) Genetic immunization is a simple method for eliciting an immune response. *Nature* **356**, 152–156.
29. Yang, N. and Sun, W. H. (1995) Gene gun and other non-viral approaches for cancer gene therapy. *Nature* **1(5)**, 481–483.
30. Burkholder, J. K., Decker, J., and Yang, N. (1993) Rapid transgene expression in lymphocyte and macrophage primary cultures after particle bombardment-mediated gene transfer. *J. Immunol. Meth.* **165**, 149–156.
31. Woffendin, C., Yang, Z., Udaykumar, Xu, L., Yang, N., Sheehy, M. J., and Nabel, G. J. (1994) Nonviral and viral delivery of a human immunodeficiency virus protective gene into primary human T cells. *Proc. Natl. Acad. Sci. USA* **91**, 11,581–11,585.
32. Ye, Z., Qiu, P., Burkholder, J. K., Turner, J., Culp, J., Roberts, T., Shahidi, N. T., and Yang, N. S. (1998) Cytokine transgene expression and promoter gene usage in primary CD34+ cells using particle-mediated gene delivery. *Hum. Gene Ther.* **9**, 2197–2205.

33. Iwasaki, A., Torres, C. A., Ohashi, P. S., Robinson, H. L., and Barber, B. H. (1997) The dominant role of bone marrow-derived cells in CTL induction following plasmid DNA immunization at different sites. *J. Immunol.* **159,** 11–14.

34. Porgador, A., Irvine, K. R., Iwasaki, A., Barber, B. H., Restifo, N. P., and Germain, R. N. (1998) Predominant role for directly transfected dendritic cells in antigen presentation to CD8+ T cells after gene gun immunization. *J. Exp. Med.* **188,** 1075–1082.

35. Klinman, D. M., Sechler, J. M., Conover, J., Gu, M., and Rosenberg, A. S. (1998) Contribution of cells at the site of DNA vaccination to the generation of antigen-specific immunity and memory. *J. Immunol.* **160,** 2388–2392.

36. Tanigawa, K., Yu, H., Sun, R., Nickoloff, B. J., and Chang, A. E. (2000) Gene gun application in the generation of effector T cells for adoptive immunotherapy. *Cancer Immunol. Immunother.* **48,** 635–643.

37. Tan, Y., Yang, N. S., Turner, J. G., Niu, G. L., Maassab, H. F., Sun, J., Herlocher, M. L, Chang, A. E., and Yu, H. (1999) Interleukin-12 cDNA skin transfection potentiates human papillomavirus E6 DNA vaccine-induced antitumor immune response. *Cancer Gene Ther.* **6(4),** 331–339.

14

Role of Cytokines in Pathology of Melanoma and Use of Biologic Response Modifiers in Melanoma

Joseph I. Clark

1. Introduction

Growth of normal cells is regulated by polypeptides that act via specific cellular receptors. Otherwise known as cytokines, these substances include the growth factors that modulate the proliferation of nonimmune cells. Lymphokines or cytokines, on the other hand, are involved in the regulation of immune cells. Advances in the last 15 yr have shown that alterations in cytokines and their receptors may play a central role in the uncontrolled proliferation of tumor cells in vitro, and such cytokine aberrations are possibly responsible for regulation of tumor growth in vivo.

A useful approach for studying the predominant in vivo effects of cytokines on melanoma cells is to analyze the growth properties and immune response to transplanted tumor cells overexpressing a cytokine gene or via exogenous addition of these cytokines to cell culture. In this setting, cytokines such as melanoma growth-stimulatory activity (MGSA) and interleukin-8 (IL-8), and growth factors including basic fibroblast growth factor (bFGF), epidermal growth factor (EGF)/transforming growth factor-α (TGF-α), TGF-β, nerve growth factor (NGF), hepatocyte growth factor (HGF), and insulin-like growth factor-1 (IGF-1) are known to stimulate growth and proliferation of melanoma cells. IL-10 is known to dampen the immune response. IL-10 mRNA is overexpressed by melanoma cell lines in vitro, which may in turn allow for the tumorigenicity of melanoma in vivo. The growth factor granulocyte macrophage colony-stimulating factor (GM-CSF) and a multitude of cytokines including interferon-α (IFN-α), IFN-β, and IFN-γ; IL-1α, IL-1β, IL-2, IL-6, IL-12, and IL-15; and tumor necrosis factor-α (TNF-α) induce an inhibitory effect on growth and progression of cutaneous melanoma.

From: *Methods in Molecular Medicine, Vol. 61: Melanoma: Methods and Protocols*
Edited by: B. J. Nickoloff © Humana Press Inc., Totowa, NJ

The clinical utility of various cytokines in the IL and IFN families (IL-2, INF-α) and growth factors such as GM-CSF has been investigated in the treatment of malignant melanoma and proven efficacious in limited instances. Ongoing and future investigations will undoubtedly expand on this small but solid base.

2. Stimulatory Cytokines and Growth Factors

2.1. Cytokine Modes of Action

Many cytokines have been found to act in a proliferative manner on melanoma tumors. These substances are produced either by the tumor cells themselves or by infiltrating host cells. The various modes of cell regulation induced by cytokines and/or growth factors include endocrine cell regulation, in which cytokines are brought through blood vessels into the circulation and act at a distant site. In the case of paracrine growth regulation, the action of the cytokine is local, whereby the producer cell affects neighboring cells by secreting the particular protein, which binds to specific receptors. Tumor cells mainly utilize the autocrine mechanism of growth; that is, they have the ability to produce cytokines with growth-stimulatory properties while expressing specific receptors for these same cytokines. In this manner, tumor cells induce an autostimulatory feedback mechanism designated as autocrine growth. Two other cytokine-mediated autostimulatory pathways have been described: the intracrine pathway describes when the cytokine interacts intracellularly with the receptor; The juxtacrine pathway delineates when the cytokine does not leave the producing cell, but may interact with the receptor on the cell membrane.

2.2. Cytokines and Malignant Potential of Melanoma

The effects of growth factors and cytokines on tumor growth in vivo are extremely complex. Cell culture systems have been developed to understand better the regulation of tumor cells by these various substances. Questions to be considered include: By what mechanisms are melanoma cells able to escape from growth control? and Do melanoma cells have an altered production and/or response to growth-regulatory cytokines or growth factors?

In vitro experiments reveal that production of autocrine growth factors is involved in the abnormal growth regulation of melanoma cells. Metastatic melanoma cells do not require mitogens for growth in culture because conditioned medium from melanoma cells possesses mitogenic properties *(1)*. The stimulatory effect of conditioned medium is probably mediated through several substances, because melanoma cells constitutively express multiple growth factors *(2)*. Several of these growth factors and cytokines have been determined to be associated with the growth of melanoma. **Table 1** summarizes the most important of these factors.

Table 1
Stimulatory Cytokines and Growth Factors[a]

Factor	Reference	Effect
MGSA	*3–8*	Autocrine growth factor; produced by nevus cells and melanoma cells; stimulates proliferation of melanoma cells and melanocytes
IL-8	*9–13*	Essential autocrine growth factor for melanoma cells; integral in melanoma progression and metastatic spread
bFGF	*17,19–22,24*	Autocrine growth factor; produced by melanoma cells but not melanocytes
EGF/TGF-α	*5,24,26–28*	Important in growth regulation of melanoma cells
TGF-β	*24,27*	Varies in effect from none to cell proliferation
NGF	*24,31,32,35*	Increases melanoma cell survival; may increase melanoma cell numbers in vitro
HGF	*36,37*	Mitogenic for melanocytes; stimulates metastatic melanoma cell lines; may have role in melanoma proliferation
IGF-1	*28*	Stimulates proliferation of melanoma cells in vitro.

[a]MGSA, melanoma growth stimulatory activity; IL, interleukin; bFGF, basic fibroblast growth factor; EGF, epidermal growth factor; TGF, transforming growth factor; NGF, nerve growth factor; HGF, hepatocyte growth factor; IGF, insulin-like growth factor.

2.2.1. Melanoma Growth-Stimulatory Activity

MGSA has been shown to have 50% homology with IL-8 and is regarded as an autocrine growth factor for melanoma cells *(3)*. Melanoma cells express transcripts for MGSA *(4,5)*; it is produced by both nevus cells and melanoma cells and stimulates the proliferation of melanoma cells as well as melanocytes *(6,7)*. Evidence for an autocrine growth loop for MGSA is demonstrated by the investigations by Lawson et al. *(8)*, which showed that antibodies against MGSA inhibited the autonomous growth of melanoma cells in vitro.

2.2.2. Interleukin-8

Using reverse transcriptase polymerase chain reaction (RT-PCR) analysis, simultaneous expression of several cytokines, including IL-8, by melanoma cells has been described *(9)*. In these experiments, mRNA for IL-8 was found more or less in all 13 melanoma cell lines tested. Others have described IL-8 mRNA production either constitutively *(10,11)* or on IL-1 stimulation *(12)*. IL-8 has been identified as an essential autocrine growth factor for human malignant melanoma cells *(11,13)*. In a study by Shadendorf et al. *(11)*, blockade of autocrine-produced IL-8 either at the mRNA level by antisense oligonucleotides or at the protein level by monoclonal antibodies (MAbs) resulted in inhibition of cell proliferation and colony formation. Besides its growth-promoting activity on melanoma cells, IL-8 acts as an immunostimulator by its chemotactic activity for neutrophils *(14)* and T-lymphocytes *(15)*. In addition, IL-8 can induce haptotactic migration of melanoma cells and thereby increase their motility *(16)*.

2.2.3. Basic Fibroblast Growth Factor

A prototypical autocrine growth factor for melanoma cells is bFGF. This growth factor is a natural mitogen for melanocytes that is found in extracts from keratinocytes *(17)*. It supports melanogenesis by influencing the commitment of neural crest-derived avian embryo cells toward transformation into melanocytes *(18)*. Yet, bFGF is produced by malignant melanoma cells and not by melanocytes *(19)*. As described for IL-8, evidence for the existence of an autocrine loop for melanoma cells is given by the fact that proliferation of these cells is inhibited by antisense oligonucleotides targeted against bFGF and its receptor *(20,21)*. Activation of transmembrane receptor kinases in melanocytes stimulates not only proliferation but also the expression of pigmentation *(22)*. Others have described the transformation of murine melanocytes with the bFGF gene resulting in autonomous growth of these cells in culture *(23)*.

Krasagakis et al. *(24)* reported their investigation of growth regulation of melanoma cells and melanocytes by bFGF, in which they cultivated melanocytes in a serum-free growth factor–reduced melanocyte medium. Melanoma cells were maintained in a similar medium. Both cell types were stimulated by this exogenous growth factor, but the growth stimulation of melanoma cells was less prominent than that of the melanocytes. Perhaps this inferior stimulation was owing to the presence of autocrine production of bFGF by melanoma cells. This conclusion was supported by the finding that exogenous bFGF had no effect on logarithmically growing dense monolayers of melanoma cell lines *(24)*.

2.2.4. Epidermal Growth Factor/Transforming Growth Factor-α

The EGF/TGF-α system is considered important in the growth regulation of melanoma cells, based on support from several lines of evidence. Both of these substances maintain similar properties and bind to the same cellular receptor, designated the EGF receptor *(25)*. Nevertheless, TGF-α is produced by melanoma cells but not melanocytes *(26,27)*.

The EGF receptor is expressed on melanoma cells either in its normal form or in a truncated form, otherwise identified as the protein product of the c-*erb*-B2 oncogene *(5)*. It has been reported that metastatic melanoma cells, but not primary melanoma cells nor normal melanocytes, respond to EGF *(24,28)*. When added to cell cultures at varying doses, exogenous EGF had no effect on melanocyte cell culture yet led to dose-dependent stimulation of metastatic melanoma cells in sparse monolayers. When EGF was added in dense monolayers of logarithmically growing cultures, no stimulation of proliferation in any cell line was observed *(24)*. By contrast, blockade of the EGF receptor by MAbs specific for this receptor did not influence melanoma cell growth *(2)*. Speculation therefore arises that an intracrine loop may exist allowing intracellular binding of EGF/TGF-α to the EGF-receptor.

2.2.5. Transforming Growth Factor-β

Three forms of TGF-β are known to exist in mammalian species: TGF-β_1, TGF-β_2, and TGF-β_3. All three have similar functions and bind to the same class of receptors *(29)*. Both melanocytes and melanoma cells produce mRNA for all three forms, and the TGF-β protein is secreted into the culture supernatant as described by Albino et al. *(27)*.

Considerable differences in the in vitro response of normal melanocytes and malignant melanoma cells to TGF-β have been observed *(24)*. Human melanocytes are strongly inhibited by exogenous TGF-β. By contrast, melanoma cells escape growth inhibition, leading to no effect, and in some cases undergo cell proliferation when this cytokine is added to cell cultures *(24)*. Similar findings describing altered sensitivity of minimally and highly metastatic melanoma cells to TGF-β have been reported in the murine system *(30)*.

2.2.6. Nerve Growth Factor

NGF is important for differentiation and survival of sympathetic and sensory neurons. Its role in human melanoma, as well as the role of other growth factors such as HGF and IGF-1, is less well understood. Much like EGF, high levels of NGF receptors are expressed on metastatic melanoma cells *(31,32)*. Low levels of this receptor are expressed on primary melanoma cells and melanocytes. Upregulation of the NGF receptor can be induced by exposure to 12-*O*-tetradecanoylphorbolacetate, a tumor promoter, or to ultraviolet radiation *(33,34)*. Under certain conditions, NGF may increase melanoma cell numbers and proliferation in vitro *(24,35)*. However, NGF mainly increases melanoma cell survival *(34)*.

2.2.7. Hepatocyte Growth Factor

It has been reported that HGF is mitogenic for melanocytes in the presence of bFGF or mast cell growth factor *(36)*. c-Met and c-Kit, the receptors for HGF, are, in contrast to the bFGF receptor, not constitutively activated in melanoma cells *(22)*. Nevertheless, several human metastatic melanoma cell lines have been shown to be stimulated by HGF, as judged by protein phosphorylation, indicating that the receptor for this ligand continues to be expressed in transformed melanocytes and may have a role in melanoma proliferation, possibly at predilected sites of metastasis. Preferential metastasis to the liver was shown to be the result of a melanoma growth factor produced by hepatocytes *(37)*. It is possible that this growth factor was HGF.

2.2.8. Insulin-Like Growth Factor-1

Exogenous IGF-1 stimulates the proliferation of melanoma cells in vitro after binding to the IGF-1 receptor present on these cells *(28)*. As of yet, no reports have described the production of IGF-1 by melanoma cells.

2.2.9. Interleukin-10

IL-10 has been shown to dampen the immune response by downregulating the secretion of several cytokines by T-cells and monocytes *(38–40)* and by reducing antigen-specific activation of T-lymphocytes by diminishing antigen-presenting capacity of monocytes *(41)*. Originally, IL-10 was found to be expressed by various normal and malignant cell types of hematopoietic origin *(42)*. Others have reported the presence of IL-10 in other malignancies, including carcinomas such as ovarian carcinoma *(43)*. Overexpression of IL-10 mRNA and production of biologically active IL-10 protein has been observed in several melanoma cell lines *(9,44,45)*. Melanocytes express IL-10 mRNA in vitro; however, levels are significantly lower than those observed in melanoma cells, and no IL-10 protein itself has been detected *(9,44,45)*. In vivo, selective expression of IL-10 mRNA has been described in tissues of primary melanomas and melanoma metastases in comparison to normal skin *(9,45)*. The production of biologically active IL-10 by melanoma cell lines suggests that IL-10 mRNA in melanoma lesions may derive, at least in part, from the tumor cells themselves. Tumor-infiltrating cells, however, could also be a source of IL-10 in melanoma tissues. The biologic relevance of IL-10 by carcinoma cells remains poorly understood, but accumulating evidence from in vitro systems supports an important role IL-10 may play not only in the suppression of T-cell-mediated responses leading to the postulated "paralysis" of an antimelanoma immune response, but also as an antiinflammatory mediator in vivo *(46)*.

3. Inhibitory Cytokines and Growth Factors

Pleiotropic cytokines and growth factors can have positive and negative effects simultaneously on various steps of tumor progression. Preclinical investigations are relatively consistent in determining a stimulatory or inhibitory role of these proteins in cutaneous melanoma; however, on occasion, contradictory results have been reported. A few examples of such contradiction follow (**Table 2**).

In 1998, Ladanyi et al. *(47)* reported on the effects of a panel of cytokines on the proliferation and type IV collagenase production in four melanoma cell lines of different origin, tumorigenicity, and metastatic capacity. TGF-β, TNF-α, and, to a lesser extent, IL-1α exhibited antiproliferative effects on the cell lines, with some lines showing varying degrees of resistance. The sensitivity did not correlate directly with the origin or the biologic behavior of the tumor lines, suggesting that cytokine resistance of advanced stage melanoma cells may be relative *(47)*. On the contrary, IL-2, IL-10, and IL-12 displayed little or no effect on proliferation. Interestingly, those cytokines that exhibited the most pronounced antiproliferative activity also proved most effective in stimulating collagenase secretion, often simultaneously, in the same line *(47)*. By contrast, it has been reported that although human melanocytes are strongly inhibited by exogenous TGF-β, melanoma cells escape growth inhibition by this cytokine *(24)*. As described above, the production of IL-10 by melanoma cells or within melanoma tissue may play an important role in immune tolerance by these malignant cells. Recombinant IL-2 possesses well-described potent antitumor activity in a number of murine tumor models, including cutaneous melanoma *(48)*. Finally, in vitro and in vivo evaluation of IL-12 in malignant melanoma models demonstrates significant antitumor activity *(49)*.

3.1. Granulocyte Macrophage Colony-Stimulating Factor

Expression of GM-CSF mRNA has been described in numerous in vitro experiments of melanoma cell lines *(9,50,51)*. Three of 13 melanoma cell lines and 4 of 7 melanocyte cultures investigated by Kruger-Krasagakes et al. *(9)* expressed GM-CSF mRNA. Two other melanoma cell line cultures were shown to produce GM-CSF mRNA and GM-CSF protein *(50,51)*; however, no reports exist on the production of GM-CSF in melanocytes. It is well known that GM-CSF was originally described as promoting the differentiation and maturation of hematopoietic precursors to mature granulocytes, macrophages, and dendritic cells *(52)*. Less well understood, but becoming clearer, are the biologic consequences of GM-CSF production by melanoma cells.

The coexistence of regions of regression and progression observed in melanoma lesions indicates that the local microenvironment strongly influences the out-

Table 2
Inhibitory Cytokines and Growth Factors[a]

Factor	Reference	Effect
GM-CSF	*9,50,51,54–56*	Augments tumor antigen presentation by APCs; stimulates specific anti-tumor immunity by lymphocytes
Interferons (IFN-α, IFN-β, IFN-γ)	*24,61–66*	Inhibits cell proliferation; immune mediators enhance effector cell activity, upregulate tumor antigens and HLA class I and II antigens; anti-angiogenic
IL-1α, IL-1β	*2,9,10,50,67–75*	Pleiotropic effects: directly augments or suppresses melanoma cell proliferation, i.e., enhances tumorigenicity and metastatic spread while causing immunostimulatory effects
IL-2	*48,54,77*	Potent immunostimulatory effects on cell-mediated immunity, both specific and nonspecific, leading to dramatic antitumor activity
IL-6	*9,10,50,78–81,88*	Both antiproliferative and growth-stimulatory effects, dependent on stage of melanoma progression; induces B-cell maturation and proliferation; induces T-cell maturation and cytotoxicity
IL-12	*49,91*	Promotes induction of a T_H1 response; stimulates NK cells and CD8+ T-cells, leading to anti-tumor immunity
IL-15	*54,93–95*	Overexpressed in regressive primary human cutaneous melanoma samples; Important regulatory mechanism for T-cell recognition of melanoma cells possibly represented by expression in melanoma cells

Table 2 (continued)

Factor	Reference	Effect
TNF-α	*9,10,66,72,96–99*	Variable effects on melanoma: cytostatic; modulates cell-surface antigens and adhesion molecules; cytotoxic: suppresses local tumor growth; enhances metastasis formation; may enhance cell-mediated immunity at tumor site

*ª*GM-CSF, granulocyte macrophage colony-stimulating factor; APCs, antigen-presenting cells; IFN, interferon; HLA, human leukocyte antigen; IL, interleukin; NK, natural killer; TNF, tumor necrosis factor.

come of this antitumor immune response *(53)*. A complex network of interacting cytokines present in the local microenvironment critically influences the outcome of immune responses. Using RT-PCR and *in situ* hybridization, higher transcript levels for GM-CSF mRNA, among other cytokines, have been observed in regressive regions of primary human cutaneous melanoma samples *(54)*.

Immunologically mediated gene therapy approaches generally use the strategy of transfecting cDNAs encoding genetic material to the malignant cells to encode a particular gene product that is capable of augmenting the host immune responses against the developing tumor. The advantage of this approach is the production of high levels of specific cytokines secreted in the vicinity of the tumor without the associated toxicities observed with systemic cytokine administration. These locally high concentrations of cytokines in the tumor environment may modulate host immune responses in several ways, including the augmentation of tumor antigen presentation by professional antigen-presenting cells (APCs) and the activation of tumor-specific lymphocytes. Immunization experiments with GM-CSF-transduced tumor cells have revealed an induction of long-lasting systemic immunity. Using a B16 melanoma model, in which irradiated tumor cells alone did not stimulate significant antitumor immunity, Dranoff et al. *(55)* found that irradiated, retrovirally transduced tumor cells expressing murine GM-CSF stimulated potent, long-lasting, and specific antitumor immunity, requiring both CD4+ and CD8+ cells. Moreover, of the 10 molecules tested GM-CSF was the most potent stimulator of systemic antitumor immunity. The possibility that localized expression of GM-CSF by vaccinating cells might specifically enhance tumor-antigen presentation by host APCs is compatible with the finding that both CD4+ and

CD8[+] cells were required for the antitumor response, because B16 cells do not express detectable amounts of class II major histocompatibility complex (MHC) molecules, even after IFN-γ treatment, and therefore are unlikely to be able to prime antigen-specific CD4[+] cells *(55)*. Using a similar technique, Armstrong et al. *(56)* evaluated the effect of melanoma-derived GM-CSF on the pathogenesis of cutaneous melanoma in a syngeneic, immunocompetent murine model system. These investigators demonstrated a dose response effect of tumor inhibition by melanoma-derived GM-CSF. Additionally, vaccination with irradiated GM-CSF-producing melanoma cells conferred optimal immunogenicity against a subsequent challenge with parental melanoma cells. Immunohistochemical studies performed on inoculation sites revealed the presence of large numbers of dendritic cells, suggesting recruitment of these APCs in the vicinity of tumor cells expressing GM-CSF *(56)*.

3.2. Interferons (IFN-α, IFN-β, IFN-γ)

IFNs are glycoproteins with diverse immunomodulatory effects on tumor cells *(57–59)*. The mechanism of action includes both direct antiproliferative and immune-mediated effects via enhanced natural killer (NK) cell activity or upregulation of tumor antigens and/or human leukocyte antigen (HLA) class I and II antigens *(57)*, and inhibition of angiogenesis induced by IFN-α *(60)*.

In vitro evaluation of these cytokines in the treatment of cultured human melanoma cells has demonstrated significant antiproliferative activity *(24,61–65)*. Whereas some investigators have observed IFN-γ to be the most potent of the interferons *(61)*, others have demonstrated IFN-β to be more efficient than IFN-α, containing well-described antitumor activity in vivo, or IFN-γ in inhibiting melanoma cell proliferation *(24,62–65)*. In fact, up to 56–80% of growth inhibition has been reported when melanoma cells have been cultured in the presence of these individual cytokines *(24)*.

The interferons are not produced directly by melanoma cells yet may be detected in tumor-involved lymph nodes in a human melanoma system. CD8[+] T-cells can be isolated from tumor-infiltrating lymphocytes from human melanoma, which are capable of producing type I cytokines, such as IFN-γ and TNF-α, in an MHC class I–restricted and tumor-specific noncytolytic interaction with the autologous melanoma cells *(66)*. Through these type I cytokines, "help" can then be provided for the process of generating as well as in maintaining an effective CD8[+] cytotoxic T-lymphocyte response. In addition, recruitment of other effector cells such as NK cells, macrophages, and others to the tumor site may then ensue, leading to a potent cell-mediated antitumor response.

3.3 Interleukin-1α and Interleukin-1β

Several studies have reported on the constitutive production of either IL-1α or IL-1β mRNA and protein by melanoma cell lines (**Table 2**) *(2,9,10,50,67–69)*. The biologic effects of IL-1 secretion by melanoma cells are complex. In vitro, some investigators have reported that IL-1 directly augments or suppresses melanoma cell proliferation *(67,70)*, whereas others have observed that IL-1 inhibits the growth of both melanoma cells and melanocytes *(71–73)*. In vivo, IL-1 exerts pleiotropic effects, and the role of melanoma-derived IL-1 is not altogether clear because it can either enhance or suppress tumorigenicity of melanoma cells. In one manner, IL-1 has been reported to induce systemic immune suppression in mice when administered via iv injection *(74)* and to enhance metastatic spread when coinjected with human melanoma cells in nude mice *(75)*. In support of the metastatic potentiation of IL-1, others have reported that melanoma-derived IL-1 mainly induces expression of intercellular adhesion molecule-1 (ICAM-1) on melanoma cells, and that treatment of melanoma cells with an anti-IL-1 antibody not only decreased the level of ICAM-1 expression but also lowered their adherence to cultured endothelium *(68)*. On the other hand, the secretion of IL-1 by melanoma cells could also act in an immunostimulatory fashion through its potential to activate other lymphoid cells, as has been observed in other tumor systems *(76)*.

3.4. Interleukin-2

Gene expression for the immunostimulatory molecule IL-2 in human melanoma cell lines is often undetectable *(9)*. Yet, other investigators have documented the presence of IL-2 mRNA by RT-PCR and *in situ* hybridization and increased transcript levels for the cytokine IL-2, in combination with GM-CSF and IL-15, in samples from regressive primary human cutaneous melanomas *(54)*. From these intriguing data, it can be hypothesized that cytokine combinations such as this may be relevant for experimental antitumor immune response studies and for immunotherapeutic and gene transfer studies in the treatment of melanoma patients.

One such study by Vile and Hart *(77)* supports this concept. In this study, they transfected B16 melanoma cells in vitro with cDNAs encoding the 5' flanking region of the murine tyrosinase gene with the murine IL-2 gene, allowing for a tissue-specific promoter to direct expression of the cytokine gene to the tumor cells. Expression of IL-2 in the murine melanoma cells completely abrogated their tumorigenicity in syngeneic mice. Injection of these constructs into established tumors resulted in efficient expression of these cytokine genes, and, although alterations in growth rates were not observed, these results suggest that direct genetic modification may be a feasible therapeutic approach for patients with advanced melanoma.

3.5. Interleukin-6

IL-6 mRNA is variably expressed by melanoma cell lines, but all cell lines that contain transcripts for IL-6 also produce biologically active IL-6 *(9,10,50)*. By contrast, melanocyte cell cultures show a more homogeneous pattern of cytokine gene expression, although generally at lower levels than melanoma cells *(9)*.

Although IL-6 is inhibitory for melanocytes *(73)*, both antiproliferative *(78–80)* and growth-stimulatory effects *(81)* have been reported on melanoma cells, depending on the stage of melanoma progression. When added to cell cultures containing melanoma cell lines, IL-6 enhances the antiproliferative effect of the potent inhibitory cytokines IL-1 and TNF-α *(78)*. Melanoma cells derived from radial growth phase or early vertical growth phase are inhibited by IL-6 *(79)*. By contrast, melanoma cells from advanced vertical growth phase lesions or metastasis are completely resistant to the IL-6-mediated growth inhibition. Subsequent work from the same group showed that endogenously produced IL-6 in metastatic melanoma cells may serve as an autocrine stimulator *(81)*.

The role IL-6 plays in host antitumor responses is multifactorial and not completely defined. IL-6 appears to serve as an inducer of B-cell maturation and proliferation and of T-cell maturation and cytotoxicity *(82,83)*. IL-6 has been shown to enhance directly the growth of B-cell lymphoma *(84)*. It has well-described autocrine growth-stimulatory functions in multiple myeloma *(85,86)*. By contrast, the administration of IL-6 to mice bearing fibrosarcomas or colon carcinomas has reduced tumor growth and metastatic colony formation *(87)*. Additionally, Sun et al. *(88)* have demonstrated decreased tumor growth in vivo by B16 melanoma cells transfected with the human IL-6 gene. Possible mechanisms for this effect included increased expression of receptor for matrix proteins and an apparent inhibition of neovascularization in the IL-6-transfected tumors.

3.6. Interleukin-12

IL-12 is a disulfide-linked heterodimeric cytokine produced primarily by "professional" APCs such as macrophages and formerly termed NK cell–stimulatory factor or cytotoxic lymphocyte maturation factor *(89,90)*. It is composed of light (p35) and heavy (p40) chains and binds to a receptor on T-cells and NK cells, promoting the induction of primarily a T_H1 response in vitro and in vivo. IL-12 has well-described antitumor activity in murine melanoma tumor models in vivo *(49,91)*.

Among a number of murine tumor models studied by Brunda et al. *(49)*, experimental pulmonary metastases or sc growth of the B16F10 melanoma was markedly reduced in mice treated intraperitoneally with IL-12, resulting in an increase in survival time. These investigators were able to demonstrate the critical role of $CD8^+$ T-cells in mediating the IL-12-induced antitumor effects against sc tumors.

Using a novel alternative approach to obtain paracrine cytokine secretion at the tumor site, Tahara et al. *(91)* transfected fibroblasts to express bioactive IL-12 and then inoculated animals using the poorly immunogenic murine melanoma cell line (BL-6) in C57Bl/6 mice. The antitumor results reported in this investigation suggest that local delivery of IL-12 inhibits tumor growth in a dose-dependent manner but leads to the development of an antitumor immune response when IL-12 is expressed at the tumor site at relatively small amounts.

3.7. Interleukin-15

Along with GM-CSF and IL-2, IL-15 mRNA and increased cytokine levels have been reported to be overexpressed in regressive primary human cutaneous melanoma samples *(54)*. IL-15 mRNA has been detected in keratinocytes, fibroblasts, macrophages, lymphocytes, and melanoma cells. The presence of IL-15 transcripts in the latter two cell types may be of particular interest. Whereas IL-15 mRNA is expressed in a variety of cell types, normal T-cells originally were suggested to lack IL-15 transcripts *(92)*. However, these results and recent reports on IL-15 mRNA expression in activated T-cells and T-cell lines *(93,94)* indicate that melanoma tumor-infiltrating lymphocytes should be included in the spectrum of IL-15 mRNA-expressing cells. Immunoreactivity of IL-15 mRNA-positive cells with anti-IL-15 antibodies indicates that these transcripts are in fact translated *(54)*. The presence of IL-15 transcripts and protein in melanoma cells may also be of particular importance. Because inhibition of endogenous IL-15 by specific antibodies results in downregulation of HLA class I expression in melanoma cells *(95)*, expression of IL-15 in melanoma cells may represent an important regulatory mechanism for T-cell recognition of melanoma cells.

3.8. Tumor Necrosis Factor-α

TNF-α mRNA is variably expressed in melanoma cell lines *(9)*. Whereas other investigators have shown TNF-α production by melanoma cells at the protein level *(10,96)*, low levels of TNF-α mRNA have been detected in cultured melanocytes as well *(9)*. The complete role of TNF-α in malignant melanoma has not yet been completely elucidated. Although melanocytes are

strongly inhibited by TNF-α *(73)*, only some melanoma cell lines are susceptible to TNF in terms of cytostatic activity *(10,97)* and modulation of cell-
surface antigens and adhesion molecules *(72)*. In addition, TNF has been shown
to possess cytotoxic properties and therefore may select for melanoma cells
with enhanced malignancy in vitro *(97)*. The in vivo effects of TNF-α are varied depending on the tumor cell line being evaluated; that is, suppression of
local tumor growth has been observed by some investigators *(98)* whereas others have reported the enhancement of metastasis formation in response to the
administration of TNF-α *(99)*. CD8[+] T-cells, isolated from tumor-infiltrating
lymphocyte cells from human melanoma, have been shown to synthesize type I
cytokines (IFN-γ and TNF-α) in an MHC class I–restricted and tumor-
specific noncytolytic interaction with autologous melanoma cells *(66)*. Such
an interaction and cytokine production may enhance cell-mediated immunity
at the tumor site. Therefore, given these variable effects, the role of TNF-α as
a modulator of melanoma growth and metastasis needs to be investigated
further.

4. Clinical Use of Cytokines and Growth Factors

Despite the vast array of preclinical information available for biologic
response modifiers and their role in the pathology of malignant melanoma, few
agents, unfortunately, have shown efficacy in the clinical treatment of patients
with this disease. This is not to say that there is a lack of clinical investigation,
but, rather, to date, most trials have been wholly negative in their outcome.
Focus, therefore, will concentrate on a relatively few such studies.

4.1. Adjuvant Treatment of High-Risk Melanoma

The prognosis for patients with cutaneous malignant melanoma worsens
considerably if the primary tumor invades deeply (>1.5 mm, American Joint
Committee on Cancer [AJCC] stage II) and/or spreads to regional lymph nodes
(AJCC stage III). Such patients are therefore appropriate candidates for studies
of postsurgical adjuvant therapy. Several observations, including the antitumor effects of biologic therapy in preclinical testing, discussed above, suggest
a role for immunologic mechanisms in controlling the proliferation and spread
of melanoma cells *(100,101)*. Therefore, specific immunomodulatory
approaches using cytokines have been evaluated.

Given the promising inhibitory effects of IFN-γ in vitro and in vivo, it was
chosen for evaluation in the treatment of patients with resected high-risk melanoma. Phase I studies showed that IFN-γ was well tolerated and favorably
affected immune parameters in patients with completely resected melanoma
(102–104). Accordingly, the Southwest Oncology Group undertook a random-

ized, phase III trial (SWOG-8642) to test whether prognosis was improved with recombinant human IFN-γ compared with observation following definitive surgery for cutaneous melanoma *(105)*. Two hundred eighty-four patients were enrolled, but, disappointingly, no statistically significant difference in disease-free or overall survival were detected.

IFN-α has undergone extensive evaluation in the adjuvant setting *(106)*, but until recently, no proven benefit was observed. In stage II patients, a recent European trial reported a benefit in disease-free survival when adjuvant IFN-α2a was compared to observation after surgical resection *(107)*. In this report, 311 patients with melanoma of a Breslow thickness ≥1.5 mm but without lymph node involvement were assigned to either adjuvant IFN-α2a administered subcutaneously for 1 yr or observation. A statistically significant improvement in disease-free survival was observed in the treatment arm, but not in overall survival. The most common side effects experienced by the treatment group were mild to moderate constitutional-type symptoms.

Stage III patients have a much higher risk of recurrence and subsequent death from malignant melanoma, therefore warranting a more aggressive approach to treatment in the adjuvant setting, in some investigator's viewpoint. In 1996, very promising results were reported from a large cooperative, randomized phase III clinical trial (E1684) evaluating very high dose IFN-α2b vs observation in patients with high-risk stage III malignant melanoma *(108)*. In this study, 287 patients with stage III resected melanoma were randomized to receive IFN-α2b at 20 mU/m^2 intravenously daily, five times per week for 4 wk, followed by 10 mU/(m^2·d) subcutaneously three times per week for 48 wk or observation. At the time of publication, median follow-up was 6.9 yr. Toxicity in the treatment arm was profound, requiring dose adjustments in the majority of patients, and consisted mainly of significant constitutional symptoms, hepatotoxicity, myelosuppression, and depression. Yet, despite this toxicity, for the first time in the treatment of malignant melanoma in the adjuvant setting, not only was an improvement in disease-free survival observed, but also an improvement in overall survival. Median disease-free survival improved from 1.0 to 1.7 yr and overall survival from 2.8 to 3.8 yr, in a statistically significant manner *(108)*. These results led to approval of IFN-α2b at this dose and schedule as adjuvant treatment for high-risk resected stage III malignant melanoma by the US Food and Drug Administration (FDA).

In an effort to confirm and extend these results, an intergroup trial was designed (E1690) and recently reported at the thirty-fifth annual meeting of the American Society of Clinical Oncology in Atlanta, GA *(109)*. This study enrolled 642 stage III patients and randomized them to one of two treatment arms or observation. The treatment arms included the same high-dose

IFN-α2b schedule outlined for E1684 vs a lower-dose regimen of IFN-α2b at 3 mU/d subcutaneously three times per week for 2 yr. Based on an intent-to-treat analysis of 608 evaluable patients, an improvement in disease-free survival was once again observed for the high-dose treatment arm when compared to observation; however, no statistically significant improvement was identified for overall survival. The low-dose arm showed no improvement in disease-free or overall survival as compared to the no-treatment arm. The explanation for this lack of advantage of overall survival is distressing and, as yet, not fully understood. Clinicians worldwide anxiously await further detailed evaluation and subsequent publication of these results to understand better the role of high-dose IFN-α2b in the adjuvant treatment of high-risk resected malignant melanoma.

4.2. Systemic Treatment of Metastatic Melanoma

Although surgery with or without adjuvant IFN-α therapy can be curative in stage I, II, or III disease, many patients will develop distant metastases. Disseminated metastatic disease is associated with a poor prognosis and a mortality rate of >95%. Several treatment options are available to patients with metastatic disease, including single-agent dacarbazine (DTIC) chemotherapy, a variety of combination chemotherapy regimens, and combinations of chemotherapy with tamoxifen or IFN-α. DTIC chemotherapy produces responses in approx 20% of patients, with a median response duration of 4–6 mo, a 5-yr survival rate of 2%, and a median survival time of 6–9 mo (110). Although single-institution phase II studies and small phase III trials have shown that combination chemotherapy, or the addition of either tamoxifen or IFN-α to DTIC chemotherapy, has potential benefit, no regimen has yet proved superior to DTIC chemotherapy alone (111–118).

Based on animal model data, a high-dose IL-2 regimen was developed in which IL-2 was administered by short iv infusion every 8 h, with or without lymphokine-activated killer cells (119,120). In 1997, the US FDA approved high-dose bolus IL-2 as a single agent for the treatment of metastatic melanoma based on a report describing the findings from an updated 270 patient database of metastatic melanoma patients treated with this same high-dose IL-2 regimen between 1985 and 1993 (121). These 270 patients were enrolled in eight phase II clinical trials during this time span conducted at 22 institutions around the United States. Patients received high-dose bolus IL-2 at 600,000–720,000 IU/kg as a 15-min iv bolus every 8 h for 14 consecutive doses over 5 d, as tolerated. After a 6- to 9-d rest period, an additional 14 doses of IL-2 were scheduled over the next 5 d. Courses of therapy were usually separated by 6- to 12-wk intervals. The overall objective response rate was 16% (95% CI, 12–21%), with 17 complete responses (6%) and 26 partial responses

(10%). Responses occurred with all sites of disease and in patients with large tumor burdens. The median response duration for patients who underwent a complete response has not been reached and was 5.9 mo for those who achieved a partial response. Twenty-eight percent of the responding patients, including 59% of the patients who achieved a complete response, remain progression free. Toxicity, although severe, inducing a capillary leak type of syndrome requiring intensive care unit type of monitoring, generally reversed rapidly after therapy was completed *(121)*. Thus, despite this relatively low overall response rate and high toxicity profile, high-dose bolus IL-2 treatment seems to benefit some patients with metastatic melanoma by producing durable complete and partial remissions and should be considered for appropriately selected patients. The only predictive factor for response was good performance status at baseline and no prior systemic therapy.

Other IL-2-based investigations, alone, at lower doses, or in combination with other cytokines and/or chemotherapy have been reported *(122–126)*. None, however, have shown the substantial durable remissions observed with the high-dose bolus IL-2 schedule described.

Few other cytokines or growth factors have been evaluated as extensively as IFN-α or IL-2 in malignant melanoma *(127,128)*, but active investigation is ongoing.

References

1. Sauvaigo, S., Fretts, R. E., Riopelle, R. J., and Lagard, A. E. (1986) Autonomous proliferation of MeWo human melanoma cell lines in serum-free medium: secretion of growth-stimulating activities. *Int. J. Cancer* **37**, 123–132.
2. Rodeck, U., Melber, K., Kath, R., Menssen, H.-D., Varello, M., Atkinson, B., and Herlyn, M. (1991) Constitutive expression of multiple growth factor genes by melanoma cells but not normal melanocytes. *J. Invest. Dermatol.* **97**, 20–26.
3. Richmond, A., Balentien, E., Thomas, H. G., Flaggs, G., Barton, D. E., Spiess, J., Bordoni, R., Franke, R., and Derynck, R. (1988) Molecular characterization and chromosomal mapping of melanoma growth stimulatory activity, a growth factor structurally related to β-thromboglobulin. *EMBO J.* **7**, 2025–2033.
4. Richmond, A., Lawson, D. H., Nixon, D. W., Stewens, J. S., and Chawia, R. K. (1983) Extraction of a melanoma growth-stimulatory activity from culture medium conditioned by the Hs0294 human melanoma cell line. *Cancer Res.* **43**, 2106–2112.
5. Chenevix-Trench, G., Martin, N. G., and Ellem, K. A. O. (1990) Gene expression in melanoma cell lines and cultured melanocytes: correlation between level of c-src-1, c-myc and p53. *Oncogene* **5**, 1187–1193.
6. Richmond, A. and Thomas, H. G. (1988) Melanoma growth stimulatory activity: isolation from human melanoma tumors and characterization of tissue distribution. *J. Cell Biochem.* **36**, 185–198.

7. Bordoni, R., Fine, R., Murray, D., and Richmond, A. (1990) Characterization of the role of melanoma growth stimulatory activity (MGSA) in the growth of normal melanocytes, nevocytes, and malignant melanocytes. *J. Cell Biochem.* **44,** 207–219.

8. Lawson, D. H., Thomas, H. G., Roy, R. G. B., Gordon, D. S., Chawla, R. K., Nixon, D. W., and Richmond, A. (1987) Preparation of a monoclonal antibody to melanoma growth stimulatory activity released into serum-free culture medium by Hs0294 malignant melanoma cells. *J. Cell Biochem.* **34,** 169–185.

9. Kruger-Krasagakes, S., Krasagakis, K., Garbe, C., and Diamantstein, T. (1995) Production of cytokines by human melanoma cells and melanocytes. *Recent Results Cancer Res.* **139,** 155–168.

10. Colombo, M. P., Maccalli, C., Mattei, S., Melani, C., Radrizzani, M., and Parmiani, G. (1992) Expression of cytokine genes, including IL-6, in human malignant melanoma cell lines. *Melanoma Res.* **2,** 181–189.

11. Schadendorf, D., Moller, A., Algermissen, B., Worm, M., Sticherling, M., and Czarniecki, B. M. (1993) IL-8 produced by human malignant melanoma cells in vitro is an essential autocrine growth factor. *J. Immunol.* **151,** 2667–2675.

12. Zachariae, C. O. C., Thestrup-Pedersen, K., and Matsushima, K. (1991) Expression and secretion of leukocyte chemotactic cytokines by normal human melanocytes and melanoma cells. *J. Invest. Dermatol.* **97,** 593–599.

13. Forster, E., Kirnbauer, R., Urbanski, A., Kock, A., and Luger, T. A. (1991) Human melanoma cells produce interleukin 8 which functions as an autocrine growth factor. *J. Invest. Dermatol.* **96,** 608.

14. Yoshimura, T., Matsushima, K., Tanaka, S., Robinson, E. A., Appella, E., Oppenheim, J. J., and Leonard, E. J. (1987) Purification of a human monocyte-derived neutrophil chemotactic factor that shares sequence homology with other host defensed cytokines. *Proc. Natl. Acad. Sci. USA* **84,** 9233–9237.

15. Larsen, C. G., Anderson, A. O., Appella, E., Oppenheim, J. J., and Matsushima, K. (1989) The neutrophil-activating protein (NAP-1) is also chemotactic for T-lymphocytes. *Science* **243,** 1464–1466.

16. Wang, J. M., Tarabolett, G., Matsushima, K., Van Damme, J., and Mantovani, A. (1990) Induction of haptotactic migration of melanoma cells by neutrophil activating protein/interleukin-8. *Biochem. Biophys. Res. Commun.* **169,** 165–170.

17. Halaban, R., Langdon, R., Birchall, N., Cuono, C., Baird, A., Scott, G., Moellmann, G., and McGuire, J. (1988) Basic fibroblast growth factor from human keratinocytes is a natural mitogen for melanocytes. *J. Cell Biol.* **107,** 1611–1619.

18. Stocker, K. M., Sherman, L., Rees, S., and Ciment, G. (1991) Basic FGF and TGF-β1 influence commitment to melanogenesis in neural crest-derived cells of avian embryos. *Development* **111,** 635–645.

19. Halaban, R., Kwon, B. S., Ghosh, S., Delli Bovi, P., and Baird, A. (1988) bFGF as an autocrine growth factor for human melanomas. *Oncogene Res.* **3,** 177–186.

20. Becker, D., Meier, C. B., and Herlyn, M. (1989) Proliferation of human malignant melanomas is inhibited by antisense oligonucleotides targeted against basic fibroblast growth factor. *EMBO J.* **8,** 3685–3691.

21. Becker, D., Lee, P. L., Rodeck, U., and Herlyn, M. (1992) Inhibition of the fibroblast growth factor receptor 1 (FGFR-1) gene in human melanocytes and malignant melanomas leads to inhibition of proliferation and signs indicative of differentiation. *Oncogene* **7,** 2303–2313.

22. Halaban, R., Fan, B., Ahn, J., Funasaka, Y., Gitay Goren, H., and Neufeld, G. (1992) Growth factors, receptor kinases, and protein tyrosine phosphatases in normal and malignant melanocytes. *J. Immunother.* **12,** 154–161.

23. Dotto, G. P., Moelmann, G., Ghosh, S., Edwards, M., and Halaban, R. (1989) Transformation of murine melanocytes by basic fibroblast growth factor cDNA and oncogenes and selective suppression of the transformed phenotype in a reconstituted cutaneous environment. *J. Cell Biol.* **109,** 3115–3128.

24. Krasagakis, K., Garbe, C., Zouboulis, C. C., and Ofanos, C. E. (1995) Growth control of melanoma cells and melanocytes by cytokines. *Recent Results Cancer Res.* **139,** 169–182.

25. Carpenter, G. and Cohen, S. (1979) Epidermal growth factor. *Annu. Rev. Biochem.* **48,** 193–216.

26. Herlyn, M., Kath, R., Williams, N., Valyi-Nagy, I., and Rodeck, U. (1990) Groth-regulatory factors for normal, premalignant and malignant human cells in vitro. *Adv. Cancer Res.* **54,** 213–234.

27. Albino, P., Davis, B. M. and Nanus, D. M. (1991) Induction of growth factor RNA expression in human malignant melanoma: markers of transformation. *Cancer Res.* **51,** 4815–4820.

28. Rodeck, U., Herlyn, M., Menssen, H. D., Furlanetto, R. W., and Koprowski, H. (1987) Metastatic but not primary melanoma cell lines grow in vitro independently of exogenous growth factors. *Int. J. Cancer* **40,** 687–690.

29. Cheifetz, S., Weatherbee, J. A., Tsang, M. L., Anderson, J. K., Mole, J. E., Lucas, R., and Massague, J. (1987) The transforming growth factor-beta system, a complex pattern of cross-reactive ligands and receptors. *Cell* **48,** 409–415.

30. Mooradian, D. L., Purchio, A. F., and Furcht, L. T. (1990) Differential effects of transforming growth factor β1 on the growth of poorly and highly metastatic murine melanoma cells. *Cancer Res.* **50,** 273–277.

31. Fabricant, R. N., DeLarco, J. E., and Todaro, G. J. (1977) Nerve growth factor receptors on human melanoma cells in culture. *Proc. Natl. Acad. Sci. USA* **74,** 565–569.

32. Herlyn, M., Thurin, J., Balaban, G., Genicelli, J. L., Herlyn, D., Elder, D. E., Bondi, E., Guerry, D., Nowell, P., Clark, W. H., and Koprowski, H. (1985) Characteristics of cultured human melanocytes isolated from different stages of tumor progression. *Cancer Res.* **45,** 5670–5676.

33. Peacocke, M., Yaar, M., Mansur, C. P., Chao, M. V., and Gilchrest, B. A. (1988) Induction of nerve growth factor receptors on cultured human melanocytes. *Proc. Natl. Acad. Sci. USA* **85,** 5282–5286.

34. Krasagakis, K., Garbe, C., Kruger-Krasagakes, S., and Orfanos, C. E. (1993) 12-O tetradecanoylphorbol-13-acetate not only modulates proliferation rates but also alters antigen expression and LAK-cell susceptibility of normal human melanocytes in vitro. *J. Invest. Dermatol.* **100,** 653–659.

35. Mather, J. P. and Sato, G. H. (1979) The growth of mouse melanoma cells in hormone-supplemented, serum-free medium. *Exp. Cell Res.* **120,** 191–200.
36. Halaban, R., Rubin, J. S., Funasaka, Y., et al. (1992) Met and hepatocyte growth factor/scatter factor signal transduction in normal melanocytes and melanoma cells. *Oncogene* **7,** 2195–2206.
37. Sargent, N. S., Oestreicher, M., Haidvogl, H., Madnick, H. M., and Burger, M. M. (1988) Growth regulation of cancer metastases by their host organ. *Proc. Natl. Acad. Sci. USA* **85,** 7251–7255.
38. Vieira, P., De Waal-Malefyt, R., Dang, M.-N., Johnson, K. E., Kastelein, R., Fiorentino, D. F., De Vries, J. E., Roncarolo, M.-G., Mosman, T. R., and Moore, K. W. (1991) Isolation and expression of human cytokine-synthesis-inhibitory-factor cDNA clones: homology to Epstein-Barr virus open reading frame BCRF1. *Proc. Natl. Acad. Sci. USA* **88,** 1172–1176.
39. De Waal-Malefyt, R., Abrams, J., Bennet, B., Figdor, C. G., and De Vries, J. (1991) Interleukin 10 (IL-10) inhibits cytokine synthesis by human monocytes: an autoregulatory role of IL-10 produced by monocytes. *J. Exp. Med.* **174,** 1209–1220.
40. Ralph, P., Nakoinz, I., Sampson-Johannes, A., Fong, S., Lowe, D., Min, H.-Y., and Lin, L. (1992) IL-10, T lymphocyte inhibitor of human blood cell production of IL-1 and tumor necrosis factor. *J. Immunol.* **148,** 808–814.
41. De Waal-Malefyt, R., Haanen, J., Spits, H., Roncardo, M.-G., Te Velde, A., Figdor, C., Johnson, K., Kastelein, R., Yssel, H., and De Vries, J. E. (1991) Interleukin 10 (IL-10) and viral IL-10 strongly reduce antigen-specific human T-cell proliferation by diminishing the antigen-presenting capacity of monocytes via downregulation of class II major histocompatibility complex expression. *J. Exp. Med.* **174,** 915–924.
42. De Waal-Malefyt, R., Yssel, H., Roncarolo, M.-G., Spits, H., and De Vries, J. (1992) Interleukin-10. *Curr. Opin. Immunol.* **4,** 314–320.
43. Pisa, P., Halapi, E., Pisa, E. K., Gerdin, E., Hising, C., Bucht, A., Gerdin, B., and Kiessling, R. (1992) Selective expression of interleukin 10, interferon-gamma, and granulocyte-macrophage colony-stimulating factor in ovarian cancer biopsies. *Proc. Natl. Acad. Sci. USA* **89,** 7708–7712.
44. Gastl, G. A., Abrams, J. S., Nannes, D. M., Oosterkamp, R., Silver, J., Liu, F., Chen, M., Albino, A. P., and Bander, N. H. (1993) Interleukin-10 production by human carcinoma cell lines and its relationship to interleukin 6 expression. *Int. J. Cancer* **5,** 96–101.
45. Kruger-Krasagakes, S., Krasagakis, K., Garbe, C., Schmitt, E., Huls, C., Blankenstein, T., and Diamantstein, T. (1994) Expression of interleukin 10 in human melanoma. *Br. J. Cancer* **70,** 1182–1185.
46. Richter, G., Kruger-Krasagakes, S., Hein, G., Huls, C., Schmitt, E., Diamanststein, T., and Blankenstein, T. (1993) Interleukin 10 transfected into Chinese hamster ovary cells prevents tumor growth and macrophage infiltration. *Cancer Res.* **53,** 4134–4137.

47. Ladanyi, A., Nagy, N. O., Jeney, A., and Timar, J. (1998) Cytokine sensitivity of metastatic human melanoma cell lines—simultaneous inhibition of proliferation and enhancement of gelatinase activity. *Pathol. Oncol. Res.* **4,** 108–114.
48. Rosenberg, S. A., Mule, J. J., Speiss, P. J., Reichert, C. M., and Schwarz, S. L. (1985) Regression of established pulmonary metastases and subcutaneous tumor mediated by the systemic administration of high-dose recombinant interleukin-2. *J. Exp. Med.* **161,** 1169–1188.
49. Brunda, J. M., Luistro, L., Warrier, R. R., Wright, R. B., Hubbard, B. R., Murphy, M., Wolf, S. F., and Gately, M. K. (1993) Antitumor and antimetastatic activity of interleukin 12 against murine tumors. *J. Exp. Med.* **178,** 1223–1230.
50. Armstrong, C. A., Tara, D. C., Hart, C. E., Kock, A., Luger, T. A., and Ansel, J. C. (1992) Heterogeneity of cytokine production by human malignant melanoma cells. *Exp. Dermatol.* **1,** 37–45.
51. Sabatini, M., Chavez, J., Mundy, G. R., and Bonewald, L. F. (1990) Stimulation of tumor necrosis factor release from monocytic cells by the A375 human melanoma via granulocyte-macrophage colony-stimulating factor. *Cancer Res.* **50,** 2673–2678.
52. Sieff, C. A., Emerson, S. G., and Donahue, R. E. (1985) Human recombinant granulocyte-macrophage colony-stimulating factor: a multilineage hematopoietin. *Science* **230,** 1171–1173.
53. Colombo, M. P., Maccalli, C., Mattei, S., Melani, S., Radrizzani, M., and Parmiani, G. (1992) Local cytokine availability elicits tumor rejection and systemic immunity through granulocyte-T lymphocyte cross-talk. *Cancer Res.* **52,** 4853–4857.
54. Wagner, S. N., Schultewolter, T., Wagner, C., Briedigkeit, L., Becker, J. C., Kwasnicka, H. M., and Goos, M. (1998) Immune response against human primary malignant melanoma: a distinct cytokine mRNA profile associated with spontaneous regression. *Lab. Invest.* **78,** 541–550.
55. Dranoff, G., Jaffee, E., Lazenby, A., Golumbek, P., Levitsky, H., Brose, K., Jackson, V., Hamada, H., Pardoll, D., and Mulligan, R. C. (1993) Vaccination with irradiated tumor cells engineered to secrete murine granuloctye-macrophage colony-stimulating factor stimulates potent, specific, and long-lasting anti-tumor immunity. *Proc. Natl. Acad. Sci. USA* **90,** 3539–3543.
56. Armstrong, C. A., Botella, R., Galloway, T. H., Murray, N., Kramp, J. M., Song, I. S., and Ansel, J. C. (1996) Antitumor effects of granulocyte-macrophage colony-stimulating factor production by melanoma cells. *Cancer Res.* **56,** 2191–2198.
57. Frank, S. J. and Meyers, M. (1995) Interferons as adjuvant therapy for high risk melanoma *Melanoma Lett.* **13,** 1–4.
58. Parkinson, D. R., Houghton, A. N., Hersey, P., et al. (1992) Biologic Therapy for Melanoma, in *Cutaneous Melanoma*, 2nd ed. (Balch, C. W., Houghton, A. N., Milton, G. W., et al., eds.), Lippincott, Philadelphia, pp. 523,524.
59. Kirkwood, J. and Ernstoff, M. (1990) Role of interferons in the therapy of melanoma. *J. Invest. Dermatol.* **95,** 180s–184s.

60. Sidky, Y. A. and Borden, E. C. (1987) Inhibition of angiogenesis by interferons: effects on tumor- and lymphocyte-induced vascular responses. *Cancer Res.* **47,** 5255–5261.

61. Tyring, S. K., Klimpel, G., and Grysk, M. (1984) Eradication of cultured human melanoma cells by immune interferon and leukocytes. *J. Natl. Cancer Inst.* **73,** 1067–1073.

62. Fisher, P. B., Miranda, A. F., and Babiss, L. E. (1986) Measurement of the effect of interferons on cellular differentiation in murine and human melanoma cells. *Methods Enzymol.* **119,** 611–618.

63. Garbe, C., Krasagakis, K., Zouboulis, C. C., Schroder, K., Kruger, S., Stadler, R., and Orfanos, C. E. (1990) Antitumor activities of interferon alpha, beta and gamma and their combinations on human melanoma cells in vitro: changes of proliferation, melanin synthesis and immunophenotype. *J. Invest. Dermatol.* **95,** 231s–237s.

64. Zouboulis, C. C., Garbe, C., Kruger, S., and Orfanos, C. E. (1990) Interferons and melanoma: comparison of the cytostatic and cytotoxic effects of natural and recombinant interferons, tumor necrosis factor-alpha and their combinations on human melanoma cells in vitro. *Skin Cancer* **5,** 137–145.

65. Krasagakis, K., Garbe, C., Kruger, S., and Orfanos, C. E. (1991) Effects of interferons on cultured human melanocytes in vitro: interferon-beta but not -alpha or -gamma inhibit proliferation and all interferons significantly modulate the cell phenotype. *J. Invest. Dermatol.* **97,** 364–372.

66. Chakraborty, N. G. and Mukherji, B. (1998) Human melanoma-specific, noncytolytic CD8+ T cells that can synthesize type I cytokine. *Cancer Res.* **58,** 1363–1366.

67. Bennicelli, J. L., Elias, J., Kern, J., and Guery, D. (1989) Production of interleukin 1 activity by cultured human melanoma cells. *Cancer Res.* **49,** 930–935.

68. Burrows, F. J., Haskard, D. O., and Bart, I. R. (1993) Influence of tumor-derived interleukin 1 on melanoma-endothelial cell interactions. *Cancer Res.* **51,** 4768–4775

69. Kock, A., Schwarz, T., Urbanski, A., Peng, Z., Vetterlein, M., Micksche, M., Ansel, J. C., Kung, H. F., and Luger, T. A. (1989) Expression and release of interleukin-1 by different human melanoma cell lines. *J. Natl. Cancer Inst.* **81,** 36–42.

70. Lachman, L. B., Dinarello, C. A., Llansa, N. D., and Fidler, I. J. (1986) Natural and recombinant human interleukin 1-β is cytotoxic for human melanoma cells. *J. Immunol.* **136,** 3098–3102.

71. Nakai, S., Mizuno, K., Kaneta, M., and Hirai, Y. (1988) A simple, sensitive bioassay for the detection of interleukin-1 using human melanoma A375 cell line. *Biochem. Biophys. Res. Commun.* **154,** 1189–1196.

72. Mortarini, R., Belli, F., Parmiani, G., and Anichini, A. (1990) Cytokine-mediated modulation of HLA-class II, ICAM-1, LFA-3 and tumor-associated antigen profile of melanoma cells: comparison with anti-proliferative activity by rIL1-beta, rTNF-alpha, rIFN-gamma, rIL4 and their combinations. *Int. J. Cancer* **45,** 334–341.

73. Swope, V. B., Abdel-Malek, Z., Kassem, L. M., and Nordlund, J. J. (1991) Interleukins 1 alpha and 6 and tumor necrosis factor-alpha are paracrine inhibitors of human melanocyte proliferation and melanogenesis. *J. Invest. Dermatol.* **96,** 180–185.

74. Robertson, B., Gahring, L., Newton, R., and Daynes, R. (1987) In vivo administration of interleukin 1 to normal mice depresses their capacity to elicit contact hypersensitivity responses: prostaglandins are involved in this modification of immune function. *J. Invest. Dermatol.* **88,** 380–387.

75. Giavazzi, R., Garofalo, A., and Bani, M. R. (1990) Interleukin 1-induced augmentation of experimental metastases from a human melanoma in nude mice. *Cancer Res.* **50,** 4771–4775.

76. Douvdevani, A., Huleihel, M., Zoller, M., Segal, S., and Apte, R. N. (1992) Reduced tumorigenicity of fibrosarcomas which constitutively generate IL-1 alpha either spontaneously or following IL-1 alpha gene transfer. *Int. J. Cancer* **51,** 822–830.

77. Vile, R. G. and Hart, I. R. (1994) Targeting of cytokine gene expression to malignant melanoma cells using tissue specific promoter sequences. *Ann. Oncol.* **5(Suppl. 4),** s59–s65.

78. Morinaga, Y., Suzuki, H., and Takatsuki, F. (1989) Contribution of IL-6 to the antiproliferative effect of IL-1 and tumor necrosis factor on tumor cell lines. *J. Immunol.* **143,** 3538–3542.

79. Lu, C., Vickers, M. F., and Kerbel, R. S. (1992) Interleukin 6: a fibroblast derived growth inhibitor of human melanoma cells from early but not advanced stages of tumor progression. *Proc. Natl. Acad. Sci. USA* **89,** 9215–9219.

80. Armstrong, C. A., Murray, N., Kennedy, M., Koppula, S. V., Tara, D., and Ansel, J. C. (1994) Melanoma-derived interleukin 6 inhibits in vivo melanoma growth. *J. Invest. Dermatol.* **102,** 278–284.

81. Lu, C. and Kerbel, R. S. (1993) Interleukin 6 undergoes transition from paracrine growth inhibitor to autocrine stimulator during melanoma progression. *J. Cell Biol.* **120,** 1281–1288.

82. Kishimoto, T. (1985) Factors affecting B cell growth and differentiation. *Annu. Rev. Immunol.* **3,** 133–157.

83. Lotz, M., Jirik, F., Kabouridis, R., Tsoukas, C., Hirano, T., Kishimoto, T., and Carson, D. A. (1988) BSF-2/IL-6 is a costimulant for human thymocytes and T lymphocytes. *J. Exp. Med.* **167,** 1253–1258.

84. Lee, C., Biondi, A., Wang, X. H., Iscove, N. N., de Sousa, J., Aarden, L. A., Wong, G. G., Clark, S. C., Messner, H. A., and Minden, M. D. (1989) A possible autocrine role for interleukin-6 in two lymphoma cell lines. *Blood* **74,** 798–804.

85. Kawano, M., Hirano, T., Matsuda, P., Taga, T., Hurii, Y., Iwato, K., Asaoku, H., Tang, B., Tanabe, O., Tanale, H., Kuramoto, A., and Kishimoto, T. (1988) Autocrine generation and general requirement of BSF-2/IL-6 for human multiple myelomas. *Nature* **332,** 83–85.

86. Kishimoto, T. (1989) The biology of interleukin-6. *Blood* **74,** 1–10.

87. Mule, J. J., McIntosh, J. K., Jablons, D. M., and Rosenberg, S. A. (1990) Antitumor activity of recombinant interleukin 6 in mice. *J. Exp. Med.* **17,** 629–636.
88. Sun, W. H., Kreisle, R. A., Phillips, A. W., and Ershler, W. B. (1992) In vivo and in vitro characteristics of interleukin 6-transfected B16 melanoma cells. *Cancer Res.* **52,** 5412–5415.
89. Kobayashi, M., Fitz, L., Ryan, M., Hewick, R. M., Clark, S. C., Chang, S., Loudon, R., Sherman, F., Perussia, B., and Trinchieri, G. (1989) Identification and purification of natural killer cell stimulatory factor (NKSF), a cytokine with multiple biologic effects on human lymphocytes. *J. Exp. Med.* **170,** 827–845.
90. Stern, A. S., Podlaski, F. J., Hulmes, J. D., Pan, Y. C. E., Quinn, P. M., Wolitzky, A.G., Familletti, P. D., Stremlo, D. L., Truitt, T., Chizzonite, R., and Gately, M. K. (1990) Purification to homogeneity and partial characterization of cytotoxic lymphocyte maturation factor from human B-lymphoblastoid cells. *Proc. Natl. Acad. Sci. USA* **87,** 6808–6812.
91. Tahara, H., Zeh, H. J., Storkus, W. J., Pappo, I., Watkins, S. C., Gubler, U., Wolf, S. F., Robbins, P. D., and Lotze, M. T. (1994) Fibroblasts genetically engineered to secrete interleukin 12 can suppress tumor growth and induce antitumor immunity to a murine melanoma in vivo. *Cancer Res.* **54,** 182–189.
92. Grabstein, K. H., Eisenman, J., Shanebeck, K., et al. (1994) Cloning of a T cell growth factor that interacts with the β-chain of the interleukin-2 receptor. *Science* **264,** 965–968.
93. Meazza, R., Verdiani, S., Biassoni, R., Coppolecchia, M., Gaggero, A., Orengo, A. M., Colombo, M. P., Azzarone, B., and Ferrini, S. (1996) Identification of a novel interleukin-15 (IL-15) transcript isoform generated by alternative splicing in human small cell lung cancer cell lines. *Oncogene* **12,** 2187–2192.
94. Onu, A., Pohl, T., Krause, H., and Bulfone-Paus, S. (1997) Regulation of IL-15 secretion via the leader peptide of two IL-15 isoforms. *J. Immunol.* **158,** 255–262.
95. Azzarone, B., Pottin-Clemenceau, C., Krief, P., Rubinstein, E., Jasmin, C., Scudeletti, M., and Indiveri, F. (1996) Are interleukin-2 and interleukin-15 tumor promoting factors for non-hematopoietic cells? *Eur. Cytokine Network* **7,** 27–36.
96. Lugassy, C. and Escade, J. P. (1991) Immunolocation of TNF-α/cachectin in human melanoma cells: studies on co-cultivated malignant melanoma. *J. Invest. Dermatol.* **96,** 238–242.
97. Zouboulis, C. C., Schroder, K., Garbe, C., Krasagakis, K., Kruger, S., and Orfanos, C. E. (1990) Cytostatic and cytotoxic effects of recombinant tumor necrosis factor-alpha on sensitive human melanoma cells in vitro may result in selection of cells with enhanced markers of malignancy. *J. Invest. Dermatol.* **95,** 223s–230s.
98. Blankenstein, T., Qin, Z., Uberla, K., Muller, W., Rosen, H., Volk, H.-D., and Diamantstein, T. (1991) Tumor suppression after tumor cell targeted tumor necrosis factor alpha gene transfer. *J. Exp. Med.* **173,** 1047–1052.
99. Qin, Z., Kruger-Krasagakes, S., Kunzendorf, U., Hock, H., Diammantstein, T., and Blankenstein, T. (1993) Expression of tumor necrosis factor by different

tumor cell lines results either in tumor suppression or augmented metastasis. *J. Exp. Med.* **178,** 355–360.

100. Shiku, H., Takahaski, T., Resnick, L. A., Oettgen, H. F., and Old, L. J. (1977) Cell surface antigens of human malignant melanoma. II. Recognition of autoantibodies with unusual characteristics. *J. Exp. Med.* **145,** 784–789.

101. Houghton, A. N., Eisinger, M., Albino, A. P., Cairncross, J. G., and Old, L. J. (1982) Surface antigens of melanocytes and melanomas: markers of melanocyte differentiation and melanoma subsets. J. Exp. Med. **156,** 1755–1766.

102. Foon, K. A., Sherwin, S. A., Abrams, P. G., et al. (1985) A phase I trial of recombinant gamma interferon in patients with cancer. *Cancer Immunol. Immunother.* **20,** 193–197.

103. Kurzrock, R., Rosenblum, M. G., Sherwin, S. A., et al. (1985) Pharmacokinetics, single-dose tolerance, and biological activity of recombinant γ-interferon in cancer patients. *Cancer Res.* **45,** 2866–2872.

104. Kleinerman, E. S., Kurzrock, R., Wyatt, D., Quesada, J. R., Gutterman, J. U., and Fidler, I. J. (1986) Activation or suppression of the tumoricidal properties of monocytes from cancer patients following treatment with human recombinant γ-interferon. *Cancer Res.* **46,** 5401–5405.

105. Meyskens, F. L., Kopecky, K. J., Taylor, C. W., Noyes, R. D., Tuthill, R. J., Hersh, E. M., Feun, L. G., Doroshow, J. H., Flaherty, L. E., and Sondak, V. K. (1995) Randomized trial of adjuvant human interferon gamma versus observation in high-risk cutaneious melanoma: a Southwest Oncology Group Study. *J. Natl. Cancer Inst.* **87,** 1710–1713.

106. Sondak, V. K. and Wolfe, J. A. (1997) Adjuvant therapy for melanoma. *Curr. Opin. Oncol.* **9,** 189–204.

107. Pehamberger, H., Soyer, H. P., Steiner, A., Kofler, R., Binder, M., Mischer, P., Pachinger, W., Aubock, J., Fritsch, P., Kerl, H., and Wolff, K. (1998) Adjuvant interferon alfa-2a treatment in resected primary stage II cutaneous melanoma. *J. Clin. Oncol.* **16,** 1425–1429.

108. Kirkwood, J. M., Strawderman, M. H., Ernstoff, M. S., Smith, T. J., Borden, E. C., and Blum, R. H. (1996) Interferon alfa-2b adjuvant therapy of high-risk resected cutaneous melanoma: the Eastern Cooperative Oncology Group trial EST 1684. *J. Clin. Oncol.* **14,** 7–17.

109. Kirkwood, J. M., Ibrahim, J., Sondak, V., Ernstoff, M., Flaherty, L., Smith, T., Richards, J., Rao, U., and Blum, R. (1999) Preliminary analysis of the E1690/ S9111/C9190 intergroup postoperative adjuvant trial of high- and low-dose IFNa2b (HDI and LDI) in high-risk primary or lymph node metastatic melanoma. *Proc. Am. Soc. Clin. Oncol.* **17,** A2072.

110. Hill, G. J. II, Krementz, E. T., and Hill, H. Z. (1984) Dimethyl triazeno imidazole carboxamide and combination therapy for melanoma: IV. Late results after complete response to chemotherapy (Central Oncology Group protocols 7130, 7131, and 7131A). *Cancer* **53,** 1299–1305.

111. McClay, E. F., Mastrangelo, M. J., Berd, D., et al. (1992) Effective combination chemo/hormonal therapy for malignant melanoma: experience with three clinical trials. *Int. J. Cancer* **50,** 553–556.

112. Falkson, C. I., Falkson, G., and Falkson, H. C. (1991) Improved results with the addition of interferon alpha-2b to dacarbazine in the treatment of patients with metastatic malignant melanoma. *J. Clin. Oncol.* **9,** 1403–1408.

113. Thompson, D., Adena, M., and McLeod, G. R. C. (1993) Interferon alfa-2a does not improve response or survival when combined with dacarbazine in metastatic malignant melanoma: results of a multi-institutional Australian randomized trial, QMP8704. *Melanoma Res.* **3,** 133–138.

114. Bajetta, E., Di Leo, A., Zampino, M., et al. (1994) Multicenter randomized trial of dacarbazine alone or in combination with two different doses and schedules of interferon alfa-2A in the treatment of advanced melanoma. *J. Clin. Oncol.* **12,** 806–811.

115. Kirkwood, J. M., Ernstoff, M. S., Giuliano, A., et al. (1990) Interferon-2a and dacarbazine in melanoma. *J. Natl. Cancer Inst.* **82,** 1062–1063.

116. Rusthoven, J. J., Quirt, I. C., Iscoe, N. A., et al. (1996) Randomized, double-blind placebo-controlled trial comparing the response rates of carmustine, dacarbazine and cisplatin with and without tamoxifen in patients with metastatic melanoma: National Cancer Institute of Canada Clinical Trials Group. *J. Clin. Oncol.* **14,** 2083–2090.

117. Falkson, C. I., Ibrahim, J., Kirkwood, J., Coates, A. S., Atkins, M. B., and Blum, R. H. (1998) Phase III trial of dacarbazine versus dacarbazine with interferon-2b versus dacarbazine with tamoxifen versus dacarbazine with interferon-2b and tamoxifen in patients with metastatic malignant melanoma: an Eastern Cooperative Oncology Group study. *J. Clin. Oncol.* **16,** 1743–1751.

118. Atkins, M. B. (1998) The role of cytotoxic chemotherapeutic agents either alone or in combination with biological response modifiers, in *Molecular Diagnosis, Prevention & Therapy of Melanoma* (Kirkwood, J. M., ed.), Marcel Dekker, New York, pp. 219–251.

119. Rosenberg, S. A., Lotze, M. T., Muul, L. M., et al. (1985) Observations on the systemic administration of autologous lymphokine-activated killer cells and recombinant interleukin-2 to patients with metastatic cancer. *N. Engl. J. Med.* **313,** 1485–1492.

120. Rosenberg, S. A., Lotze, M. T., Muul, L. M., et al. (1987) A progress report on the treatment of 157 patients with advanced cancer using lymphokine-activated killer cells and interleukin-2 or high-dose interleukin-2 alone. *N. Engl. J. Med.* **316,** 889–897.

121. Atkins, M. B., Lotze, M. T., Dutcher, J. P., et al. (1999) High-dose recombinant interleukin 2 therapy for patients with metastatic melanoma: analysis of 270 patients treated between 1985 and 1993. *J. Clin. Oncol.* **17,** 2105–2116.

122. Atkins, M. B., O'Boyle, K. R., Sosman, J. A., et al. (1994) Multiinstitutional phase II trial of intensive combination chemoimmunotherapy for metastatic melanoma. *J. Clin. Oncol.* **12,** 1553–1560.

123. Keilholz, U., Conradt, C., Legha, S. S., et al. (1998) Results of interleukin-2-based treatment in advanved melanoma: a case record-based analysis of 631 patients. *J. Clin. Oncol.* **16,** 2921–2929.

124. Legha, S. S., Ring, S., Eton, O., Bedikian, A., Buzaid, A. C., Plager, C., and Papadopoulos, N. (1998) Development of a biochemotherapy regimen with concurrent administration of cisplatin, vinblastine, dacarbazine, interferon alfa, and interleukin-2 for patients with metastatic melanoma. *J. Clin. Oncol.* **16,** 1752–1759.

125. McDermott, D. F., Trehu, E. G., Mier, J. W., Sorce, D., Rand, W., Ronayne, L., Kappler, K., Clancy, M., Klempner, M., and Atkins, M. B. (1998) A two-part phase I trial of high-dose interleukin 2 in combination with soluble (Chinese hamster ovary) interleukin 1 receptor. *Clin. Cancer Res.* **5,** 1203–1213.

126. Richards, J. M., Gale, D., Mehta, N., and Lestingi, T. (1999) Combination of chemotherapy with interleukin-2 and interferon alfa for the treatment of metastatic melanoma. *J. Clin. Oncol.* **17,** 651–657.

127. Bajetta, E., Vecchio, M. D., Mortarini, R., Nadeau, R., Rakhit, A., Rimassa, L., Fowst, C., Borri, A., Anichini, A., and Parmiani, G. (1998) Pilot study of subcutaneous recombinant human interleukin 12 in metastatic melanoma. *Clin. Cancer Res.* **4,** 75–85.

128. Chachoua, A., Oratz, R., Liebes, L., Alter, R. S., Felice, A., Peace, D., Vilcek, J., and Blum, R. H. (1994) Phase Ib trial of granulocyte-macrophage colony-stimulating factor combined with murine monoclonal antibody R24 in patients with metastatic melanoma. *J. Immunother.* **16,** 132–141.

15

Surgical Techniques for Treatment of Primary Cutaneous Melanoma

June K. Robinson

1. Incidence and Mortality

The incidence and mortality rates of melanoma increased dramatically from 1973 to 1994, rising 120.5 and 38.9%, respectively (*1*). From 1990 to 1994, men had higher incidence (17.3/100,000) and mortality rates (3.5/100,000) than women (incidence: 11.6/100,000; mortality: 1.7/100,000) and had more melanomas on the trunk or the head and neck; women had more on the lower limbs, but the largest increases for an anatomic site were for the trunk. Incidence rates for birth cohorts born after 1945 seem to be stabilizing. Mortality rates of melanoma are declining for women born in the 1930s or later and men born since the 1950s.

In the United States, a large proportion of the melanomas detected in recent years were in the local stage and had a thickness <0.75 mm (*2*). Thus, in recent years, a large proportion of the melanomas were treated with ambulatory office-based surgery procedures with a local excision having 1-cm margins. The median depth of melanoma has decreased in association with public education campaigns in a number of developed countries. The fraction of melanomas presenting as thick primary melanomas is dwarfed by the intermediate thickness group that is clinically node negative with a Breslow depth of 1.0–4.0 mm.

2. Staging

In 1988, the American Joint Committee on Cancer (AJCC) (*3*) adopted a four-stage classification for melanoma based on Breslow thickness (*4*), Clark levels (*5*), and metastases, with the stage predicting the prognosis (*6*) (**Table 1**).

From: *Methods in Molecular Medicine, Vol. 61: Melanoma: Methods and Protocols*
Edited by: B. J. Nickoloff © Humana Press Inc., Totowa, NJ

Table 1
Staging System for Cutaneous Melanoma Adopted by the AJCC

Stage	Description[a]
0	Melanoma *in situ*, not an invasive lesion Clark's level I $T_{is}N_0M_0$
IA	Localized, tumor ≤0.75 mm in thickness and invades the papillary dermis Clark's level II $T_1N_0M_0$
IB	Localized, tumor >0.75 mm but not >1.5 mm in thickness and/or invades to papillary-reticular dermal interface Clark's level III $T_2N_0M_0$
IIA	Localized, tumor >1.5 mm but not >4 mm in thickness and/or invades the reticular dermis interface Clark's level IV $T_3N_0M_0$
IIB	Localized, tumor >4 mm in thickness Clark's level V $T_4N_0M_0$
IIIA	Regional lymph node(s) metastasis ≤3 cm in greatest dimension Any T, N_1, M_0
IIIB	Regional lymph node(s) metastasis >3 cm in greatest dimension and/or in transit metastasis Any T, N_2, M_0
IV	Distant metastasis Any T, any N, M_1

[a]is, *in situ*; N, lymph node; T, tumor; M_1, distant metastasis.

Approximately 85% of patients present with melanoma in stages 0, I, and II. The distribution in 1995 was 14.9%, stage 0; 47.7%, stage I; 23.1%, stage II; 8.9%, stage III; and 5.3%, stage IV, which favors better survival than two decades ago *(7)*. Stages I and II divide localized disease into low risk (≤1.5 mm) and high risk (>1.5 mm), with Breslow tumor depth being the most important prognostic factor in stage II disease. In a review of 5093 cases, the 10-year survival rate was reported as high as 97% for melanomas having a thickness of ≤1.00 mm (thin melanoma, localized to skin) and as low as 14% for those with melanoma >4.00 mm thick (thick melanoma, localized to skin) *(7)*. The average 5-year survival rate for patients with stage II melanoma (intermediate and

Table 2
Five-Year Disease-Free Survival for Primary Melanoma
by Thickness

Thickness (mm)	Five-year disease-free survival (%)
<0.76	96
0.76–1.49	87
1.50–2.49	75
2.50–3.99	66
≥4.00	47

thick melanoma localized to the skin) is between 27 and 42% *(6,8)* (**Table 2**). It is probable that the mortality rate in stage II disease is owing to the presence of clinically silent nodal or distant metastases.

Those with nodal disease (stage III disease), which includes both microscopic disease found on elective regional node dissection and macroscopic disease removed by therapeutic lymph node dissection, have an overall 5-year survival rate of about 30% *(9)*. Individuals with a single involved node have a more favorable outcome than those with four or more positive nodes. Once distant metastases form (stage IV), the disease is rarely curable and median survival time is approx 6 mo. It remains to be seen whether sentinel node biopsy with detection of submicroscopic nodal disease by polymerase chain reaction (PCR) for tyrosinase mRNA and therapeutic intervention with node dissection or adjuvent therapy with high-dose interferon α-2b therapy will change the prognosis *(10–12)*.

As the prognostic accuracy of the Breslow tumor depth has evolved over the years since the AJCC staging system began, a convenient way to classify patients with stage 0, I, and II melanoma has evolved using the terms *thin*, *intermediate*, and *thick* *(13)*. The concept of *in situ* (limited to the epidermis), thin (<1 mm), intermediate (1–4 mm), and thick (>4 mm) melanoma is an artificial segmentation of the neoplastic continua made by those who study melanoma to manipulate the available information to make predictions about the disease's anticipated future biologic behavior and make treatment recommendations. The assessment of the significance of the segmentation (thin, intermediate, thick) changes as new information becomes available and always recognizes that the prognosis for an individual may be affected by other risk factors. Other independent risk factors include increasing age, male gender, tumor ulceration, neurotropism, and regression in thinner (<1 mm) tumors *(14)*. Melanomas on the hands and feet carry a worse prognosis than those on the trunk and head, and those on the extremities have a better prognosis *(15)*.

The AJCC melanoma staging being developed has major changes to the current scheme (**Table 1**). The changes in the 2000 staging sysem (**Table 3**) include:

1. use of thickness and ulceration to classify primary melanoma;
2. employment of the number of positive lymph nodes, and differentiating between microscopic vs macroscopic disease, to classify stage III patients;
3. grouping of satellite metastases and in-transit lesions into stage III;
4. inclusion of serum lactate dehydrogenase (LDH) and site of metastasis into the M classification in stage IV; and
5. use of intraoperative lymphosciatigraphy and sentinel node biopsy within the classification *(16)*.

3. Treatment of Primary Tumor

Historically, a wide excision with 5-cm margins with regional lymph node dissection was recommended for all melanomas *(17)*. This margin of excision was based on a single 1907 autopsy examination performed by Dr. W. S. Handley on a patient with advanced melanoma. The theoretical basis for this recommendation was to remove any hidden foci of melanoma cells that may give rise to local recurrences or metastasis *(18)*. The recommendation to excise tissue to the underlying fascia was based on the desire to remove the superficial vasculature and lymphatics in the sc tissue. This sole report formed the basis for the treatment of melanoma until 1977, when Breslow and Macht *(19)* described 35 patients with melanomas treated with narrow margins.

The definitive treatment for primary melanoma is surgical excision. The margin for surgical treatment of melanoma and the decision to perform selective lymph node dissection is defined by the Breslow depth. Although Breslow's tumor thickness is of primary importance, Clark's level of tumor invasion may provide additional prognostic value for thin melanomas. As a lesion gets thicker, the risk of microsatellitosis increases; therefore, the margins of wide local excision increase. Head and neck lesions have been exempt from the large databases used to derive the recommendations for treatment of cutaneous melanoma (**Table 4**). For thin lesions (≤1 mm), 1-cm margins of excision are recommended *(20)*. For intermediate thickness lesions (1.1–4.0 mm), excision of 2-cm margins when feasible is recommended *(21,22)*. If direct primary closure is not possible, a skin graft or rotation flap is employed. This reduction in the margin of resection for thin and intermediate thickness melanomas resulted in significant cost savings because fewer patients required hospitalization. The margin of resection for thick melanomas remains controversial but is generally accepted as 2 to 3 cm, which usually requires a skin graft. Although patients with tumors >4 mm in thickness have a relatively high risk of local recurrence (10–20%), there is little evidence to support extending

Table 3
American Joint Committee on Cancer—Proposed Staging
for Cutaneous Melanoma: 2000

Clinical staging				Pathologic staging
Stage 0	Tis: *in situ*	N0	M0	same
Stage IA	T1^a: < or = 1.0 mm without ulceration	N0	M0	same
Stage IB	T1^b: < or = 1.0 mm with ulceration	N0	M0	same
	T2^a: 1.01–2.0 mm without ulceration	N0	M0	same
Stage IIA	T2^b: 1.01–2.0 mm with ulceration	N0	M0	same
	T3^a: 2.01–4.0 mm without ulceration	N0	M0	same
IIB	T3^b: 2.01–4.0 mm with ulceration	N0	M0	same
	T4^a: > 4.0 mm without ulceration	N0	M0	same
IIC	T4^b: > 4.0 mm with ulceration	N0	M0	same
Stage IIIA	any T1–4^a (1 node, macrometastasis)	N1^b	M0	T1–4^a N1^a M0 (1 node, micrometatasis)
IIIB	any T1–4^a (2–3 nodes, macromet)	N2^b	M0	T1–4^a N1^b M0 (1 node, macromet) T1–4^a N2^a M0 (2–3 nodes, micromet)
Stage IIIC	any T [in transit met/sattelite(s), without nodes]	N2^c	M0	any T N2^b,N2^c, M0 [N2^b:2–3 nodes, macromet N2^c: in transit met/ satellite(s), no node]
	any T [4 or > nodes, in transit met/satellite(s)]	N3	M0	any T N3 M0
Stage IV	any T	any N	any M	any T any N any M

^{a}Micrometastases are diagnosed after elective or sentinel lymphadenectomy.
^{b}Macrometastases are defined as clinically detectable lymph node metastases confirmed by therapeutic lymphadenectomy or when any lymph node metastasis exhibits gross extracapsular extensions.
^{c}In-transit met(s)/satellites(s) without lymph nodes.
Adapted from: Balch CM, Buzaid AC, Atkins MB, et al. (2000) A new American Joint Committee on Cancer Staging system for cutaneous melanoma. *Cancer* **88**, 1484–1491.

the width of local excision beyond 2 cm. Wide local excisions may reduce the incidence of local recurrence but are unlikely to have a survival benefit when the risk of preexisting systemic metastasis is so high.

Recently, Piepkorn and Barnhill *(23)* recommended lateral 1-cm margins for melanomas of all depths; however, margins <1 cm are associated with too

Table 4
Margin of Excision Recommendations by Tumor Thickness

Tumor thickness	Surgical margin[a] (cm)
In situ	0.5
<1 mm (thin)	1
>1–4 mm (intermediate)	2
>4 mm (thick)	2–3[b,c]

[a]The surgical margin is measured from the clinical edge of the lesion and consists of clinically normal skin, which is particularly difficult to obtain for lentigo maligna in chronically sun-damaged skin of the head and neck.
[b]Narrower margin not widely accepted.
[c]As the 2000 staging system is accepted, margins of excision may change to 1.0 cm for thickness < 2mm and 2.0 cm for ≥ 2 mm tumor thickness.

great a risk for local recurrence *(18,22,24–27)*. In usual clinical practice, margins are generally identified without using a Wood's light to help identify the border of pigmentation. In lentigo maligna melanoma and superficial spreading melanoma, the fading border makes it difficult to discern with visual inspection. Wood's light examination of the lesion helps delineate the margins. For example, for a thin melanoma, the margin of resection is inked at multiple points measured radially 1.0 cm from the edge of pigmentation. If a primary closure is anticipated, the surgeon orients an ellipse about this circle and excises directly down to the fascia, removing the epidermis, dermis, and the entire sc layer in a "block." If a graft is planned, the circular incision is excised down to fascia, and the graft is harvested and placed into the defect **(Fig. 1)**. If the lentigo maligna melanoma arises in extensively actinically damaged skin, atypical melanocytes may remain at the margins of resection and a local recurrence may represent progression of the atypical melanocytes to melanoma *in situ* and not an inadequate initial margin of resection.

Certain areas require modification of the usual guidelines for wide local excision. Excision of thick melanomas of the face may require margins that would necessitate sacrifice of vital structures, such as the anterior orbit. In this situation, some recommend the use of a somewhat narrower margin. Postoperative radiation therapy may reduce the risk of local recurrence *(28,29)*. Subungual melanoma of the finger requires resection proximal to the distal interphalangeal joint or ray amputation. Subungual melanoma of the toe necessitates amputation at the metatarsophalangeal joint. Excision of melanoma overlying the breast should include superficial mammary fascia; mastectomy is not indicated *(30)*.

4. Follow-up

Long-term follow-up for patients with melanoma is important because metastasis may be quite delayed. Ten to 15% of recurrence appears after 5 yr. Late recurrences have occurred predominately in women with thin primary tumors on the extremities *(31)*, which is in contradistinction to the short disease-free interval for thin melanoma of the head and neck in men *(32)*. The disease-free interval in a series of nine cases of melanoma of the head and neck was 3 yr or less. This difference may be owing to the histologic subtype of melanoma; for example, lentigo maligna melanoma and superficial spreading melanoma recurred locally in the skin in the early period and nodal and visceral metastasis was within 10 yr. Although the risk of progressive disease is low for thin melanoma, which has a rate of metastasis of up to 5% of thin melanomas (<0.75 mm in Breslow thickness), it appears to increase slightly over time *(33)*.

Another reason to maintain long-term follow-up is detection of second or multiple primary tumors. Patients with a history of melanoma, clinically atypical nevi, and familial melanoma are at especially increased risk of developing multiple primary tumors (estimated relative risk of 500) *(34)*. Having a prior melanoma confers an estimated relative risk of 9 of developing another melanoma. Monthly skin self-examination and examination by a dermatologist is necessary to detect the new primary lesions or local recurrences (**Table 5**). Although there are currently no universally accepted guidelines for further radiologic and laboratory evaluation of all stages of melanoma patients, a consensus exists for stage 0 and I patients *(20)*. The majority of physicians order the following tests: no tests for melanoma *in situ*, baseline chest X-ray and liver function studies for stage I patients, and no additional diagnostic studies unless the patient becomes symptomatic *(35)*. In asymptomatic stage II patients, there is no clear indication for further radiologic studies, but many physicians order initial computed tomography (CT) scans of the brain, chest, and abdomen. Stage III and IV disease warrant further radiologic studies, directed by symptomatology, physician findings, and sites of recurrence. These modalities may include CT, magnetic resonance imaging, bone scans, ultrasound, and FDG scans *(36)*.

5. Lymph Node Dissection

Lymph nodes are the most common site of initial metastasis. Although the management of nonpalpable regional lymph nodes is controversial, there is consensus that thin melanomas (stage IA) do not require lymph node dissection *(37)*. At the other extreme, patients with tumors >4 mm in thickness have a very high incidence of distant as well as local and regional metastasis. The sur-

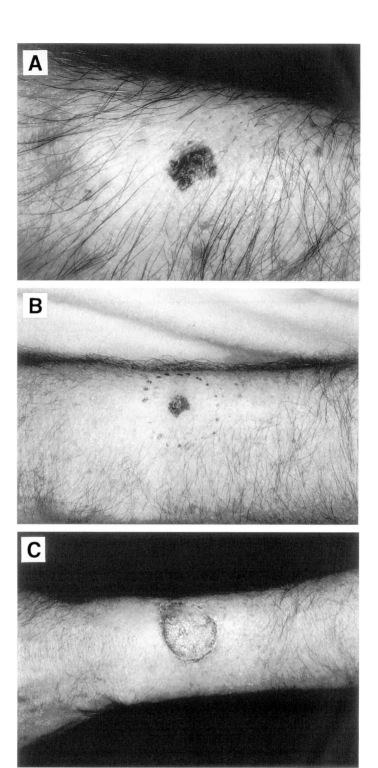

Table 5
Follow-up Guidelines

Breslow depth	History and physical examination	Chest X-ray/laboratory studies[a]
Stage I/II (<1.0 mm, thin)	6 mo × 2 yr; 12 mo thereafter	None
1.0–4.0 mm (intermediate)	4–6 mo × 3 yr; 12 mo thereafter	Initial: CXR, optional CBC, LFTs Follow-up: yearly CXR, optional CBC, LFTs
>4.0 mm (thick)	4–6 mo × 3 yr; 12 mo thereafter	Initial: CXR, optional CBC, LFTs Follow-up: yearly CXR, optional CBC, LFTs
Stage III/IV	3–4 mo × 5 yr; 12 mo thereafter	Initial: CXR and CT scans[b] Initial: CBC, LFTs Follow-up: every 6–12 mo CXR, LFTs

[a]LFTs (liver function tests) are LDH, AST, ALT, Alk Phos.
[b]CT scans and blood studies based on physical examination findings. FDG whole-body scan can replace the battery of imaging tests performed on high-risk patients (*28*).
CXR = chest x-ray, CBC = complete blood count

vival of this group is not improved by elective lymph node dissection (ELND). Thus, the intermediate thickness group with nonpalpable nodes is the group that logically could benefit from ELND because the incidence of regional node metastasis is significantly greater than the incidence of distant metastasis.

In the past, some surgeons excised lymph nodes only when they were clinically palpable (therapeutic lymph node dissection), and others preferred to remove the nodes in high-risk (intermediate or thick melanomas) patients even when they were not palpable because of the likelihood of microscopic node metastases. Complete lymph node dissection is associated with significant

---

Fig. 1. (*previous page*) (**A**) This pigmentation varies over the surface of this lesion of the left forearm, which has irregular borders and is 7 × 5 mm in diameter. A 3-mm punch biopsy of the darkest portion of the lesion reveals a melanoma. Breslow depth = 0.43 mm. (**B**) Surgical margins were plotted using a Woods light to define the border of the pigmentation and then a 1.0-cm was margin marked from the end of the pigmentation of the lesion. (**C**) Two weeks after the resection, the split thickness graft, which was applied to the fascia over the muscle, is depressed; however, this will rise to the level of the surrounding skin over the next few months.

morbidity but provides useful staging information in melanoma because lymph node metastasis is an important prognostic factor. Palpable lymph nodes are strongly associated with distant metastasis (70–85%) and a 5-yr survival rate of only 30%. Any palpable lymph node should be initially examined by fine-needle aspiration. An open lymph node biopsy is performed subsequently if the aspirate result is positive or inconclusive. Patients with occult disease in the lymph node have a more favorable prognosis *(9)*.

Early retrospective reviews of ELND *(9,37,38)* did demonstrate a survival benefit, but prospective randomized trials *(39,40)* did not. A concern with these studies is that the nodal basins that were dissected were not identified by lymphoscintigraphy, and, thus, they may not have included the ones to which the region preferentially drained. Although these studies were noted to have design flaws, recent results from the Intergroup Melanoma Trial have also demonstrated no survival advantage. The Intergroup Melanoma Trial has found an apparent survival advantage in patients under age 60 with primary melanomas 1 to 2 mm thick *(41)*. In a randomized trial of patients with truncal melanoma ≥1.5 mm in thickness, there was no survival advantage after immediate ELND *(42)*. Lymphoscintigraphy using technetium sulfur colloid, which is concentrated in the nodes within minutes after id injection, is an accurate preoperative method to map lymph node basins at risk for melanoma metastasis. Initial studies showed surprisingly different drainage patterns than would have been predicted by anatomic guidelines. A study of 82 patients with intermediate thickness melanomas found discordant drainage in 63% of head and neck cases and in 32% of truncal cases *(43)*. The timing of the lymphoscintigraphy is important. It should be conducted before wide local excision to avoid disruption of the lymphatic drainage and obstruction of the true location of the draining nodes.

6. Intraoperative Mapping and Sentinel Lymph Node Biopsy

Melanoma metastasis spreads via the lymphatics in an orderly fashion, and, therefore, the sentinel node is the first lymph node a metastasis encounters before entering into "higher" or more "proximal" nodes. Morton et al. *(44)* introduced the sentinel lymph node (SLN) biopsy for cutaneous melanoma patients in 1991. Studies since then have indicated that the SLN is representative of all nodes in the basin, particularly if the SLN is negative. The SLN biopsy technique has evolved from the use of lymphazurin blue vital dye injected around the site of the primary melanoma to localize the SLN identified by preoperative lymphoscintigraphy with a tattoo placed on the skin over the node. Now, the SLN is isolated in vivo by a handheld gamma probe based on the level of radioactivity of a "hot" SLN compared with background *(10,45)*. Ideally, intraoperative mapping should be performed after initial biopsy and before wide local excision. After injecting the radiolabeled tracer, mapping is delayed for 4 h to allow maximal localization in the nodes.

An advantage of SLN biopsy is that it can be performed under local anesthesia for most groin dissections and some head and neck dissections. Usually, axillary SLNs require general anesthesia because the nodes are buried under considerable fat. Because node dissection can be expected only to increase survival in patients with node metastases, SLN biopsy could become a tool to identify patients with occult node metastasis, who could then undergo node dissection. Specialized pathology techniques may reduce the already low false negative rate of SLN biopsies performed by serially sectioning the nodes and routine processing with hematoxylin and eosin (H&E), which detects 1 melanoma cell in 10,000 normal cells *(46)*. Some centers use S-100 immunoperoxidase staining to improve the accuracy of diagnosis to 1 abnormal cell in 100,000 normal cells *(47)*. However, a possible pitfall of S-100 antibody staining of melanoma cells is confusion with other cells, such as interdigitating dendritic cells, nevus cells, and certain macrophages within lymph nodes. Newer methods of PCR testing for tyrosinase mRNA are able to detect about 3 melanoma cells in a background of 10 million normal lymphocytes *(12)*. PCR has been shown to detect micrometastases in SLNs originally negative by routine histology *(12)*. With continued study, the sensitivity of PCR technology may yield an unacceptable false positive rate by detecting normal nevus cells within lymph node capsules. Capsular nevi are present within 25% of SLN *(48)*.

SLN biopsy and PCR analysis of the node remain in the realm of research, and the benefit to the patient in terms of prolonging the disease-free interval is not known. A national multicenter trial is currently studying the survival advantage of complete lymph node dissection based on SLN and the possible advantage to SLN-positive patients of qualifying for adjuvant therapy protocols. At present, the ability of adjuvent therapy to prolong life has been questioned, and the scientific community awaits the publication of the Eastern Co-operative Oncology Group Trial 1690 by Kirkwood et al. *(49)*, which is the study designed to confirm the encouraging results reported in their earlier trial. The suggestion and hope is that early detection of occult nodal metastasis may substantially affect the final outcome of these patients. Currently, the technique of SLN biopsy should be considered a staging procedure.

7. Lentigo Maligna Treated with Mohs Surgery

The management of lentigo maligna ([LM] melanoma *in situ*) is now as controversial as the margin of resection for intermediate thickness melanoma was prior to the results of the prospective randomized trials. The answer to the controversy could be provided by a prospectively randomized trial of Mohs surgery vs surgical margins of 5 mm or 1 cm. The challenge of LM treatment is

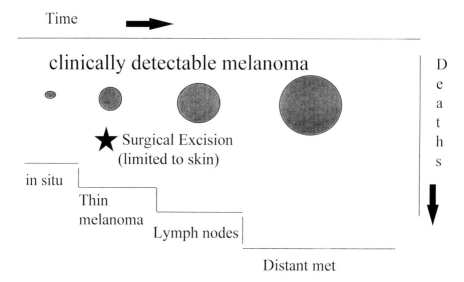

Fig. 2. Clinical progression of melanoma.

that the disease commonly occurs on extensively actinically damaged skin of the head and neck, which is a field of atypical melanocytes. Even after excision of the lesion using a Wood's light to define the edge of the pigmentation and 0.5-cm margins (**Table 4**), there are often scattered atypical melanocytes at or near the lateral edge of the specimen. Repeated reexcisions may show similar results. These atypical melanocytes have been observed to extend as far as 10 cm beyond the clinical border of an LM *(50)*, which brings into question the clinical relevance of this finding *(51)*. When deciding whether the margin of resection is free of tumor, the Mohs surgeon interprets the presence of atypical melanocytes in frozen sections prepared with H&E. The interpretation is guided by whether the atypical melanocytes are present as scattered single cells (interpreted as a negative margin) or clumps of three or more cells (a positive margin) as well as whether they rise above the basal layer or extend down adnexal structures (a positive margin) *(52)*. Methods used to assist in this interpretation include rush permanent paraffin sections *(53)*, immunoperoxidase staining with HMB-45 *(52,54,55)* and Mel-5 *(56)*. Given the "field effect" and histologic "skip areas" in LM, careful long-term clinical monitoring of the excision site is needed to detect any possible recurrence.

8. Conclusion

The optimal lateral surgical margins for melanoma are still being investigated. However, several studies have shown that more conservative margins have not resulted in higher recurrence rates. Furthermore, the advantages of

Mohs micrographic surgery, the SLN biopsy technique, and early dissection of occult disease with or without postsurgical adjuvent therapy are still under discussion. Even with this array of promising new therapeutic strategies, the importance of early detection in melanoma should not be underestimated. Melanoma progresses to metastatic disease in a variable period of time (**Fig. 2**). Metastatic melanoma remains resistant to all currently available therapy. At this time and for the foreseeable future, successful treatment depends on detection in the *in situ* or thin phase of the disease.

References

1. Hall, H. I., Miller, D. R., Rogers, J. D., and Bewerse, B. B. (1999) Update on the incidence and mortality from melanoma in the United States, *J. Am. Acad. Dermatol.* **40**, 35–42.
2. Fremgen, A. M., Bland, K. I., McGinnis, L. S., Eyre, H. J., McDonald, C. J., and Menck, H. R. (1999) Clinical highlights from the national cancer data base. *Cancer* **49**, 145–148.
3. Beahrs, O. H., Henson, D. E., Hutter, R. V. P., et al. eds. (1992) *Manual for Staging of Cancer*, 4th ed. JB Lippincott, Philadelphia, pp. 143–147.
4. Breslow, A. (1970) Thickness, cross-sectional areas and depth of invasion in the prognosis of cutaneous melanoma. *Ann. Surg.* **172**, 902–908.
5. Clark, W. H. Jr., From, L., Bernardino, E. A., et al. (1969) The histogenesis and biologic behavior of primary human malignant melanoma of the skin. *Cancer Res.* **29**, 705–727.
6. Balch, C. M., Soong, S. J., Shaw, H. M., et al. An analysis of prognostic factors in 8500 patients with cutaneous melanoma, in *Cutaneous Melanoma*, 2nd ed. (Balch, C. M., Houghton, A. N., Milton, G. W., et al., eds.),. JB Lippincott, Philadelphia, pp. 165–199.
7. Garbe, C., Buttner, P., Bertz., J, et al. (1995) Primary cutaneous melanoma: identification of prognostic groups and estimation of individual prognosis for 5093 patients. *Cancer* **75**, 2484–2491.
8. Balch, C. M., Cascinelli, N., Drzewiecki, K. T., et al. (1992) A comparison of prognostic factors worldwide, in *Cutaneous Melanoma*, 2nd ed. (Balch, C. M., Houghton, A. N. A., Milton, G. W., et al., eds.), JB Lippincott, Philadelphia, pp. 188–199.
9. Balch, C. M., Soong, S. J., Murad, T. M., et al. (1981) A multifactorial analysis of melanoma. III. Prognostic factors in melanoma patients with lymph node metastases (stage II). *Ann. Surg.* **193**, 377–388.
10. Albertini, J. J., Cruse, C. W., Rapport, D., et al. (1996) Intraoperative radiolymphoscintigraphy improves sentinel lymph node identification for patients with melanoma. *Ann. Surg.* **223**, 217–224.
11. Ross, M., Reintgen, D. S., and Balch, C. (1993) Selective lympadenectomy: emerging role of lymphatic mapping and sentinel node biopsy in the management of early stage melanoma. *Semin. Surg. Oncol.* **9**, 219–223.

12. Shivers, S. C., Wang, X., Li, W., et al. (1998) Molecular staging of malignant melanoma. *JAMA* **280,** 1410–1415.
13. Urist, M. M. (1996) Surgical management of primary cutaneous melanoma. *CA* **46,** 217–224.
14. Barnhill, R. L., Mihm, M. C., and Fitzpatrick, T. B. (1993) Neoplasms: malignant melanoma, in *Dermatology in General Medicine,* 4th ed., (Fitzpatrick, T. B., Eisen, A. Z., Wolff, K., et al., eds.), McGraw-Hill, New York, pp. 1078–1115.
15. Brown, M. (1997) Staging and prognosis of melanoma. *Semin. Cutan. Med. Surg.* **16(2),** 113–121.
16. Balch C. M., Buzaid, A. C., Atkins, M. D., et al. (2000) A new American joint committee on cancer staging system for cutaneous melanoma. *Cancer* **88,** 1484–1491.
17. Handley, W. S. (1907) The pathology of melanocytic growths in relation to their operative treatment. *Lancet* **1,** 927–996.
18. Kelly, J. N., Sagabiel, R. W., Calderon, W., et al. (1984) The frequency of local recurrence and microsatellitosis as a guide to re-excision margins for cutaneous malignant melanoma. *Ann. Surg.* **200,** 759–763.
19. Breslow, A. and Macht, S. P. (1977) Optimal size for resection margin for thin cutaneous melanoma. *Surg. Gynecol. Obstet.* **145,** 691–702.
20. Goldsmith, L. A., Askin, F. B., Chang, A. E., Cohen, C., Dutcher, J. P., Gilgor, R. S., Green, S., Harris, E. L., Havas, S., Robinson, J. K., Swanson, N. A., and Tempero, M. A. (1992) Diagnosis and treatment of early melanoma. NIH consensus development panel on early melanoma. *JAMA* **268,** 1314–1319.
21. Balch, C. M., Urist, M. M., Karakousis, C. P., et al. (1993) Efficacy of 2 cm surgical margins for intermediate-thickness melanomas (1 to 4 mm): results of a multi-institutional randomized surgical trial. *Ann. Surg.* **218,** 262–269.
22. Veronesi, U. and Cascinelli, N. (1991) Narrow excision (1 cm margin): a safe procedure for thin cutaneous melanoma. *Arch. Surg.* **126,** 438–441.
23. Piepkorn, M. and Barnhill, R. L. (1996) A factual, not arbitrary, basis for choice of resection margins in melanoma. *Arch. Dermatol.* **132,** 811–814.
24. Bagley, F. H., Cady, B., Lee, A., et al. (1981) Changes in clinical presentation and management of malignant melanoma. *Cancer* **47,** 2126–2134.
25. Schmoeckel, C., Bockelbrink, A., Bockelbrink, H., et al. (1983) Low-risk and high-risk malignant melanoma, III. *Eur. J. Cancer Clin. Oncol.* **19,** 245–249.
26. Zeitels, J., La Rossa, D., Hamilton R., et al. (1988) A comparison of local recurrence and resection margins for stage I primary cutaneous malignant melanomas. *Plast. Reconstr. Surg.* **81,** 688–693.
27. O'Rourke, M. G. E. and Altmann, C. R. (1993) Melanoma recurrence after excision: is a wide margin justified? *Ann. Surg.* **217,** 2–5.
28. Thorn, M., Pouten, F., Berstrome, R., et al. (1994) Clinical and histopathologic predictors of survival in patients with malignant melanoma: a population-based study in Sweden. *J. Natl. Cancer Inst.* **86,** 761–769.
29. Ang, K. K., Byers, R. M., Peters, L. J., et al. (1990) Regional radiotherapy as adjuvant treatment for head and neck malignant melanoma. *Arch. Otolaryngol. Head Neck Surg.* **116,** 169–172.

30. Storm, F. K. and Mahvi, D. M. (1994) Treatment of primary melanoma, in *Malignant Melanoma*, 1st ed., (Lejeune, F. J., Chaundhuri, P. K., and Das Gupta, T. K., eds.), McGraw-Hill, New York, pp. 193–204.
31. Levy, E., Silverman, M. K., Vossaert, K. A., et al. (1991) Late recurrence of malignant melanoma: a report of five cases, a review of the literature and a study of associated factors. *Melanoma Res.* **1**, 63–67.
32. Vilmer, C., Bailly, C., Le Doussal, V., et al. (1999) Thin melanomas with unusual aggressive behavior: a report of nine cases. *J. Am. Acad. Dermatol.* **34**, 439–444.
33. Slinguff, C. L., Dodge, R. K., Stanley, W. E., et al. (1992) The annual risk of melanoma progression: implications for the concept of cure. *Cancer* **70**, 1917–1927.
34. Rhodes, A. R. (1995) Public education and cancer of the skin: what do people need to know about melanoma and non-melanoma skin cancer. *Cancer* **75(Suppl)**, 613–636.
35. Provost, N., Marghoob, A. A., Kopf, A. W., DeDavid, M., Wasti, Q., and Bart, R. S. (1997) Laboratory test and imaging studies in patients with cutaneous malignant melanomas: a survey of experienced physicians. *J. Am. Acad. Dermatol.* **36**, 711–720.
36. Rinne, D., Baum, R. P., Hor, G., and Kaufman, R. (1998) Primary staging and follow-up of high risk melanoma patients with whole-body ^{18}F-fluorodeoxyglucose positron emission tomography. *Cancer* **82**, 1664–1671.
37. Morton, D. L., Wanek, L., Nizze, J. A., Elashoff, R. M., and Wong, J. H. (1991) Improved long-term survival after lymphadenectomy of melanoma metastatic to regional lymph nodes. *Ann. Surg.* **214**, 491–501.
38. Das Gupta, T. K. (1977) Results of treatment of 269 patients with primary cutaneous melanoma: a five-year prospective study. *Ann. Surg.* **186**, 201–209.
39. Sim, F. H., Taylor, W. F., Ivins, J. C., Pritchard, D. J., and Soule, E. H. (1978) A prospective randomized study of the efficacy of routine elective lymph node lymphadenectomy in management of malignant melanoma: preliminary results. *Cancer* **41**, 948–956.
40. Veronesi, U., Adamus, J., Bandiera, D. C., et al. (1977) Inefficacy of immediate node dissection in stage I melanoma of the limbs. *N. Engl. J. Med.* **297**, 627–631.
41. Balch, C. M., Soong, S. J., Bartolucci, A. A., et al. (1996) Efficacy of an elective regional lymph node dissection of 1 to 4 mm thick melanomas for patients 60 years of age and younger. *Ann. Surg.* **224**, 255–266.
42. Cascinelli, N., Marabito, A., Santinani, M., et al. (1998) Immediate or delayed dissection of regional nodes in patients with melanoma of the trunk: a randomized trial. *Lancet* **351**, 793–796.
43. Norman, J., Wells, K., Kearney, R., Cruse, C. W., Berman, C., and Reintgen, D. S. (1993) Identification of lymphatic basins in patients with cutaneous melanoma. *Semin. Surg. Oncol.* **9**, 224–227.
44. Morton, D. L., Wen, D. R., Wong, J. H., et al. (1992) Technical details of intraoperative lymphatic mapping for early stage melanoma. *Arch. Surg.* **127**, 392–399.
45. Alex, J. C. and Krag, D. N. (1993) Gamma-probe guided localization of lymph nodes. *Surg. Oncol.* **2**, 137–143.

46. Cochran, A. J., Wen, D., and Morton, D. L. (1988) Occult tumor cells in lymph nodes of patients with pathological stage I malignant melanoma. *Am. J. Surg. Pathol.* **12,** 612–618.
47. Gershenwald, J. E., Colome, M. I., Lee, J. E., et al. (1998) Patterns of recurrence following a negative sentinel lymph node biopsy in 243 patients with Stage I or II melanoma. *J. Clin. Oncol.* **6,** 2253–2260.
48. Carson, K. F., Wen, D. R., Li, P. X., Lana, A. M., Bailly, C., Morton, D. L., and Cochran, A. J. (1996) Nodal nevi and cutaneous melanoma. *Am. J. Surg. Pathol.* **20,** 834–840.
49. Kirkwood, J. M., Strawderman, M. H., Ernstoff, M. S., et al. (1996) Interferon alfa-2b adjuvant therapy of high-risk resected cutaneous melanoma: the Eastern Co-operative Oncology Group Trial EST 1684. *J. Clin. Oncol.* **14,** 7–17.
50. Dhawan, S. S., Wolfe, D. J., Rabinowitz, H. S., et al. (1990) Lentigo maligna. *Arch. Dermatol.* **126,** 928–930.
51. de Berker, D. (1991) Lentigo maligna and Mohs. *Arch. Dermatol.* **127,** 421.
52. Robinson, J. K. (1994) Margin control for lentigo maligna. *J. Am. Acad. Dermatol.* **31,** 79–85.
53. Cohen, L. M., McCall, M. W., Hodge, S. J., et al. (1994) Successful treatment of lentigo maligna and lentigo maligna melanoma with Mohs' micrographic surgery aided by rush permanent section. *Cancer* **73,** 2964–2970.
54. Stonecipher, M. R., Leshin, B., Patrick, J., et al. (1993) Management of lentigo maligna and lentigo maligna melanoma with paraffin-embedded tangential sections: utility of immunoperoxidase staining and supplemental vertical sections. *J. Am. Acad. Dermatol.* **29,** 589–594.
55. Griego, R. D. and Zitelli, J. A. (1998) Mohs micrographic surgery using HMB-45 for a recurrent acral melanoma. *Dermatol. Surg.* **24,** 1003–1006.
56. Gross, E. A., Andersen, W. K., and Rogers, G. S. (1999) Mohs microscopic excision of lentigo maligna using Mel-5 for margin control. *Arch. Dermatol.* **135,** 15–17.

IV

MONITORING

16

Utility of Fine-Needle Aspiration Biopsy for Prospective Analysis of Patients Undergoing Therapy for Metastatic Melanoma

Adam I. Riker

1. Introduction

Many of the recent advancements in the area of tumor immunobiology have allowed us to focus our efforts on the experimental treatment of patients with metastatic melanoma. It has been both a frustrating and often a seemingly futile effort on the parts of physicians and researchers alike in treating such patients. The last decade of research has resulted in a paradigm shift in our understanding of the immunologic interactions between a tumor cell and the host immune response. The discovery and clinical application of tumor-associated antigens has allowed for a selective and highly specific approach to the treatment of patients with stage IV metastatic melanoma (*1*).

However, no matter what approach is utilized, there will always remain an absolute need to follow carefully and thoroughly all patients who receive either experimental or standard therapy. Follow-up visits must include a thorough physical examination noting changes such as any degree of tumor regression (or growth), side effects or drug-related toxicity possibly related to the treatment, or possible changes on serologic or immunologic evaluation. This last aspect of treatment, the immunologic evaluation and response of the patient, has become an integral part of the prospective analysis of experimental treatments of the patient with metastatic melanoma.

Our early experience in treating patients with peptide-based immunotherapy has made us acutely aware of our shortcomings in terms of truly understanding the complex molecular and immunologic interactions that occur within the in vivo tumor microenvironement. Thus, to overcome the difficulties associated

From: *Methods in Molecular Medicine, Vol. 61: Melanoma: Methods and Protocols*
Edited by: B. J. Nickoloff © Humana Press Inc., Totowa, NJ

with the analysis of sequential changes in melanoma-associated antigen (MAA) expression, we developed a method of fine-needle aspiration biopsy (FNAB) of metastatic melanoma nodules that provides for the serial analysis of the same lesion over time *(2)*.

There has been renewed enthusiasm in our attempts to understand the cellular immune response to melanoma. This has translated into the development of peptide-based vaccinations based on the utility of small peptide fragments derived from the so-called MAAs, which are recognized by T-lymphocytes. This has provided us with a basis for the rational design of many of the current antitumor and T-cell-based vaccine trials. These MAAs are specifically recognized by human leukocyte antigen (HLA) class I–restricted cytotoxic T-lymphocytes (CTLs). Such immunologic responses remain a vital key to our understanding of the true interactions between the host immune system and the tumor cell.

2. Materials

1. For immunocytochemistry, the following monoclonal antibodies (Mabs) are utilized: W6/32 (Sera Labs, Westbury, NY) for HLA class I *(3)*; IVA-12 (American Type Culture Collection, Rockville, MD) for HLA class II; KS-I *(4)* for HLA-A2 fluorescein isothiocyanate (FITC) antihuman CD8 and FITC anti-human CD4 (Pharmingen, San Diego, CA); and anti-MART-1/Melan-A murine IgG_{2b} (M2-7C10) *(5,6)* and anti-gp100 mAbHMB-45 (Enzo Diagnostics, Farmingdale, NY).

2. The secondary antibody is goat anti-mouse IgG (FITC). For secondary staining, biotinylated goat anti-mouse IgG (Kirkergaard & Perry, Gaithersburg, MD) is used followed by avidin-biotin-peroxidase (Vectasin Elite Kit; Vector, Burlingame, CA) *(5)*.

3. For reverse transcriptase polymerase chain reaction (RT-PCR), a set of two primers is selected to amplify each MAA cDNA. Each PCR reaction is composed of 10X PCR buffer, 1.5 mM $MgCl_2$, 200 μM dNTP, 1.25 U of AmpliTaq Gold, and 0.5 μL of cDNA for a final reaction volume of 20 μL. Ten microliters of light mineral oil covers the reaction mixture.

4. Primer selection for all experiments is based on the known genomic sequence of all genes of interest. All primers amplify a fragment that spans a known intron. The following primers are used:
   a. gp100: 5′-CTTGGTGTCTCAAGGCAACT (sense) and 5′-TCCAGGTA AGTATGAGTGAC (antisense).
   b. MART-1: 5′-ATGCCAAGAGAAGATGCTCAC (sense) and 5′-AGCATG TCTCAGGTGTCTCG (antisense).
   c. Tyrosinase: 5′-TTGGCAGATTGTCTGTAGCC (sense) and 5′-GCTATCCC AGTAAGTGGACT (antisense).
   d. β-Actin: 5′-TGGGCCGCTCTAGGCACCA (sense) and 5′-GTTGGCCTTA GGGTTCAGGGGG (antisense).

Table 1
Establishment of Melanoma Cell Lines from FNAB Samples

	Lesions	Patients	
Total number	39	23	
Established cell lines	26	16	
Success (%)	67	70	
	Positive Growth[a]	Negative Growth[b]	χ^{2c}
Size of lesion (cm^2) (SEM)	29.5 ($\pm$ 7.1)	17.6 ($\pm$ 3.8)	0.06
Total cells in FNAB sample	$7.8 \pm 3.2 \times 10^7$	$1.3 \pm 5.1 \times 10^7$	0.03
(before ACK lysis buffer)			
(median)	(20)	(10)	
Total cells in FNAB sample	$4 \pm 3.2 \times 10^6$	$0.5 \pm 0.2 \times 10^6$	0.006
(after ACK lysis buffer)			
(median)	(2)	(0.2)	

[a]Positive growth is defined as a melanoma cell line that expanded in vitro for greater than five consecutive passages and expanded for cryopreservation of at least 1×10^7 cells.
[b]Negative growth is defined as no appreciable expansion of melanoma cells after 30 d in culture.
[c]χ^2, variance of melanoma cell growth.

3. Methods

An overall success rate in the range of 60–80% can be expected with the utilization of FNAB samples for in vitro culturing and establishment of long-term melanoma cell lines. More recently, this success rate has improved to be about 80%, with the establishment of more than 40 long-term melanoma cell lines. Each lesion aspirated represents a distinct lesion, with some lesions aspirated from the same patient at different time points. In several patients, multiple lesions were simultaneously aspirated and analyzed separately. All established cell lines should be analyzed for the expression of MAA as determined by FACS analysis.

The average size of metastases from which cell lines originated was larger than that of metastases from which we could not establish a cell line (29.5 ± 7.1 cm^2 vs 17.6 ± 3.8 cm^2, $\chi^2 = 0.06$). There was a direct correlation between the total number of cells obtained (RBCs and viable nucleated cells) from FNAB and the ability to establish successfully a melanoma cell line in vitro ($7.8 \pm 3.2 \times 10^7$ vs $1.35 \pm 5 \times 10^7$, respectively, without RBC lysis buffer; $\chi^2 = 0.03$). Lysis of RBCs from the starting samples resulted in a lower cell number ($4.2 \pm 1.7 \times 10^6$ vs $0.5 \pm 0.25 \times 10^6$, respectively, with lysis buffer; $\chi^2 = 0.006$).

It is also feasible to establish autologous tumor/TIL pairs and solitary TIL cultures. Analysis of several of these pairs has revealed that autologous TIL cells were able to recognize autologous, HLA-matched tumor cell lines. Several TIL cultures exhibited growth of primarily CD8+ lymphocytes with other T-cell cultures of primarily CD4+ cells. Thus, much data have shown that autologous tumor/TIL pairs, solitary TIL, and melanoma cell lines can be readily generated from samples obtained by FNAB. These samples are extremely important reagents in determining the nature and identification of new melanoma antigens as well as further defining the specificity of the TIL cells from the autologous tumor samples.

A comparison of the levels of expression of gp100 and MART-1 utilizing immunocytochemistry was performed on cytospins from the original FNAB and from 10 subsequently established cell lines (by FACS) obtained from the same specimens. There was a strong correlation in MAA expression between fresh tumor explants and cultured cell lines using the two staining methods. In general, cell lines generated from metastases with high expression of gp100 were found to have high levels of gp100 by FACS analysis compared with the expression of the same antigens as detected by immunocytochemistry on freshly explanted tumor cells. In all cell lines, there was a high level of HLA-A2 expression, indicating that the loss or decreased expression of the HLA molecule was not a major factor in determining the level of either gp100 or MART-1 expression.

Occasionally, it was noted that if the fresh tumor explant was positive for gp100, subsequent in vitro culturing of this sample resulted in the loss of this MAA by FACS analysis. This selective pressure is known to occur, because the loss of these tumor antigens is not essential for the survival of the tumor cell. Remember that MAA expression is of no known importance to the tumor cell and bears no relationship to the neoplastic process. Thus, MA expression in melanoma cells is a remnant of the melanocytic origin, and its loss of expression may occur without significant repercussions on cancer cell survival. Therefore, these antigens could be particularly sensitive to immune selection during disease progression, under the effects of antigen-specific immunization and, of course, in vitro culturing.

3.1. Sample Collection by FNAB

1. Begin with a 23-gage needle attached to a 10-cc syringe that can be placed within a commercially available "pistol grip" device. This allows for its use with a single hand, allowing the second hand to stabilize the lesion to be aspirated.
2. Ensuring that the tip of the needle is firmly within the tumor nodule, apply a slight suction to the syringe while maintaining a slow, continuous back and forth motion. Always ensure that the tip of the needle remains within the tumor nodule during aspiration.

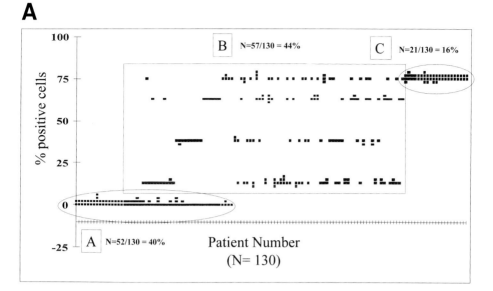

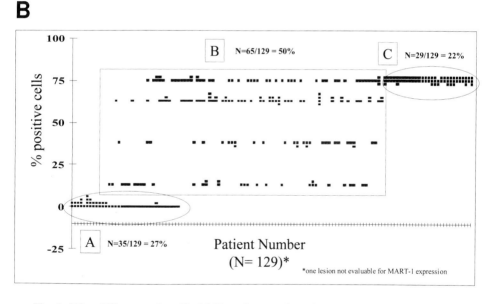

Fig. 1. (A) gp100 expression: Variability of expression of gp100 in multiple synchronous lesions within a patient. A total of 130 sets of synchronous lesions were evaluated for expression of gp100 and MART-1, demonstrated as the percentage of positive cells within a tumor population. (B) MART-1 expression: The same set of lesions (the order of patients is not the same from left to right; they are ranked according to the level of antigen expression) is evaluated for MART-1 expression. A, The overall percentage of lesions (all lesions, or at least one lesion of a synchronous set of lesions) evaluated by immunohistochemistry/immunocytochemistry negative for gp100 or MART-1 antigen expression; B, heterogeneity of melanoma antigen expression among multiple synchronous lesions; C, data sets representing lesions that were strongly positive and homogeneous for antigen expression (>75% positive).

3. Prior to removing the needle, discontinue suction and remove the collected specimen in the hub and lumen of the needle. Place a small sample on a slide and staine (DIFF-QUIK®) and evaluate at the bedside utilizing a standard light microscope to ascertain the adequacy of the sample.

3.2. Cell Culture Techniques

1. Once an adequate sample is obtained for both diagnosis and immunostaining by the cytopathology department, carry out a second pass under sterile conditions for subsequent in vitro culturing.
2. Place samples immediately into complete media at the bedside consisting of Iscove's media (Biofluids, Rockville, MD) supplemented with 10 mM HEPES buffer, 100 U/mL of penicillin (Biofluids), 100 µg/mL of streptomycin (Biofluids), 10 µg/mL of ciprofloxacin (Bayer, West Haven, CT), 0.03% L-glutamine (Biofluids), and 0.5 µg/mL of amphotericin B (Mediatech, Cellgro, VA) with 10% heat-inactivated human AB serum (Gemini Bioproducts, Calabasas, CA).
3. A total cell count is performed to include all nucleated and red blood cells (RBCs).
4. Place and expand all samples in either 24- or 48-well plates (Costar®; Corning, Calabasas, NY) at 4×10^6 or 2×10^6 cells/well, respectively. If RBC contamination remains a problem, ACK red blood cell lysing buffer (Biofluids) may be utilized first.
5. In separate wells, attempt to generate tumor-infiltrating lymphocytes (TILs) by adding interleukin-2 (IL-2) (Chiron, Emeryville, CA) every other day (1000 Cetus U/mL).
6. Maintain all cultures at 37°C in 5% CO_2 and replenish fresh media every 3 d. Split tumor cells and TILs as needed and expand based on the rapidity of cell growth.

3.3. Fluorescent Activated Cell-Sorting Analysis

Cell-surface expression of HLA and other surface antigens (CD8 and CD4) is performed utilizing previously described methods (5). Intracellular staining for detecting MA is performed as previously described, reported as the mean equivalence of fluorescence, which is the mean fluorescent channel number normalized between experiments utilizing standardized fluorescent beads (7).

3.4. Immunocytochemistry of Cytospin Preparations

Immunocytochemistry is performed on cytospin preparations from the original FNA sample and on subsequent established cell lines. The cytospins are fixed in acetone and stained with the same MAbs used for the FACS analysis (Biogenex, San Ramon, CA).

3.5. Polymerase Chain Reaction

1. PCR is performed with obvious dependency on the primer selection and melting temperatures of the primers. The protocol used in most reactions is as follows: Ten high-stringency cycles of initiation at 94°C for 9 min, denaturation at 94°C

Table 2
FNAB-Established Autologous Tumor/TIL Pairs and TIL Cultures

	Autologous TIL	
Cell line	CD4 (%)	CD8 (%)
F001	<1	99
F015	12	82
F035	<1	99
F005	89	10
F020	98	<1
F045	6	94
F046	94	3
TIL line	CD4 (%)	CD8 (%)
T001	70	28
T002	8	90
T003	17	64
T004	11	74
T005	4	95
T006	1	99
T007	24	86
T008	87	10
T009	98	2

for 30 s, annealment at 65°C for 1 min, and extension at 72°C for 1 min. This is followed by 20 low-stringency cycles of 94°C for 30 s, 60°C for 1 min, 72°C for 1 min, and a final extension at 72°C for 10 min.

2. For each sample, mix 6 µL of PCR product and 3 µL of bromophenol blue 5X loading buffer and run on a 1.3% agarose gel for 45 min at 150 V. Stain the gel with Vistra Green (Amersham Life Sciences, Arlington Heights, IL) 1:10,000 dilution in 1X TBE for 50 min and analyze on a FluoroImager 595 (Molecular Dynamics, Sunnyvale, CA).

3.6. HLA Typing

An HLA phenotype of each sample is determined by using sequence-specific primer-PCR *(8,9)*

4. Notes

1. Currently, there are no standardized methods of monitoring the response to treatment of patients with metastatic melanoma. However, the clinical response of patients, in both terms of increased overall and disease-free survival, seems to be

Table 3
Correlation of Antigen Expression Between Melanoma Samples

	Fresh Tumor Explant[a]			Daughter Cell Lines[b]		
	Immunocytochemistry			FACS analysis[c]		
Tumor	gp100 (%)	MART-1 (%)	HLA-A2	gp100 MEFc/(%)	MART-1 MEF/(%)	HLA-A2 (MEF/(%)
F007	50–75	>75	+	382/94	1039/93	642/94
F013	>75	>75	+	214/70	279/67	261/98
F009	50–75	>75	+	189/44	348/84	418/97
F017	>75	50–75	+	57/19	251/76	253/99
F020	50–75	<25	+	22/9	246/51	226/90
F026	50–75	50–75	+	23/37	67/73	70/99
F023	Negative	Negative	+	12/5	76/32	133/84
F001	<25	50–75	+	0/0	29/12	266/99
F002	25–50	50–75	+	0/0	114/35	166/97
F003	<25	50–75	+	0/0	84/30	161/99

[a]The expression of MAA by fresh tumor explants was analyzed by immunocytochemistry utilizing the same antibodies for FACS analysis with the results evaluated by a single pathologist and graded on overall percentage of positive cells.
[b]FACS analysis was performed on established cell lines for the same MAA expression using intracellular staining with the MAb HMB-45 for gp100, anti-MART-1/Melan-A murine IgG$_2$b for MART-1, and MAb W6/32 for HLA-A2 expression.
[c]mEF, mean equivalence of fluorescence (7).

the ultimate clinical end point. There remain many questions about the proper form of surveillance for patients undergoing peptide-based vaccination. The clinical relevance of in vitro data has always been a confounding factor in determining its in vivo relevance. On the other hand, the evaluation of the immunologic response to therapy by serial FNAB of the same lesion will provide much needed information about the molecular mechanisms, which are so poorly understood at present.

2. The limited success of establishing melanoma cell lines from tumor digests obtained from excisional biopsies is most commonly attributed to contamination of fibroblasts within the sample. This results in a rapid overgrowth and contamination of the tumor cell population of interest. Thus, it remains a challenge to obtain a pure population of tumor cells for in vitro culture and expansion, with only a few authors examining the utility of FNAB for the establishment of neoplastic cell cultures. FNAB of melanoma lesions provides numerous advantages for the analysis of primary and metastatic tumors. It is a minimally invasive procedure with almost no associated morbidity well described elsewhere (10,11). The specimen can be evaluated immediately at the bedside to determine the quality, quantity, and overall cellular morphology of the FNAB specimen.

Table 4
Tissue Procurement in Melanoma Patients

Method	Potential advantages	Potential disadvantages
Excisional biopsy	minor procedure	Surgical procedure
	Complete removal of lesion	Possible morbidity
	Adequate tissue obtained	In vitro culturing difficult
	High sensitivity/specificity	Loss of prospective analysis
Incisional/core biopsy	Minor procedure	Architectural disruption
	Adequate tissue obtained	Potential wound breakdown
	Prospective analysis of lesion	Possible morbidity
	High sensitivity/specificity	

3. The establishment of melanoma cell lines in vitro from FNAB samples poses relatively few difficulties, with an appreciable success rate. In other histologies, such as renal cell carcinoma, breast cancer, ocular melanoma, colon cancer, small-cell lung cancer, and mesothelioma, it was much more difficult to establish long-term cultures in vitro. Several could be grown to two or three cell passages only to perish soon thereafter. It is likely that certain solid tumors may require supplemental growth factors that are not present in the standard media or sera utilized. Li et al. *(12)* demonstrated that only a relatively small number of tumor cells obtained by FNAB were required for the successful propagation of primary breast cancer cell lines in vitro. Of 25 attempted cases, 12 were passageable, resulting in up to 10^7 viable tumor cells. In all cell lines examined, the cultured cells closely resembled the original tumor tissue and displayed one or more tumor phenotypes.

4. It cannot be stressed enough that a true dedication to meticulous cell culture techniques is absolutely required in order to achieve this success rate. Sterile methods must be utilized during each step of growth and cell expansion, with extreme care taken to ensure that the media and other reagents such as IL-2 are changed at least every third day. Complacency with cell culture will most assuredly result in contamination by fungus, bacteria, or fibroblasts.

5. Some minor points to consider are that in performing all molecular procedures involved with the isolation of either total or messenger RNA, extreme care must be taken to ensure purity of the reagents, and all procedures should be performed only in an area that has been exclusively designated for RNA isolation alone. In addition, all reagents should be of molecular grade, with diethylpyrocarbonate-water used in all cases. Any number of commercially available RNA isolation kits that result in the isolation of high-quality total RNA are available. Similarly, the conversion of total RNA to complementary DNA has been performed with a standard kit (Gibco-BRL, Rockville, MD).

6. It is important that your PCR cycler be optimized and that samples be amplified previously in a reproducible manner. Although each experiment results in slightly different cycling parameters resulting in slightly different PCR products, it is

Table 5
Advantages of FNAB of Metastatic Melanoma

1. Immediate sample assessment
2. Easy to perform/tolerable without local anesthesia
3. Low morbidity
4. Minimal disruption of tumor architecture
5. Preferential sampling of tumor/lymphocytes
6. Efficient and effective method of tissue procurement
7. High sensitivity/specificity
8. No evidence of architectural or functional disruption
9. Minimal collection of stromal cells/minimal fibroblast overgrowth
10. Accurate measurement of immunologic and cellular changes that occur within the tumor microenvironment of the same lesion or from multiple synchronous or metachronous lesions from the same patient
11. Prospective analysis of melanoma lesions prior to, during, and after treatment

essential that the same PCR settings (*Tm*, time of extension and annealment) are used for each PCR amplification. Each set of primers has been designed with an appropriate *Tm* for each set of cycling conditions.

7. The literature suggests that because of the marked heterogeneity of MAA expression in synchronous melanoma lesions, one metastatic melanoma tumor nodule obtained by wide local excision is inadequate in terms of formulating generalized conclusions about the overall response of all lesions to treatment *(13–15)*. It is essential that each lesion be evaluated as its own entity, realizing that each is composed of different clones of tumor cells, with each expressing variable amounts of the target MAA. It is only through the separate and thorough evaluation of each melanoma lesion that we can expect to understand the complex interactions that are occurring within the tumor microenvironment.

8. In terms of those patients currently enrolled in peptide-based vaccinations, FNAB has evolved into an efficient method of sequentially analyzing all metastatic nodules from a single patient. In one of the largest analyses of multiple synchronous melanoma samples all obtained by FNAB, there appears to be a marked heterogeneity in the expression of the MAA, gp100, and MART-1. An in-depth analysis of more than 500 melanoma lesions has revealed that MAA expression of tumors treated with peptide-based immunotherapy is owing, in part, to a process of immunoselection *(16)*. Such selection may be the specific result of the immune pressure placed on the tumor cells as a direct result of peptide-based vaccination. This is most likely owing to the result of antigen-specific cytotoxic T-cells destroying those tumor cells that are expressing the appropriate MAA in an HLA-restricted fashion. However, because of the heterogeneity of MAA expression of melanoma cells, a small percentage of cells that have never expressed the target MAA will remain.

9. Jager et al. *(17)* demonstrated an inverse relationship of MAA expression in lesions and cytotoxic T-cell responses in response to repeated intradermal vaccination with peptides derived from the MART-1 and tyrosinase antigens. In all cases investigated, there was no detectable CTL response against these peptides when the respective tumor expressed the corresponding antigen. By contrast, there were frequent antigen-specific CTL responses in those patients whose tumors did not express the antigen. Thus, the expression of MAA seemed to be associated with the lack of antigen-directed CTL responses in vivo, suggesting that CTL responses against MAA may mediate regression of antigen-positive tumors, resulting in the immunoselection of melanoma lesions negative for the expression of MAA.

10. An important aspect of treating patients with immunotherapeutic vaccines is the selection of patients for therapy based on the MAA expression in tumor nodules. Currently, such a strict criterion is not formally utilized in choosing those patients who possess the highest levels of expression of the target MAA. Despite our current understanding of the importance of the high expression of MAA by tumor cells, patients are not denied enrollment in peptide-based vaccination trials even if the MAA expression of their tumor is minimal or completely negative. Jager et al. *(18)* propose that patients be selected for therapy with antigen-specific immunotherapy according to antigen expression as assessed by immunohistochemistry staining rather than by mRNA, thus providing valuable information about cellular antigen localization, heterogeneity and intensity of antigen staining, and overall percentage of cellular MAA positivity. Future studies will indeed call attention to the fact that MAA expression by tumor cells is essential for a clinical response to peptide-based immunotherapy, obviating the importance of screening melanoma patients for MAA expression prior to such treatment.

11. Caution should be applied in utilizing vaccines designed only to elicit a CTL response exclusively against gp100 positive tumor nodules because most, if not all, melanoma tumors are extremely heterogeneous in their expression of gp100. It is the homogeneity of MAA expression that seems to play a critical role in the proper recognition and lysis of tumor cells by specific TIL populations, possibly preventing the development of antigen-loss variants in vivo.

12. One must keep in mind that a selection bias occurs whenever a population of tumor cells is placed in vitro for further expansion and characterization. Many consider a freshly prepared tumor cell digest as being a superior representation of the in vivo situation, but success rates with such methods remain poor, often struggling to overcome the incessant problem of fibroblast overgrowth. FNAB is a fast and extremely efficient method, allowing for the analysis of all aspects of tumor cell activity. Obtaining a pure melanoma culture from tumor cell digests of excised specimens remains a formidable task, often resulting in contaminating fibroblasts and other cells infiltrating the tumor microenvironment.

13. The added complexity of patient heterogeneity also needs to be taken into account when analyzing tumor escape mechanisms. Patients who exhibit lower precursor frequencies toward a particular HLA/MAA combination could exert

decreased immunologic pressure toward that combination, and, therefore, detection of a specific escape mechanism may prove to be much more difficult to document. It is also possible that the level of immune competence of a patient toward a particular MAA/HLA allele is a reflection of the level of epitope availability in that patient. This could have extremely important implications in the selection of patients for a particular treatment protocol. We have recently noted a strong correlation between the expression of gp100 and the response of HLA-A*0201 melanoma patients treated with a gp100-specific peptide vaccination *(2)*. Only patients exhibiting high levels of gp100 expression, as analyzed by immunohistochemistry for gp100 from cytospins, were found to respond to the vaccine.

References

1. Rosenberg, S. A., Yang, J. C., Schwartzentruber, D., et al. (1998) Immunologic and therapeutic evaluation of a synthetic tumor associated peptide vaccine for the treatment of patients with metastatic melanoma. *Nat. Med.* **4,** 321–327.
2. Riker, A. I., Panelli, M. C., Kammula, U. S., et al. (1999) Development and characterization of melanoma cell lines established by fine needle aspiration biopsy: advances in the monitoring of patients with metastatic melanoma. *Cancer Detection Prevention* **23(5),** 387–396.
3. Brodsky, F. M. and Parham, P. (1982) Monomorphic anti-HLA-A,B,C monoclonal antibodies detecting molecular subunits and combinatorial determinants. *J. Immunol.* **128,** 129–135.
4. Tsujisaki, M., Sakaguchi, K., Igarashi, M., et al. (1988) Fine specificity and idiotype diversity of the murine anti-HLA-A2, A28 monoclonal antibodies CR11-351 and KS1. *Transplantation* **45,** 632–639.
5. Marincola, F. M., Hijazi, Y. M., Fetsch, P., et al. (1996) Analysis of expression of the melanoma associated antigens MART-1 and gp100 in metastatic melanoma cell lines and in in situ lesions. *J. Immunother.* **19,** 192–205.
6. Kawakami, Y., Battles, J. K., Kobayashi, T., et al. (1997) Production of recombinant MART-1 proteins and specific antiMART-1 polyclonal and monoclonal antibodies: use in the characterization of the human melanoma antigen MART-1. *J. Immunol. Methods* **202,** 13–25.
7. Cormier, J. N., Panelli, M. C., Hackett, J. A., et al. (1999) Natural variation of the expression of HLA and endogenous antigen modulates CTL recognition in an *in vitro* melanoma model. *Int. J. Cancer* **80,** 271–280.
8. Bunce, M., O'Neill, C. M., Barnardo, M. C., et al. (1995) Phototyping: comprehensive DNA typing for HLA-A, B, C, DRB1, DRB3, DRB4, DRB5 & DQB1 by PCR with 144 primer mixes utilizing sequence-specific primers (PCR-SSP). *Tissue Antigens* **46,** 355–367.
9. Player, M. A., Barracchini, K. C., Simonis, T. B., et al. (1996) Differences in frequency distribution of HLA-A2 sub-types between American and Italian

Caucasian melanoma patients: relevance for epitope specific vaccination protocols. *J. Immunother.* **19**, 357–363.

10. Zajdela, A., Ennuyer, A., Bataini, P., et al. (1976) Value of the cytologic diagnosis of adenopathies by aspiration biopsy: cytohistologic comparison of 1756 cases. *Bull. Cancer* **63**, 327–340.

11. Engzell, U., Jakobsson, P. A., Sigurdson, A., et al. (1971) Aspiration biopsy of metastatic carcinoma in lymph nodes of the neck: a review of 1101 consecutive cases. *Acta Otolaryngol. (Stockh.)* **72**, 138–147.

12. Li, Z., Bustos, V., Miner, J., et al. (1998) Propagation of genetically altered tumor cells derived from fine-needle aspirates of primary breast carcinoma. *Cancer Res.* **58**, 5271–5274.

13. Scheibenbogen, C., Weyers, I., Ruiter, D. J., et al. (1996) Expression of gp100 in melanoma metastases resected before and after treatment with IFN and IL-2. *J. Immunother.* **19**, 375–380.

14. de Vries, T. J., Fourkour, A., Wobbes, T., et al. (1997) Heterogeneous expression of immunotherapy candidate proteins gp100, MART-1, and tyrosinase in human melanoma cell lines and in human melanocytic lesions. *Cancer Res.* **57**, 3223–3229.

15. Lehmann, F., Marchand, M., Hainaut, P., et al. (1995) Differences in the antigens recognized by cytolytic T cells on two successive metastases of a melanoma patient are consistent with immune selection. *Eur. J. Immunol.* **25** 340–347.

16. Riker, A. I., Kammula, U. S., Panelli, M. C., et al. (1999) Immune selection following antigen specific immunotherapy of melanoma. *Surgery* **126**, 112–118.

17. Jager, E., Ringhoffer, M., Karbach, M., et al. (1996) Inverse relationship of melanocyte differentiation antigen expression in melanoma tissues and CD8+ cytotoxic T-cell responses: evidence for immunoselection of antigen-loss variants in vivo. *Int. J. Cancer* **66**, 470–476.

18. Jager, E., Ringhoffer, M., Altmannsberger, M., et al. (1997) Immunoselection in vivo: independent loss of MHC class I and melanocyte differentiation antigen expression in metastatic melanoma. *Int. J. Cancer* **71**, 142–147.

17

A Molecular Technique Useful in the Detection of Occult Metastases in Patients with Melanoma

RT-PCR Analysis of Sentinel Lymph Nodes and Peripheral Blood

James S. Goydos and Douglas S. Reintgen

1. Introduction

When cutaneous melanoma is confined to the skin, simple excision with adequate margins will usually cure the patient *(1,2)*. Local recurrences do occur but reexcision still results in a very high cure rate. When cutaneous melanoma spreads beyond the primary site, the metastases are predominantly by way of the lymphatics. If in-transit disease or regional lymph node involvement is present, the 5-yr survival rate drops to approx 60% *(1–3)*. Accurate staging of the locoregional lymphatic basin is thus extremely important. Preoperative lymphoscintigraphy followed by selective lymphadenectomy has revolutionized the staging of cutaneous melanoma by delivering to the pathologist only those nodes that are most likely to contain metastatic cells *(4)*. A close examination of these sentinel lymph nodes (SLNs) by serial sectioning and immunohistochemical staining can detect very minute quantities of melanoma. This type of detailed examination is impossible in standard lymphadenectomy specimens that can contain 20–40 lymph nodes. The standard technique used to examine large numbers of lymph nodes is to examine only 1–5% of each node using hematoxylin and eosin staining. This can obviously miss micrometastatic disease and understage the patient.

Multiple prospective studies have validated the concept and utility of selective lymphadenectomy and the World Health Organization Melanoma Committee has declared it to be a standard of care for nodal staging of melanoma

From: *Methods in Molecular Medicine, Vol. 61: Melanoma: Methods and Protocols*
Edited by: B. J. Nickoloff © Humana Press Inc., Totowa, NJ

(5–9). However, serial sectioning and immunohistochemical staining of even a few SLNs is still time-consuming and expensive. Furthermore, optical resolution and the experience and patience of the dermatopatholgist limit light microscopy. Patients with histologically negative SLNs still have an unacceptably high rate of recurrence, ranging from 10 to 15% *(10,11)*. A method is needed to examine SLNs and detect microscopic and "submicroscopic" disease that is cost-effective and highly sensitive and specific.

Another instance in which detection of subclinical disease would be useful is the detection of circulating tumor cells in peripheral blood. Clinical studies have shown that tumor cells can be detected in the peripheral blood and bone marrow of patients with no clinical evidence of disease *(12)*. A rapid and highly sensitive and specific detection system that could detect low volumes of circulating tumor cells would be useful for staging and prognosis. Patients could be monitored with simple blood tests instead of the expensive, time-consuming, and often uncomfortable methods that are now employed for surveillance, such as computed tomography scans. Patients could also be stratified into different risk groups, which would make the clinical trials more uniform and interpretable.

Reverse transcriptase polymerase chain reaction (RT-PCR) is a technique that may be able to detect clinically occult metastatic disease *(11,13,14)*. This technique is based on the fact that even though every nucleated cell in an organism contains a complete copy of genomic DNA, each type of cell transcribes only certain genes. If one could identify a unique protein produced by the target cell, one could search for the messenger RNA (mRNA) coding for that protein. If this unique mRNA is present in the tissue sample, the cell producing this marker protein must also be present. The reason to search for the mRNA instead of the actual protein is that proteins are relatively stable and could travel to the target tissue whereas mRNA is rapidly degraded and only transiently present in its cell of origin *(15)*. Recent studies have shown that marker mRNAs can be detected in SLNs and peripheral blood in patients with melanoma *(11,13,14,16,17)*. Furthermore, a recent study by Shivers et al. *(10)* suggests that the detection of melanocyte-specific mRNA in SLNs may be clinically significant.

Marker proteins must have certain characteristics if they are to be employed in RT-PCR studies. The protein would ideally be specific for the cell type of interest. However, few tumor-specific proteins are known, and most marker proteins are specific for the tumor's cell of origin. An example would be tyrosinase, the first enzyme in the melanin synthesis pathway, which is present in normal melanocytes as well as most melanomas. Because lymphocytes do not normally produce melanin, tyrosinase should not be present in a normal lymph node. If tyrosinase mRNA is detected in a sample of SLNs from a patient with melanoma, then we assume that melanoma cells (or normal melanocytes *[18]*) are present in that lymph node. The second requirement for a marker protein is that the gene sequence must be known. Tyrosinase also fulfills this requirement because its DNA sequence is well studied. Finally, the protein must not be too long or too short because this could make analysis and primer selection difficult. Tyrosinase is a medium-sized protein with unique regions that fulfills the aforementioned requirements.

Once the marker protein is chosen, five steps are necessary to run an RT-PCR analysis. First, the tissue must be harvested and preserved to inactivate RNases that would rapidly degrade the mRNA. Second, the mRNA must be extracted from the tissue and first-strand cDNA produced using the enzyme RT. cDNA is the preferred molecule to examine because it is much more stable than mRNA. Third, the cDNA sequence of the protein must be examined and PCR primers chosen. Fourth, the cDNA must be combined with the preselected primers and PCR then performed using DNA polymerase and a thermocycler. Fifth, the cDNA PCR product must be examined to detect the marker. Many different techniques have been proposed to carry out each of these steps; we outline one method herein.

2. Materials
2.1. Harvest and Preservation of Tissue

1. Liquid nitrogen in an appropriate container for transport (Thermo-Flask; Lab-line, Melrose Park, IL).
2. Freezer (–80°C) for storage of specimens.

2.2. Harvest and Preparation of Peripheral Blood

1. Ficoll (LSM; Organon Teknika, Durham, NC).
2. Blood collection tubes with EDTA.
3. Freezer (–80°C) for storage of specimens.

2.3. Extraction of Total RNA

1. Trizol Reagent (Life Technologies, Grand Island, NY) (store at –20°C).
2. Chloroform (no additives) (store at room temperature).
3. Isopropyl alcohol (store at room temperature).
4. 75% Ethanol (RNase free) (store at room temperature).
5. RNase-free water or 0.5% sodium dodecyl sulfate (SDS) solution (store at room temperature).

2.4. First Strand cDNA Synthesis

1. First-strand cDNA synthesis kit (Life Technologies) (store kit at –20°C).
2. Oligo(dT) (0.5µg/µL).
3. 10X PCR buffer: 200 mM Tris-HCl (pH 8.4), 500 mM KCl.

4. 25 m*M* MgCl$_2$.
5. 0.1 *M* Dithiothreitol (DTT).
6. 10 m*M* dNTP mix (10 m*M* each of dATP, dCTP, dGTP, and dTTP).
7. Reverse transcriptase (200 U/μL).
8. RNase H (2 U/μL).
9. Diethylpyrocarbonate (DEPC)-treated water.

2.5. Polymerase Chain Reaction

1. PCR Super Mix (Life Technologies) (store at –20°C).
2. Specific forward and reverse primers (store at –20°C).
3. Licensed thermocycler.
4. Thin-walled reaction tubes that fit the thermocycler.

2.6. Gel Electrophoresis

1. Agarose (Ultra Pure; Gibco-BRL) (stored as a powder at room temperature until mixed).
2. TBE buffer (Gibco-BRL) (store at 15–30°C).
3. Horizontal gel electrophoresis apparatus.
4. Ethidium bromide.
5. Ultraviolet (UV) transillumination apparatus.
6. DNA ladder (100 bp) (store at –20°C).

3. Methods

An example for the processing of lymph nodes and peripheral blood to detect the enzyme tyrosinase is illustrated. This technique will work equally well with other markers when used with the proper primers and PCR reaction temperatures appropriate for the primers.

3.1. Harvesting and Preservation of Tissue and Peripheral Blood

Because RNases are ubiquitous, it is important to preserve tissues quickly to limit mRNA degradation. Transient mRNAs can be destroyed within a few minutes of harvesting, and, therefore, rapid excision and immediate preservation in the operating room is necessary *(10,11,13,14)*. When preserving SLNs, excise the node, immediately transport the node to the back table in the operating room, bivalve the node, and place one quarter to one half in a sterile plastic container. Immediately place this container in liquid nitrogen, which halts enzymatic degradation. Transport the specimens to the laboratory and store at –80°C until processed. In this way, specimens are snap-frozen in less then 5 min after excision. If specimens are not to be processed within a few days, transfer them to a liquid nitrogen storage tank for long-term banking (*see* **Notes 1** and **2**). Collect peripheral blood in a sterile glass tube containing EDTA. Separate the blood on a Ficoll gradient by placing 8 mL of room temperature Ficoll in a 50-mL centrifuge tube and layering 10 cc of whole blood with EDTA, mixed 1:2 with warm phosphate-buffered saline (PBS), on top of the Ficoll. Care should be taken not to mix the blood and Ficoll at the interface. Centrifuge the preparation at room temperature for 10 min at 405*g* and remove the layer on top of the Ficoll and wash twice with PBS. The cell pellet can then be stored at –80°C until RNA extraction *(17,19)*.

3.2. Extraction of Total RNA from Nodal Tissue

Total RNA is extracted from lymph node samples using a modification of the method first described by Chomczynski and Sacchi *(20)* using a monophasic solution of phenol and guanidine isothiocyanate (Trizol reagent) (*see* **Notes 3** and **4**). The RNA extraction protocol is as follows:

1. Homogenize the sample: Place 100–200 mg of lymph node tissue in 2 mL of Trizol reagent in a 15-mL centrifuge tube and grind using a Teflon rod. The frozen tissue thaws rapidly, so it is important to homogenize the tissue quickly. The Trizol reagent has anti-RNase activity.
2. Separation of phases: Incubate the 15-mL tube at room temperature (15–30°C) for 5 min after homogenization and then add 0.5 mL of chloroform (0.25 mL/mL of Trizol used). Cap the tube tightly and shake vigorously by hand for 15–20 s and then let sit at room temperature for 2 to 3 min. Centrifuge the sample at 12,000*g* for 15 min at 2–8°C. This will separate the sample into a lower phenol-chloroform phase containing DNA and protein, an interphase, and an upper aqueous phase containing the RNA. The aqueous phase should be about 1 mL in volume. Pipet 0.8–1 mL of the aqueous phase into a 2-mL centrifuge tube, avoiding contamination by the interphase.
3. Precipitation of RNA: The RNA can now be precipitated from the aqueous phase by adding isopropyl alcohol. Add approx 0.8–1 mL of isopropyl alcohol to the tube and incubate the sample at room temperature for 10–15 min. Next, centrifuge the sample at 12,000*g* for 10 min at 2–8°C; the RNA should form a pellet on the bottom of the tube. Discard the supernatant and wash the RNA pellet once in 1.8 mL of 75% ethanol. Dissolve the pellet by vortexing and then centrifuge at 7500*g* for 5 min at 2–8°C.
4. Prepare the RNA for reverse transcription: Discard the supernatant and air-dry the RNA pellet for 5–10 min. Do not let the pellet completely dry out or redissolving the RNA will be difficult. Dissolve the RNA in RNase-free water or a 0 5% SDS solution by gentle pipeting and incubation at 55°C for 5–10 min. The RNA is now ready for first-strand DNA synthesis.

3.3. Extraction of Total RNA from Peripheral Blood

The extraction of total RNA from peripheral blood is the same as for nodal tissue except the homogenization step is simpler. Pipeting the cell pellet in 1 mL of the Trizol reagent for every 10^7 cells in the pellet will homogenize the cells and ready them for phase separation.

3.4. First-Strand cDNA Synthesis

mRNA is converted into a cDNA copy before performing PCR to amplify the marker. One strand of the cDNA is first synthesized by priming the RNA with an oligonucleotide and then using the enzyme RT to produce cDNA. Total RNA has been extracted from the lymph node cells and peripheral blood but only the mRNA, which makes up about 1–2% of total RNA, is of interest. To produce cDNA from total mRNA, one can exploit the fact that the vast majority of eukaryotic RNAs contain a 3′ poly(A) tail. An oligo(dT) primer is used to bind to this poly(A) tail and selectively convert the mRNA to cDNA. Once the first-strand cDNA has been produced, treat the mixture with RNase to eliminate residual RNA that can interfere with the PCR reaction. Because very small volumes of the reagents are required for each synthesis reaction, it is best to prepare master mixes containing enough of the reagents to perform several reactions. The incubations are best carried out in water baths preheated to 70, 42, and 37°C (*see* **Note 5**).

1. Determine the concentration of the isolated mRNA spectrophotometrically by absorption at 260 and 280 nm.
2. Add 1–5 µg of the total RNA (approx 1 µL) and 1 µL of oligo(dT) (0.5 µg/µL) solution to a sterile 1.5-mL tube. Incubate at 70°C for 10 min and then place on ice for 1 min.
3. Make a master mix of the reaction components added in the following order: In a 1.5-mL sterile tube combine 8 µL of the 10X PCR buffer, 8 µL of 25 mM MgCl$_2$, 4 µL of the 10 mM dNTP mix, and 8 µL of the 0.1 M DTT. This will make enough reaction mix for four reactions. Larger amounts of reaction mix can be made and stored at +4°C for short periods.
4. Place 7 µL of the master reaction mix into the tube containing the RNA/oligo(dT) mixture and gently mix. Collect the mixture in the bottom of the tube by gentle centrifugation for a few seconds and then incubate for 5 min at 42°C.
5. Add 1 µL (200 U) of the RT to the tube, mix gently, recollect at the bottom of the tube by gentle centrifugation for a few seconds, and then incubate at 42°C for 50 min.
6. Terminate the RT reaction by incubating at 70°C for 15 min and then chilling the specimen on ice for 5 min.
7. A mixture of RNA and cDNA is now present in the tube. Destroy the RNA because it will interfere with the PCR reaction. Recollect the specimen at the bottom of the tube by gentle centrifugation for a few seconds, and then add 1 µL

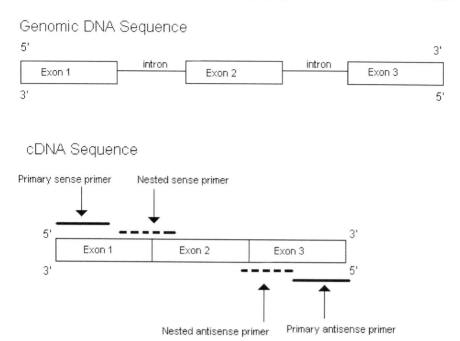

Fig. 1. Genomic DNA is made up of exons and introns. The introns are spliced out of the mRNA message and therefore the cDNA ends up with no introns. First-strand cDNA synthesis produces antisense cDNA, which reacts with the sense primers to produce the sense cDNA sequence. The antisense primers then react with the newly produced sense cDNA sequence and produce a new antisense cDNA. This produces very large amounts of cDNA specific for the primers used. Nested primers are used to amplify a smaller segment cDNA by reacting with cDNA produced in the primary PCR reaction. Because both sense and antisense cDNA strands are present in the primary PCR product, less cDNA is needed in the nested reaction. Note that the primary primers are on different exons. This would result in a much larger DNA product if contaminating genomic DNA was used as the template. The nested primers cross between exons and would probably not bind to genomic DNA

of RNase H to the tube and incubate at 37°C for 20 min. The cDNA is now ready for PCR amplification or it can be stored at –20°C.

3.5. Selection and Production of Primers (see Note 6)

The cDNA sequences of tyrosinase and many other proteins are available from several sources, including Genbank, Genetic Sequence Database, which can be found at <www.ncbi.nlm.nih.gov/Genbank/GenBankOverview.html.> To amplify the specific marker cDNA of interest, primers that have certain characteristics must be produced (**Fig. 1**).

Choose primers that will give a PCR product between 200 and 2000 bp in length. Primers and primer artifacts will obscure shorter products during gel electrophoresis, and longer products are less efficiently amplified because the polymerase tends to fall off the template during long extensions. To decrease the possibility of the primers amplifying contaminating genomic DNA, choose primers that span an intron. One should attempt to choose primers that are located on separate exons so that the genomic DNA amplification product will be larger than the cDNA product. Avoid primers that may form secondary structures because this could greatly impede the PCR reaction. An algorithm is available to determine when a primer may have the propensity to form secondary structures *(21)*. Try to avoid complementary 3′ ends in the two primers because this can lead to the formation of primer dimers. If possible, choose primers that have annealing temperatures of about 55–65°C. Nested primers increase the sensitivity and specificity of the reaction. Nested primers amplify a region of the cDNA that lies between your first set of primers (**Fig. 1**). Nested primers are used in a second PCR reaction that utilizes the product of the first reaction as the cDNA substrate.

Computer programs are now available to choose the optimal primers for a given cDNA. Many universities also maintain Web sites that will obtain the cDNA sequence from GenBank for you and pick primers based on your requirements. Once the primers have been chosen, they will need to be synthesized for you. Commercial firms are available that will synthesize the primers to your specifications and many universities maintain DNA synthesis core facilities *(13)*.

3.6. Polymerase Chain Reaction (see Notes 7, 8, and 9)

PCR is carried out using a thermostable DNA polymerase, such as *Taq* polymerase, using a thermocycle apparatus that cycles the reaction temperature among primer annealing temperature, primer extension temperature, and denaturation or melting temperature. The optimum temperatures for the three steps in the cycle depend on the primers you choose and the length of the cDNA. The temperatures in our example are optimized for the tyrosinase primers used in the example (**Fig. 2**). To verify the integrity of the mRNA isolated from the specimen, an ubiquitous housekeeping gene is also amplified from each cDNA sample. β-Actin is the most commonly used housekeeping gene, and primers to amplify β-actin are easily obtainable from commercial sources or the sequence of appropriate primers is available in GenBank as well as in the literature *(22)*. If the cDNA sample is negative for β-actin, it is considered to be unreliable and should not be used.

1. Use thin-walled reaction tubes for the PCR reaction. The tubes you use will partially determine the profile of the cycling. We use 0.2-mL, thin-walled, RNase-

Tyrosinase Primers

Human tyrosinase PCR primer HTYR1 (primary sense): ttggcagatt gtctgtagcc

Human tyrosinase PCR primer HTYR2 (primary antisense): aggcattgtg catgctgctt

Human tyrosinase PCR primer HTYR3 (nested sense): gtctttatgc aatggaacgc

Human tyrosinase PCR primer HTYR4 (nested antisense): gctatcccag taagtggact

Fig. 2. Genbank copy of the human tyrosinase PCR primers known as HTYR1-4. Human tyrosinase PCR primers: HTYR1 (primary sense), ttggcagatt gtctgtagcc; HTYR2 (primary antisense), aggcattgtg catgctgctt; HTYR3 (nested sense), gtctttatgc aatggaacgc; HTYR4 (nested antisense), gctatcccag taagtggact.

and DNase-free, polypropylene dome-topped tubes that work with the heated lid of our thermocycler (Labscientific, Livingston, NJ).

2. Place the reaction tubes on ice and add the individual components using aerosol-resistant barrier pipet tips. A separate area should be set aside in the laboratory for setting up the reaction because cross-contamination with environmental DNA can be a problem.

3. A premixed PCR reaction mix that contains 22 mM Tris-HCl (pH 8.4), 55 mM KCl, 1.65 mM MgCl$_2$, 220 µM dGTP, 220 µM dATP, 220 µM dCTP, 220 µM dTTP, 22 U of recombinant *Taq* DNA polymerase, and stabilizers can be used (PCR SuperMix; Life Technologies). Add 45 µL of this mix to each reaction tube.

4. Add 0.5 µL of each primer (200 nM concentration) and 4 µL of the cDNA solution to each tube. The thermocycler should be prewarmed to approx 80°C. Cap the reaction tubes and place in the thermocycler.

5. Start the cycling program: An initial denaturation step of 95°C for 2 to 3 min is followed by the first cycle of denaturation at 94°C for 30 s, primer annealing at 56°C for 30 s, and primer extension at 72°C for 60 s.

6. Repeat the cycle 35 times. Use a final extension step of 72°C for 5–15 min at the end of the run to promote completion of partial extension products and annealing of single-stranded complementary products.

7. Remove the reaction tubes and place on ice for a few minutes before opening the tubes to avoid aerosolization. Centrifuge the tubes for a few seconds to collect the mixture and store the tubes at +4°C until they are analyzed.

8. Now run the nested PCR using the same reagents in **Subheadings 3.6.3.** and **3.6.4.** except use 2 µL of the cDNA from the first PCR reaction instead of the primary cDNA. The denaturation and primer extension temperatures and times are the same as for the first reaction. The annealing temperature is determined by your choice of nested primers. The same annealing temperature and time for both the first and the nested reactions is often appropriate (56°C for 30 s in this example).

3.7. Gel Electrophoresis (see Notes 10, 11, and 12)

The samples and a 100-bp DNA ladder (used to determine the size of the bands) can now be run on a 2% agarose gel containing ethidium bromide. The agarose gel is produced by mixing agarose power in TBE buffer and heating (in a microwave oven or hot plate) to dissolve the agarose. As the agarose solution cools it forms a gel. The cooling agarose is placed in a mold to produce a horizontal gel of the correct thickness (about 1 cm thick) and the cDNA is run on the gel to separate the bands. One to two microliters of ethidium bromide (10 mg/mL) can be placed directly in the gel before it cools, or the gel can be stained after the cDNA has been run. The bands are detected using UV transillumination and photographed using a digital camera, video unit, or a Polaroid camera (**Fig. 3**). In most applications, this method is sufficient to detect the cDNA marker product from your PCR reaction and the nested PCR product *(10,17,23)*. If bands of the correct size for your primary and nested PCR products are present, and the β-actin housekeeping band is also present, you can assume that you have the correct cDNA and that the marker is present in your tissue. If the β-actin band is present but the primary and nested bands are missing, you can assume that the marker is not present in your sample. If the primary PCR product band is present but the nested marker is absent, you may have amplified an unrelated cDNA or contaminating genomic DNA. If the β-actin band is not present, you cannot rely on the quality of the extracted mRNA even if a band does show up in the marker or nested PCR product lanes *(10,13,17,22,23)*, *See* **Notes 13, 14,** and **15** for same thoughts on the clinical utility of this RT-PCR analysis.

4. Notes

1. The use of liquid nitrogen for tissue preservation is an easy and rapid method that stops RNase reactions and allows delayed transport to the laboratory while the operation is in progress. However, not all facilities have ready access to liquid nitrogen stores and the personal needed to maintain them. An alternative method of lymph node preservation is the use of dry-ice slurries. Dry ice is often easily obtainable from the pathology department and the addition of 70% ethanol to the dry ice makes for an acceptable freezing medium. The specimen is transported immediately to the back table in the operating room and bivalved as before. The portion to be used for RT-PCR is placed in a plastic container and then submerged in the dry ice/ethanol slurry. This will rapidly drop the temperature of the specimen to –20 to –30°C, and it can then be transferred to the laboratory. Problems with this technique are that the freezing temperature is less than ideal and that the mixture is flammable. This limits the time the specimen can sit before transfer and increases the risk that the mRNA will be degraded. Another alternative method for preserving the lymph node tissue is the immediate immersion of

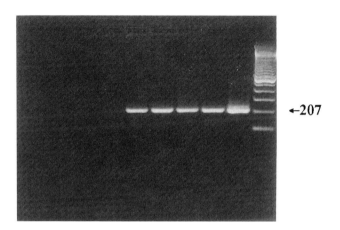

Fig. 3. An ethidium bromide–stained gel electrophoresis of the PCR products from lymph node and cell line mRNA using nested tyrosinase primers and a DNA ladder (M). The nested primers should produce a product with a band at 207 bp. Lane 2, breast cancer cell line; lane 3, colon cancer cell line; lane 4, normal lymph node; lanes 5 and 6, histologically positive SLNs from patient with melanoma; lanes 7 and 8, histologically negative SLNs from patient with melanoma; lane 9, melanoma cell line. Lane 1 is blank.

    the tissue in the Trizol solution, in the operating room, and immediate processing. This technique decreases the possibility that the mRNA will be degraded but requires that a toxic substance be transported to and from the operating room as well as someone to be available for the transport and immediate processing of the tissue.

2. Another potential problem with the harvesting and preservation of the tissue is that excess fat and connective tissue may interfere with the extraction of the nodal RNA. We believe that it is important that all excess fat and surrounding tissue be carefully dissected away from the nodal tissue in the operating room prior to preservation. This can be distracting and time-consuming and is often neglected in the midst of an ongoing operation. However, with practice the lymph node tissue in the operating room can be processed expediently and will yield better results.

3. When working with RNA and DNA, several environmental issues need to be addressed. RNases and DNases are ubiquitous—they are present on your hands, on the bench top, on glassware and plasticware, and just about any other surface in your laboratory. It is very easy to inadvertently introduce these enzymes into your reactions, with often devastating results. In addition, DNA can contaminate your specimens and reaction mixtures and lead to erroneous results. Several pre-

cautions and environmental isolation techniques are necessary in any laboratory that intends to perform RT-PCR *(11,15)*:

a. Physical isolation of the separate parts of the process should be a routine procedure and can not be overemphasized. The tissue processing should be carried out as far away as possible from the area designated for reverse transcription and PCR reactions. Gel electrophoresis should be done in a third location using dedicated equipment.

b. All glassware should be processed to ensure freedom from RNases and DNases and plasticware should be certified RNase and DNase free. This includes pipet tips, tubes, and storage containers.

c. Dedicated pipets, water baths, and benchtop areas should be used when possible. Alternatively, these instruments and areas can be cleaned with reagents that destroy RNases and DNases.

d. If erroneous or uninterpretable results are obtained during the RT-PCR process, the first thing that should be done is to search for a breach in these environmental rules. A pipet that was borrowed by a colleague or a contaminated work space is often the culprit.

4. The method that we describe to extract total RNA from lymph nodes and blood utilizes a common technique first described by Chomczynski and Sacchi *(20)*. The Trizol method works well because the tissue is liquified in the same tube as the separation of the RNA from the other cellular elements. The mixture has strong anti-RNase activity, and, thus, the frozen tissue is thawed in an environment that preserves the RNA. However, the Trizol reagent is extremely toxic and must be handled carefully. The manual grinding of the tissue can produce splashing and contamination and needs to be performed in a chemical hood. An alternative method of extracting the RNA from the tissue is to use a closed system that utilizes the same extraction schema. We have found that the FastRNA-Green Kit in conjunction with the FastPrep Tissue lysis apparatus (BIO 101, Vista, CA) extracts RNA as efficiently as the Trizol reagent but without the added danger of handling the reagents during processing. With this kit you place a chaotropic RNA stabilizing agent, a phenol acid reagent, and chloroform isoamyl alcohol in a tube containing a matrix material that is used to grind the tissue. The frozen specimen is then placed in the tube and the tube is placed in an apparatus that agitates the tube. The tissue is lysed within 20–40 s and the heat of the reaction further denatures contaminating RNases. The total RNA is then extracted from the mixture in a similar fashion as in the Trizol reaction. We have found that this is an excellent method to extract RNA from tissues, especially when multiple samples need to be processed at once. Drawbacks include the need to purchase the FastPrep machine and the need to transfer the material from tube to tube during processing, which can add pipeting errors and contamination risks to the procedure *(24)*.

5. First-strand cDNA synthesis is one of the least demanding portions of the RT-PCR process but is also the part that can lead to the most problems. First, the

mRNA is very susceptible to degradation by contaminating RNases and precautions must be taken to minimize this risk (*see* **Note 3**). Second, mRNA transcripts that contain a high GC content can have secondary structures that limit the reverse transcription process. To avoid secondary mRNA structure, you may need to increase the reaction temperatures and avoid cooling the mixture until the cDNA is transcribed. Using the First-Strand Synthesis Kit, you can change the reaction as follows:

   a. Transfer the RNA/oligo(dT) mixture from the initial 70°C water bath to a 50°C water bath instead of cooling on ice.
   b. Prewarm the reaction mix to 42°C before adding it to the RNA/primer mix (which is at 50°C). The components of the reaction mix are increased in volume and DEPC-treated water is added to increase the volume of the reaction. Use 30 µL of DEPC-treated water, 30 µL of 10X PCR buffer, 30 µL of 25 mM MgCl$_2$, 10 µL of 10 mM dNTP mix, and 30 µL of 0.1 M DTT. Add 25 µL of this mix to the RNA/oligo(dT) mixture.
   c. The RT reaction will now take place at 50°C for 50 min.

   Third, if you detect the possible contamination of the cDNA with genomic DNA, you need to treat the mRNA with DNase prior to the RT reaction. To do this you need an amplification grade DNase I (available from Gibco-BRL) or you need to use an RNase inhibitor because some DNases also degrade RNA. For 1 to 2 µg of total RNA, use 1 µL of a 10X reaction buffer (200 mM Tris-HCl [pH 8.4], 500 mM KCl, and 20 mM MgCl$_2$), 1 µL of DNase, and 10 µL of DEPC-treated water. Incubate at room temperature for 15 min. Add 1 µL of 25 mM EDTA and then terminate the reaction at 65°C for 15 min. Chill on ice for 1 min and then proceed with the RT reaction.

6. As stated in the **Subheading 3.**, you can obtain the cDNA sequence of the marker protein of interest and produce primers using one of a number of computer programs. However, even though the primers look good on paper, this does not mean that they will work well in your application. If the primers you choose do not work as well as planned, you may need to start from scratch and redesign the primers. If the marker you are interested in is unique, and has never before been used in RT-PCR reactions, then this is the best process to follow to obtain the best primers. However, if the marker protein has been amplified previously with primers that have worked well, it is always easier and more cost-effective to use these same primers in your reactions. The primer sequences that amplify cDNA from a number of common marker proteins including tyrosinase, MART-1, and gp100 are available in the literature and some are even available from GenBank. The tyrosinase primers that we describe in **Subheading 3.** have been published previously *(19)*. We found that a slightly different PCR cycle worked best for these primers in our particular thermocycler. This is often the case, and experimentation with even well-characterized primers is usually necessary.

7. We like to use a premixed combination of components for our PCR reaction because this saves time and eliminates pipeting errors and the chance of contamination. The components in the mixture include the *Taq* polymerase, the dNTPs,

and the magnesium-containing reaction buffer. An alternative to the use of this PCR mix is to use separate components added one at a time. The advantages of the separate component method is that you have more flexibility in the composition of your mix. You can use a different polymerase, such as Vent or Pwo polymerase, either of which may work better in your PCR reaction. You also have more flexibility in the amount of magnesium you add, which is an important component of the mixture. If you have too much primer and cDNA template in your mixture, you may deplete the magnesium, which could lead to low yields.

8. Two other problems that plague some PCR reactions are evaporation of the reaction mix owing to the high temperatures and uneven heating of the reaction tubes. We use a thermocycler with a heated top and also use domed reaction tubes. This decreases the possibility of either of these two problems occurring. If you have an older thermocycler, you may need to add a layer of mineral or silicone oil to the top of the contents of the tubes to decrease evaporation. Some thermocyclers also require the use of oil around the tubes to heat the reaction mix evenly. However, this is rarely used today because the thin-walled tubes fit well in the thermocycler wells and heated tops also even out the heating cycle.

9. What we have described in **Subheading 3.** is the traditional two-tube, two-enzyme method that first produces the cDNA from the mRNA and then uses a separate tube and enzyme to perform the PCR. There are advantages to this method: flexibility, because different conditions and enzymes can be used for the different steps; decreased cost, because only small amounts of the enzymes are needed; the ability to stop after the RT step and store the cDNA for long periods of time; the ease of troubleshooting, because the reactions are separated; and the long track record in the literature that this method enjoys. However, the two-tube, two-enzyme method is time-consuming and multiple tubes and pipet steps increase the likelihood that contamination will occur. In an attempt to minimize the possibility of contamination and to make the reactions easier to perform, several one-tube RT-PCR kits have been developed. Two main techniques have been described *(23,25–27)*:

   a. The one-enzyme, one-tube technique utilizes the *Tth* DNA polymerase. This unique DNA polymerase has intrinsic RT activity and can be used for both the RT and the PCR portions of the reaction. The biggest advantage, beyond the use of fewer pipet steps and the use of only one tube, is that the RT reaction can be carried out at higher temperatures, which decreases problems with secondary structure formation by the mRNA *(26)*. One disadvantage to this system is that the RT reaction requires the presence of manganese ions and the PCR reaction requires the presence of magnesium ions. This requires the opening of the tube for the addition of a different buffer prior to the PCR portion of the reaction. This problem has been partially alleviated by the development of buffers that can be used for both the RT and PCR portions of the reaction. Another problem is the limit *Tth* places on the length of the RT-PCR product; generally, *Tth* can produce only a 1-kb product, but further refinements of the technique are also addressing this limitation. Finally, this is the most expensive method because a large amount of the *Tth* polymerase is needed.

b. The second technique is the two-enzyme, one-tube reaction. This technique uses different enzymes for the RT and PCR portions of the reaction. It also uses RT and one or sometimes multiple DNA polymerases in a reaction buffer optimized for both types of enzyme. Advantages include amplification of longer products and the ability to use DNA polymerases with lower error rates. Disadvantages include the use of lower temperatures for the RT portion of the reaction, which could lead to interference by mRNA with secondary structure (*see* **Note 5**), and the inability to store the cDNA for any period of time because of the possible degradation of the DNA polymerase during storage *(27)*.

A recent comparison of these three methods was reported by Sellner and Turbett *(23)*. They found that the one-tube, two-enzyme method was the most sensitive, followed by the two-tube, two-enzyme method, and then the one-tube, one-enzyme method. We have successfully used the uncoupled two-tube, two-enzyme method and the one-tube, two-enzyme method and have found no difference in the sensitivity of these techniques. The one-tube methods are certainly faster and less cumbersome but lack flexibility. If you are using a standard primer set to detect a marker in a large number of different specimens, we suggest that you try one of the one-tube methods.

10. This is a straightforward method for isolating DNA fragments for identification. The only important things to remember during gel electrophoresis concern safety precautions and interpretation of the bands. Ethidium bromide is used to tag the DNA fragments in the gel by binding to the DNA and fluorescing under UV light. Ethidium bromide is toxic and should be handled with care. Gels should be discarded in the proper containers, and gloves should always be worn when working with this substance. The determination of the size of the DNA fragments is done by comparing the location of the band on the gel to the standard DNA ladder that is run on the same gel. Different running speeds of the bands can occur if the gel is not uniform in thickness and density. Letting the agarose cool to a temperature that allows you to handle the container with only latex gloves prior to pouring the gel will keep the gel from warping the gel apparatus and decrease inconsistencies in the density of the gel. Use a voltage that slowly separates the DNA fragments and a gel that is long enough to easily discern the different bands.

11. When using nested primers, it is only really necessary to run the PCR product from the nested run. We usually run both the nested and primary PCR products to determine whether we are getting the proper results in both PCR steps as a quality control device. If we detect a band of the correct size in the primary reaction but not in the nested reaction, we repeat the nested reaction and run a Southern blot on the primary band (*see* **Note 12**).

12. To determine more accurately that you have amplified the correct marker cDNA and to detect very small amounts of the PCR products, it is often necessary to

employ a more sensitive and specific detection method than ethidium bromide–stained agarose gel electrophoresis. One method that can be used is Southern blotting. In this technique, an oligonucleotide probe is manufactured that can hybridize to the cDNA of interest. The cDNA is transferred by capillary action by blotting the agarose gel with a filter membrane made of nitrocellulose or nylon. UV crosslinking or baking fixes the cDNA to the membrane, and then labeled oligonucleotide probe is hybridized to the cDNA in the membrane. The probe is then detected by exposing X-ray film. The traditional method utilizes a radio-labeled oligonucleotide produced using a sample of the marker cDNA and specific primers. The PCR reaction is carried out as before except a radiolabeled deoxynucleoside, such as tritiated thymidine, is used in the reaction. We generally us a nonradioactive, chemiluminescent Southern blot technique that does not require the production of radioactive PCR products. The advantage of this method, aside from avoiding the use of radioactive compounds, is that the labeled oligonucleotide probe can be manufactured in large quantities and stored for long periods. We employ a method that adds digoxigenin-11-dUTP residues to the 3′ end of our oligonuclotide using the enzyme terminal transferase (3′ Tailing Kit; Roche Molecular Biochemicals). Digoxigenin is a chemiluminescent compound that produces a light signal that can be detected on X-ray films using a detection kit. Use a 25- to 30-bp homologous DNA sequence, produced in the same way as the PCR primers, as the oligonucleotide probe. Examine the section of cDNA that you will be amplifying and pick an appropriate region that will be present in both the primary PCR product and the nested product. The oligonucleotide can be produced by a university's DNA synthesis facility or by a commercial facility. The use of Southern blotting adds an order of magnitude to the sensitivity and specificity of the detection of marker cDNA. Southern blotting should be used as an adjunct to ethidium bromide gel electrophoresis.

13. The usefulness of RT-PCR analysis of peripheral blood and lymph node tissue for the detection of clinically significant metastatic cancer is being studied. Muhlbauer et al. *(28)* have shown that they can detect melanoma-inhibitory activity mRNA in the peripheral blood of melanoma patients. They found a correlation between positive samples and tumor burden in stage III and IV patients but concluded that melanoma-inhibitory activity RT-PCR was of little value as a surrogate marker for clinical staging or the detection of metastatic disease. Mellado et al. *(29)* reported that they could detect tyrosinase mRNA in peripheral blood and that a positive tyrosinase RT-PCR result correlated with a significantly shorter disease-free and overall survival in patients with stage III and IV disease. Keilholz *(30)* summarized the results of seven studies of RT-PCR detection of circulating melanoma cells. Although most of the studies were able to use RT-PCR analysis of the peripheral blood to detect circulating melanoma cells, some found a correlation with stage of disease *(11,12,19,31,32)*, whereas others did not *(33,34)*. He concluded that there was too wide a variation in the reported incidence of circulating cells in patients of similar stage and that quality control

standards need to be designed and implemented. It is probably too soon to know whether the detection of circulating melanoma cells by RT-PCR will be clinically useful, and larger trials, such as the ongoing Sunbelt Melanoma Trial, are needed to answer this important area of question *(35)*.

14. The clinical significance of the detection of melanoma markers in SLNs is also under study. Palpable lymph nodes often contain grossly visible melanoma metastases but SLNs are, by definition, nonpalpable and should contain much smaller amounts of melanoma. A recent study by Wagner et al. *(36)* examined the typical tumor burden found in histologically positive SLNs. They found that most SLNs contain minute tumor volumes but that primary tumor thickness and the pattern of SLN metastases may not be predictive of tumor burden or the presence of positive non-SLNs. Another area that needed to be investigated was whether or not the minute amounts of tumor found in SLNs represented active metastatic disease or simply shed tumor cells of little malignant potential. Scheunemann et al. *(37)* addressed this area of question by detecting minute quantities of tumor cells in lymph nodes and then showing that these cells could produce progressive tumor nodules in severe combined immunodeficiency disease mice. They concluded that minute amounts of tumor sometimes found in lymph nodes could represent clinically significant disease. Several groups have now shown that they can detect melanoma markers in SLNs using RT-PCR *(10,13,38,39)*. These studies have shown that histologically positive SLNs are almost universally positive by RT-PCR for tyrosinase and other melanoma markers. The incidence of histologically negative but RT-PCR positive lymph nodes varied between 12 and 65%. The clinical significance of these histologically negative but RT-PCR positive lymph nodes has recently been examined by Shivers et al. *(10)*. They found that patients with histologically positive SLNs (all of which were also positive by RT-PCR analysis for tyrosinase) had a 61% recurrence rate with a mean follow-up of 28 mo. Patients with histologically negative and RT-PCR negative SLNs had a 1% recurrence rate and those who were histologically negative but RT-PCR positive had a 13% recurrence rate within the same follow-up period. This shows a statistically significant increase in recurrence detected solely by RT-PCR analysis *(10)*.

15. Large prospective, randomized trials are under way that will address the clinical significance of RT-PCR analysis of peripheral blood and SLNs in patients with melanoma. Until the results of these trials are available we must continue to develop quality standards and search for more specific and sensitive markers for melanoma and other malignancies *(35,40,41)*. RT-PCR analysis is poised to become a significant component of staging systems, and treatment protocols and standards are needed to ensure comparable results.

References

1. Balch, C. M., Murad, T. M., and Soong, S. J. (1979) Tumor thickness as a guide to surgical management of clinical stage I patients. *Cancer* **43**, 883–888.

2. Balch, C. M., Soong, S. J., Bartolucci, A. A., et al. (1996) Efficacy of an elective regional lymph node dissection of 1–4 mm thick melanomas for patients 60 years of age and younger. *Ann. Surg.* **224,** 255–266.

3. Ross, M. I. (1992) The case for elective lymphadenectomy. *Surg. Oncol. Clin. North Am.* **1,** 205.

4. Morton, D. L., Wen, D.-R., Wong, J.H., et al. (1992) Technical details of intraoperative lymphatic mapping for early stage melanoma *Arch. Surg.* **127,** 392–399.

5. Morton, D. L. and Chan, A. D. (1999) Current status of intraoperative lymphatic mapping and sentinel lymphadenectomy for melanoma: is it standard of care? *J. Am. Coll. Surg.* **189,** 214–223.

6. Ross, M. I., Reintgen, D., and Balch, C. M. (1993) Selective lymphadenectomy: emerging role for lymphatic mapping and sentinel node biopsy in the management of early stage melanoma. *Semin. Surg. Oncol.* **9,** 219–223.

7. Krag, D. N., Meijer, S. J., Weaver, D. L., et al. (1995) Minimal-access surgery for staging of malignant melanoma. *Arch. Surg.* **130,** 654–660.

8. Essner, R., Conforti, A., Kelley, M. C., et al. (1999) Efficacy of lymphatic mapping, sentinel lymphadenectomy, and selective complete lymph node dissection as a therapeutic procedure for early-stage melanoma. *Ann. Surg. Oncol.* **6,** 442–449.

9. Emilia, J. C. D. and Lawrence, W. J. (1997) Sentinel lymph node biopsy in malignant melanoma: the standard of care? *J. Surg. Oncol.* **65,** 153,154.

10. Shivers, S. C., Xiangning, W., Weiguo, L., et al. (1998) Molecular staging of malignant melanoma: correlation with clinical outcome. *JAMA* **280,** 1410–1415.

11. Mellado, B., Colomer, D., Castel, T., et al. (1996) Detection of circulating neoplastic cells by reverse-transcriptase polymerase chain reaction in malignant melanoma: association with clinical stage and prognosis. *J. Clin. Oncol.* **14,** 2091–2097.

12. Brossart, P., Keilholz, U., Willhauck, M., et al. (1993) Hematogenous spread of malignant melanoma cells in in different stages of disease. *J. Invest. Dermatol.* **101,** 887–889.

13. Goydos, J. S., Ravikumar, T. S., Germino, F. J., et al. (1998) Minimally invasive staging of patients with melanoma: sentinel lymphadenectomy and detection of the melanoma-specific proteins MART-1 and tyrosinase by reverse transcriptase polymerase chain reaction. *J. Am. Coll. Surg.* **187,** 182–190.

14. Wang, X., Heller, R., Van Voorhis, N., et al. (1994) Detection of submicroscopic lymph node metastases with polymerase chain reaction in patients with malignant melanoma. *Ann. Surg.* **220,** 768–774.

15. Sarantou, T., Chi, D. D. J., Garrison, D. A., et al. (1997) Melanoma-associated antigens as messenger RNA detection markers for melanoma. *Cancer. Res.* **57,** 1371–1376.

16. Waldmann, V., Deichmann, M., Bock, M., et al. (1999) The detection of tyrosinase-specific mRNA in bone marrow is not more sensitive than in blood for the demonstration of micrometastatic melanoma. *Br. J. Dermatol.* **140,** 1060–1064.

17. Schittek, B., Blaheta, H.-J., Florchinger, G., et al. (1999) Increased sensitivity for the detection of malignant melanoma cells in perpheral blood using an improved protocol for reverse transcription-polymerase chain reaction. *Br. J. Dermatol.* **141,** 37–43.

18. Carson, K. F., Wen, D. R., Li, P. X., et al. (1996) Nodal nevi and cutaneous melanomas. *Am. J. Surg. Pathol.* **20,** 834–840.

19. Smith, B., Selby, P., Southgate, K., et al. (1991) Detection of melanoma cells in peripheral blood by means of reverse transcriptase and polymerase chain reaction *Lancet* **338,** 1227–1229.

20. Chomczynski, P. and Sacchi, N. (1987) Single-step method of RNA isolation by acid guanidinium thiocyanate-phenol-chloroform extraction. *Anal. Biochem.* **62,** 156–159.

21. Pallansch, L., Beswick, H., Talian, J., et al. (1990) Use of an RNA folding algorithm to choose regions for amplification by the polymerase chain reaction. *Anal. Biochem.* **185,** 57–62.

22. Kwon, B. S., Haq, A. K., Pomerantz, S. H., et al. (1987) Isolation and sequence of a cDNA clone for human tyrosinase that maps at the mouse c-albino locus. *Proc. Natl. Acad. Sci. USA* **84,** 7473–7477.

23. Sellner, L. N. and Turbett, G. R. (1998) Comparison of three RT-PCR methods. *BioTechniques* **25,** 230–234.

24. Dana, R. C., Saghbini, M., Lippman, D., et al. (1995) Isolating RNA using the new FastPrep system. *NIH Res.* **7,** 61.

25. Seller, L. N., Coelen, R. J., and Mackenzie, J. S. (1992) A one-tube, one manipulation RT-PCR reaction for detection of Ross River virus. *J. Virol. Methods.* **40,** 255–264.

26. Myers, T. W. and Gelfand, D. H. (1991) Reverse transcription and DNA amplification by a Thermus thermophilus DNA polymerase. *Biochemistry* **30,** 7661–7666.

27. Mallet, F., Oriol, G., Mary, C., et al. (1995) Continuous RT-PCR using AMV-RT and Taq DNA polymerase: characterization and comparison to uncoupled procedures. *BioTechniques* **18,** 678–687.

28. Muhlbauer, M., Langenbach, N., Stolz, W., et al. (1999) Detection of melanoma cells in the blood of melanoma patients by melanoma-inhibitory activity (MIA) reverse transcriptase-PCR. *Clin. Cancer Res.* **5,** 1099–1105.

29. Mellado, B., Gutierrez, L., Castel, T., et al. (1999) Prognostic significance of the detection of circulating malignant cells by reverse transcriptase-polymerase chain reaction in long-term clinically disease-free melanoma patients. *Clin. Cancer Res.* **5,** 1843–1848.

30. Keilholz, U. (1999) Debate: is RT-PCR useful for monitoring of the melanoma tumor burden in blood? in *Perspectives in Melanoma III* (John M. Kirkwood, ed.), New Orleans, LA, pp. 21–23.

31. Hoon, D. S. B., Wang, Y., Dale, P. S., et al. (1995) Detection of occult melanoma cells in blood with a multiple-marker polymerase chain reaction assay. *J. Clin. Oncol.* **13,** 2109–2116.

32. Battyani, Z., Grob, J., Xerri, L., et al. (1995) PCR detection of occult melanoma cells in blood with a multiple-marker polymerase chain reaction assay. *J. Clin. Oncol.* **131,** 443–447.

33. Foss, A. J., Guille, M. J., Occleston, N. L., et al. (1995) The detection of melanoma cells in peripheral blood by reverse transcriptase-polymerase chain reaction. *Br. J. Cancer* **72,** 155–159.

34. Reinhold, U., Ludtke-Handjery, H. C., Schnautz, S., et al. (1997) The analysis of tyrosinase-specific mRNA in blood samples of melanoma patients by RT-PCR is not a useful test for metastatic tumor progression. *J. Invest. Dermatol.* **108,** 166–169.

35. Buzaid, A. C. and Balch, C. M. (1996) Polymerase chain reaction of melanoma in peripheral blood: too early to assess clinical value. *J. Natl. Cancer Inst.* **88,** 569–570.

36. Wagner, J. D., Davidson, D., Coleman, J. J., et al. (1999) Lymph node tumor volumes in patients undergoing sentinel lymph node biopsy for cutaneous melanoma. *Ann. Surg. Oncol.* **6,** 398–404.

37. Scheunemann, P., Izbicki, J. R., and Pantel, K. (1999) Tumorigenic potential of apparently tumor-free lymph nodes. *N. Engl. J. Med.* **340,** 1687.

38. Bieligk, S. C., Ghossein, R., Bhattacharya, S., et al. (1999) Detection of tyrosinase mRNA by reverse transcription-polymerase chain reaction in melanoma sentinel nodes. *Ann. Surg. Oncol.* **6,** 232–240.

39. Blaheta, H. J., Schittek, B., Breuninger, H., et al. (1999) Detection of melanoma micrometastasis in sentinel nodes by reverse transcription-polymerase chain reaction correlates with tumor thickness and is predictive of micrometastatic disease in the lymph node basin. *Am. J. Surg. Pathol.* **23,** 822–828.

40. Keilholz, U., Willhauck, M., Rimoldi, D., et al. (1998) reliability of RT-PCR-based assays for detection of circulating tumor cells. *Eur. J. Cancer* **34,** 750–753.

41. Keilholz, U. (1996) Diagnostic PCR in melanoma: methods and quality assurance. *Eur. J. Cancer* **32,** 1661–1663.

18

Immunoscope Analysis of T-Lymphocytes Infiltrating Melanocytic Tumors

Philippe Musette, Jos Even, Louis Dubertret, Philippe Kourilsky, and Gabriel Gachelin

1. Introduction

Melanomas are most frequently infiltrated by actively proliferating T-lymphocytes (1). Some of these T-cells are cytolytic and recognize peptide antigens derived from melanoma-specific antigens (2). However, with the noteworthy exception of rare immune-mediated, sponaneous regressions of melanomas (3), or in the particular case of the halo nevus phenomenon in which normal melanocytes are killed by CD8$^+$-specific T-cells (4), the ongoing melanocyte-specific T-cell responses are most frequently incapable of controlling the growth of the tumor, resulting in the malignant melanocytic tumors escaping an otherwise specific immune T-cell response. The understanding of the mechanisms that underlie the switch of efficient to inefficient (and vice versa) T-cell responses is thus of primary importance in conceiving specific immunotherapies of melanomas.

In recent years, research has focused on the identification of melanoma-specific antigens (reviewed in **refs. 5** and **6**) and on the identification of the melanoma-specific T-cell clones infiltrating melanocytic tumors that are potentially able to drive an efficient killer response (2). Concerning the identification of melanoma-specific T-cells, several strategies have been used, ranging from extensive T-cell cloning to systematic sequencing of all polymerase chain reaction (PCR) products derived from the mRNAs encoding the T-cell receptor (TCR) α- and β-chains of the T-cells that infiltrate the tumor. The various biases to representativity introduced by cell cloning are well known. Only the direct identification of T clones undergoing local expansions is able

From: *Methods in Molecular Medicine, Vol. 61: Melanoma: Methods and Protocols*
Edited by: B. J. Nickoloff © Humana Press Inc., Totowa, NJ

to avoid or minimize the numerous biases introduced by cell culture and cloning *(7)*. The quantification of the TCRBV and AV uses by fluorescence-activated cell sorter (FACS) analysis does not generate an accurate picture of antigen-driven T-cell responses because the number of cells recovered from the tumors is usually low, and it identifies only those T-cell populations that exceed 0.1–0.5% of the total at best, a value sufficient for identifying marked T-cell expansions, but insufficient for monitoring specific T-cell responses in blood, and *a fortiori* for monitoring circulating memory T-cells. Finally, the monitoring of specific T-cell clones is nearly impossible if one excepts the growing use of peptide-loaded major histocompatibility complex (MHC) I and II tetramers *(8)*, whose sensitivity, however, is in the same range as FACS analysis. Alternative techniques have thus been designed to describe the T-cell repertoire in tumor-infiltrating lymphocytes (TILs) and in various other pathologic conditions. In view of our present knowledge of the size of T-cell clonal populations in peripheral blood in humans *(9)*, only PCR-derived techniques are sensitive and versatile enough to identify small-scale T-cell expansions. In these circumstances, most, but not all, the alternative techniques used to define the locally expanded T-cell clone candidates for further functional investigation are thus PCR based. We developed the Immunoscope® technique *(10–12)*, a semiquantitative method aimed at approaching the overall diversity of the CDR3 region length of the β-chain of the TCR of T-cells contained in as few as 10,000 T-cells. The methods used in achieving this goal are discussed next.

1.1. Proper Sampling

The Immunoscope technique was developed to generate some kind of a "snapshot" of T-cell populations by minimizing the number of steps between the biopsy and the experiment. To avoid the selective pressures owing to T-cell culture in vitro and also to prevent degradation of mRNA, the biopsies are immediately frozen in liquid nitrogen following surgery. Peripheral blood lymphocytes (PBLs) are harvested by Ficoll fractionation, or after red blood cell lysis, and immediately frozen in liquid nitrogen. The samples are kept at –78°C. Alternatively, the tissues can be homogenized in the lysing buffer (*see* **Subheading 3.2.2.**) and kept frozen.

1.2. Exhaustive RNA Extraction

Minimize losses of infrequent mRNAs, total RNA (in order to better protect the mRNA) is preferred over polyA+ mRNA *(13)*.

1.3. Adequate cDNA Synthesis

The unstable mRNA is reverse transcribed into more stable cDNA. The quality of the cDNA and its relative amount are determined by assaying the actin of

HGPRT mRNA contents, and the amount of mRNA related to T-cells is determined by assaying the CD3δ mRNA content by quantitative PCR *(12,14)*.

1.4. PCR Amplification of BV-BC cDNA Sequences

The resulting cDNAs are PCR amplified slightly below saturation, using each of the BV-specific primers and a unique BC-primer.

1.5. Analysis of BV-BC PCR Products by Runoff Elongations Using Specific Primers

The preceding procedure generates 24 independent samples. Each BV-BC amplification product is subjected to a primer extension reaction using either an internal fluorescently labeled BC-specific primer or each of the 13 fluorescently labeled BJ-specific primers. The fluorescent "runoff" DNA encompasses the CDR3 region of the β-chain of the TCR, the region that recognizes the antigenic peptides bound to MHC molecules. The runoff products are analyzed in an automated DNA sequencer to determine the length of the spectrum of the CDR3 regions, as well as the intensity of fluorescence of each peak. The distribution of the intensity of fluorescence as a function of the CDR3 length yields a Gaussian pattern in complex T-cell populations such as PBLs, whereas antigen-driven responses yield preeminent peaks, which distort the Gaussian distribution and are indicative of expanded T-cell populations *(10)*. This generates up to 2000 independent signals (i.e., 2000 independent peaks) out of as few as 10,000 T-cells. The signals can be made quantitative by quantitating the genuine T-cell-specific mRNA content on the basis of the CD3δ mRNA content of the crude extract *(15)* or any other quantitative PCR-based method.

1.6. Generation of Clone-Specific (Clonotypic) Primers for In Vivo Follow-up of Clones

The DNA of the β-chains of the T-cells undergoing expansion (expanded peaks of a given CDR3 size) can be eluted from the gels, PCR amplified, cloned, and sequenced (the second generation of the Immunoscope is based on the additional systematic sequencing of the PCR products of interest, a technique not described herein). Alternatively, the DNA contained in expanded peaks can be directly sequenced or cloned and the clones sequenced without an additional PCR step. From the nucleotide sequence of the expanded β-chains, clonotypic probes extending from BJ into the CDR3 sequence can be designed, labeled with a fluorescent dye, and used instead of a LB2 J-specific primer in a primer extension reaction: these more selective primers provide a 10-fold increase in the resolution power of the technique *(11,16)*. Clonotypes have been used to monitor T-cells in a variety of pathologic conditions *(16–18)* and to identify the T-cells that share the same TCR β-chain, i.e, either individual clones if a unique α-chain is associated to the thus defined TCR β-chain, or a maximum of 25 different T-cell clones, since, according to recent data obtained in the laboratory, an average of 25 different α-chains can associate to a given β-chain in peripheral T-cells *(9)*.

1.7. Previous Uses of Immunoscope Technique

The Immunoscope technique has been routinely used for identifying T-cell clones in a variety of human diseases, such as rheumatoid arthritis *(14,18)*, multiple sclerosis *(16)*, renal cell carcinoma *(19)*, bladder carcinoma *(20)*, infection by Epstein-Barr virus *(14)*, human immunodeficiency virus *(21)*, and influenza virus *(22)*. Several studies on the T-cells that infiltrate melanocytic tumors have been conducted using the Immunoscope approach (reviewed in **ref. 23**). The complex behavior of the T-cells infiltrating melanomas was studied and T-cell clones undergoing expansion were characterized, some of which were found infiltrating all tumor sites of the same patient *(24)*. We have recently analyzed the diversity of the β-chains of the TCR used by the T-cells that infiltrate nevi undergoing immune-mediated regression *(25)*. An Immunoscope-based strategy aimed at the description of the T-cells relevant to the specific antimelanoma response has been recently discussed *(26)*. Finally, the same strategy, although made more complex by the number of AV and AJ segments, is applicable to the study of the TCR α-chains.

The Immunoscope approach has been adapted to any system showing a highly complex diversity of genetic origin relative to human γ/δ T-cells in normal and pathologic conditions *(27)*. The only prerequisite for such analyses is the availability of exhaustive data sets of the nucleotide sequences of the system under study.

2. Materials
2.1. Preparation of Samples

1. Liquid N$_2$
2. Ficoll PBL fractionation kit.

2.2. Extraction of Rna

1. Poly A$^+$ or total RNA extraction kit.
2. Extraction solution: 4 *M* guanidinium isothiocyanate, 25 m*M* sodium citrate, pH 7.0, 0.5% Na *N*-laurylsarcosinate, 0.1 *M* 2-mercaptoethanol.
3. 5.7 *M* CsCl in 25 m*M* Na acetate, pH 5.2, 10 m*M* Na EDTA, pH 8.0.
4. 2.4 *M* CsCl in 25 m*M* Na acetate, pH 5.2, 10 m*M* Na EDTA, pH 8.0.
5. Diethylpyrocarbonate (DEPC).
6. DEPC-treated water.

7. 2 *M* Na acetate, pH 4.0.
8. Isopropanol.
9. 70% Ethanol.
10. Tissue grinder.
11. High-speed ultracentrifuge.
12. Low-speed centrifuge.
13. Speed-vac or equivalent.

2.3. Reverse Transcription

1. Kit for reverse transcription (e.g., Boehringer-Mannheim, Germany).
2. AMV reverse transcriptase (Boehringer Mannheim) and its proper buffer.
3. 15-mer Oligo dT primer, 50 µ*M* solution in water.
4. RNAsin (Promega or other sources).
5. dNTP (Pharmacia) mix: 10 m*M* final each.
6. Water bath.
7. Low-speed centrifuge.

2.4. cDNA Amplification: Generation of Primary BV-BC PCR Products

1. Set of all BV-specific primers (available in a kit developed by Applied BioSystems, Foster City, CA, or designed according to **Table 1**).
2. BC-specific primer.
3. *Taq* polymerase and its proper buffer.
4. *Pfu* polymerase and its proper buffer.
5. dNTP stock solutions (10 m*M*) (Pharmacia).
6. Stock solution of $MgCl_2$ (25 m*M*).
7. PCR thermocycler accepting 96-well plates.
8. 96-well plates and plate covers.
9. Multichannel pipet (12-tip).
10. Setup for agarose gel electrophoresis.

2.5. Runoff Elongations and Analysis of TCR β-Chain Diversity

1. Stock solution of 10 m*M* dNTP (Pharmacia).
2. $MgCl^{2+}$ stock solution (25 m*M*).
3. Fluorescently labeled BC primer.
4. Fluorescently labeled BJ primers.
5. EDTA (20 m*M*).
6. Formamide.
7. *Taq* polymerase and its buffer.
8. PCR thermocycler accepting 96-well plates.
9. 96-well plates and sealers (Costar, Cambridge MA).
10. Multichannel pipet.

Table 1
BV and BC PCR Primers

Primer	Sequence	Distance (bases) to codon 95
BV1	5'-CCGCACAACAGTTCCCTGACTTGC-3'	86
BV2	5'-CACAACTATGTTTTGGTATCGTC-3'	199
BV3	5'-CGCTTCTCCCTGATTCTGGAGTCC-3'	63
BV4	5'-TTCCCATCAGCCGCCCAAACCTAA-3'	89
BV5	5'-GATCAAAACGAGAGGACAGC-3'	247
BV6A	5'-GATCCAATTTCAGGTCATACTG-3'	214
BV6B	5'-CAGGG(C/G)CCAGAGTTTCTGAC-3'	163
Mixed with		
	5'-CAGGG C TCAGAGGTTCTGAC-3'	
BV7	5'-CCTGAATGCCCCAACAGCTCT-3'	84
BV8	5'-GGTACAGACAGACCATGATGC-3'	182
BV9	5'-TTCCCTGGAGCTTGGTGACTCGC-3'	43
BV11	5'-GTCAACAGTCTCCAGAATAAGG-3'	91
BV12	5'-TCC(C/T)CCTCACTCTGGAGTC-3'	59
BV13A	5'-GGTATCGACAAGACCCAGGCA-3'	179
BV13B	5'-AGGCTCATCCATTATTCAAATAC-3'	150
BV14	5'-GGGCTGGGCTTAAGGCAGATCTAC-3'	162
BV15	5'-CAGGCACAGGCTAAATTCTCCCTG-3'	75
BV16	5'-GCCTGCAGAACTGGAGGATTCTGG-3'	43
BV17	5'-TCCTCTCACTGTGACATCGGCCCA-3'	58
BV18	5'-CTGCTGAATTTCCCAAAGAGGGCC-3'	86
BV20	5'-TGCCCCAGAATCTCTCAGCCTCCA-3'	101
BV21	5'-GGAGTAGACTCCACTCTCAAG-3'	69
BV22	5'-GATCCGGTCCACAAAGCTGG-3'	49
BV23	5'-ATTCTGAACTGAACATGAGCTCCT-3'	62
BV24	5'-GACATCCGCTCACCAGGCCTG-3'	51
BC1	5'-GGGTGTGGGAGATCTCTGC-3'	(reverse primer)

2.6. Separation of Runoff Elongation Products

1. Acrylamide (*see* **Note 1**).
2. Bisacrylamide.
3. Urea.
4. 10X Tris-borate buffer (pH 8.0).
5. Fluorescently labeled size standard markers (Applied Biosystems) in automated DNA sequencer such as Applied Biosystems 373A DNA sequencing system or ABI prism 377 DNA sequencing system.

2.7. Immunoscope Analysis

1. Immunoscope 3.0 software package (Applied BioSystems) or GeneScan software package (Applied BioSystems).
2. A MacIntosh (for use with Immunoscope 3.0) or a PC (for use with GeneScan) bench computer.

3. Methods

A few general safety rules should be enforced. Cells and samples should be handled under P2 safety conditions and potential infectious hazard should be considered from the sample collection stage to the extraction of RNA. Gloves and laboratory coats should be worn and the guidelines for good laboratory practice followed. Finally, all steps from the collection of the samples to the preparation of the PCR reaction should be performed in rooms in which no PCR products are handled. This greatly reduces the risk of contamination. Alternatively, the dUTP Uracyl DNA Glycosylase system is helpful to prevent contamination.

3.1. Samples

After surgical resection, the melanocytic tissue samples must immediately be frozen in liquid N_2 and stored at $-80°C$ or in liquid N_2, until RNA is extracted. If the sample is small or the lymphocyte count is low, the surgical sample can be briefly (2–4 d) grown in vitro in the proper culture medium and the lymphocytes collected afterward and either frozen or immediately processed toward the RNA extraction step. PBLs were harvested following Ficoll fractionation.

3.2. Extraction of RNA

3.2.1. Principles

Various kits for the preparation of both polyA$^+$ mRNA and total RNA are commercially available (*see* **Note 2**). Kits are particularly useful when several samples have to be treated at the same moment. In the laboratory, we prefer to use the Chirgwin technique *(13)*, which gives high yields of total RNA and is carried out throughout in denaturing conditions, thus minimizing the risk of degradation of infrequent mRNAs. Also, inhibitors contained in some tissues are removed by CsCl centrifugation used to fractionate RNA. Briefly, the tissue is homogenized in guanidinium isothiocyanate. RNA is separated by centrifugation through a discontinuous gradient of CsCl, precipitated, washed, and dried.

3.2.2. Procedure

1. Make the denaturing solution: The denaturing solution consists of 4 *M* guanidinium isothiocyanate; 25 m*M* sodium citrate, pH 7.0; and 0.5% Na

N-laurylsarcosinate. The solution is made by stirring and mild heating. It is then filtered on Whatman no. 1 paper and kept at room temperature in brown bottles and is stable for several months. Just before use, 0.1 *M* final 2-mercaptoethanol is added and the resulting extraction solution is unstable.

2. Grind the tissue in 7.5 mL of denaturing solution and homogenize until the DNA is sheared. This volume is sufficient for up to 5×10^8 cells. Add carrier cells to small samples, e.g., insect cells (*see* **Note 3**). Low-speed centrifugation (3000*g* for 5 min at room temperature) eliminates the unground tissues.

3. Prepare SW41 (or equivalent) centrifuge tubes by adding 3 mL of 5.7 *M* CsCl, followed by carefully layering 0.7 mL of 2.4 *M* CsCl solution (*see* **Note 4**).

4. Layer the extract on top of the discontinuous gradient.

5. Weight balance the tubes by adding denaturing solution.

6. Centrifuge for 24 h in the SW41 rotor at 110,000*g* and 20°C. RNA is pelleted (hardly visible) and DNA (recoverable using a Pasteur pipet) is visible at the interphase between the two CsCl layers.

7. Aspirate off all the solution.

8. Resuspend the pellet in 0.5 mL of denaturing solution and transfer in an 1.5-mL Eppendorf tube.

9. Total RNA is recovered by precipitation. Add 50 µL of 2 *M* Na (pH 4.0) and 0.5 mL of isopropanol. Allow the RNA to precipitate for a minimum of 30 min at –20°C and collect as a white precipitate by centrifugation (15,000*g* at 5°C for 30 min).

10. Discard the supernatant.

11. Wash the pellet with 1 mL of 70% ethanol, and collect by centrifugation under the same conditions as in **step 9**. Then vacuum-dry the pellet and dissolve it in 100–200 µL of DEPC-treated water.

12. The RNA concentration is determined by the absorbance at 260 and 280 nm: 1 OD_{260} is 40 µg/mL. The OD_{260}/OD_{280} ratio should be close to 2. Keep the RNA solution at –20°C or better at –78°C. The mRNA content of the samples can be standardized on the basis of their HGPRT mRNA content (thus on the basis of all cells in the sample), or on the basis of the CDR3δ mRNA content (only T-cells).

3.3. Reverse Transcription: Synthesis of cDNA

3.3.1. Principles

Only a single-strand reverse transcription is performed, sufficient for PCR amplification. The AMV reverse transcriptase (RT) is the most commonly used enzyme. However, depending on the fidelity of transcription needed, other enzymes can be used (*see* **Note 5**).

3.3.2. Procedures

The use of the reverse transcription kit developed by Boehringer-Mannheim is described next.

1. Mix 10 µL of total RNA in water (1–10 µg) with 2 µL of dNTP mix and 2 µL of the oligo dT primer solution.
2. Place the mixture in a preheated water bath at 70°C for 10 min to ensure the destruction of RNA secondary structures. Then centrifuge the heated tube briefly to collect the liquid and cool on ice for 1 min.
3. Add 4 µL of the 5X reverse transcriptase buffer, 1 µL of RNAsin, and 1 µL of Boehringer AMV RT.
4. Incubate the mixture for 1 h at 42°C, and then centrifuge and store at –20°C.

3.4. cDNA Amplification: Generation of Primary BV-BC PCR Products

3.4.1. Principles

The proper PCR amplification of each BV-BC-encoding single-strand cDNA is the critical step of the Immunoscope approach of T-cell diversity. The PCR products will be used for further analysis based on the diversity of the BJ regions used and the CDR3 length. It is therefore of primary importance to avoid any sampling error. Thus, care should be taken to carry out the amplification step using a sufficient number of cDNA molecules. This can be computed by assuming that each T-cell possesses about 200 mRNA molecules coding for its TCR β-chain and also by taking into account the number of subsequent runoff reactions that will be carried out on each PCR product. Also, enough cDNA should be retained for quantitative PCR (standardization processes) and possible additional analyses (e.g., cytokines, chemokine receptors, AV chains etc).

3.4.2. Procedure

The reaction is carried out either in tubes or in 96-well Costar plates, in a final volume of 20 µL, using a Perkin-Elmer thermocycler (*see* **Note 6**). It is suggested to PCR amplify all the BV segments of interest (ideally all BVs) in a unique experiment (e.g., same mix, buffer, enzyme, thermal conditions). The PCR kit produced by Promega has been satisfactorily used in the laboratory. The use of this kit is described next and follows the specifications of the supplier. **Table 1** lists the sequences of the primers. Several thermostable polymerases are used in the laboratory—*Taq* polymerase from Promega or Goldstar polymerase of Eurogentec—depending on the experiments to follow PCR amplification reaction. If the polymerase adds an untemplated A, the addition should be systematic for the runoff experiments to be analyzable on the automatic sequencer. This explains the use of the Promega enzyme, which systematically adds an untemplated A nucleotide. The following protocol is adapted to the study of four different cDNA preparations.

Table 2
Positions of BV Primers in 96-Well Plates

Well	Row 1 BV	Row 1 BV size	Row 2 BV	Row 2 BV size
1	9	146	18	189
2	23	165	6B	266
3	16	146	4	192
4	3	166	13A	282
5	22	152	11	194
6	21	172	8	285
7	24	154	20	204
8	15	178	2	302
9	17	161	13B	253
10	7	187	6A	317
11	12	162	14	265
12	1	189	5	350

1. Prepare a 2.5 µ*M* stock solution of the BV primers in rows A and B. To manage the different length of the PCR products and avoid spilling over of the signals into the improper lanes, the oligonucleotide primers should be put in a precise order (**Table 2**) defined by a rule of increasing size of the PCR products. The stock plate can be stored for months in a freezer.

2. Dispense the BV primers into a 96-well plate: row A into rows A, C, E, and G; row B into rows B, D, F, and H.

3. Prepare a reaction mix for each cDNA and one for the negative control; 327 µL of water, 50 µL of 25 m*M* MgCl$_2$; 62 µL of 2 m*M* dNTP; 50 µL of 10X *Taq* polymerase buffer; 3 µL of 100 µ*M* BC primer; 3 µL (5 U/µL) of *Taq* polymerase; cDNA or 5 µL of water.

4. Distribute 20 µL of the mix into the plate (mix one into rows A and B, and so on) using a multichanel pipet.

5. Seal the plate and place it in the thermocycler.

6. Amplify DNA using the following standard amplification program: 30 s at 94°C; 40 cycles of 25 s at 94°C, 45 s at 60°C, and 45 s at 72°C; 5 min at 72°C.

7. After the run has been completed, check amplification (and the absence of amplification in the negative controls) by running 5 µL of the reaction mixture on a 2% agarose gel. The PCR plate can be stored for months at –20°C.

3.5. Runoff Elongations and Analysis of TCR β-Chain Diversity

3.5.1. Principles

The crude BV-BC PCR products appear as a single band on an agarose gel, owing to a mixture of β-chains differing in their BD and BJ uses as well as by the length and sequences of the CDR3 regions. This diversity cannot be

Table 3
Fluorescent Runoff Primers

Primer	Sequence[a]	Distance (bases) to codon 106
BC2	5′-F-ACACAGCGACCTCGGGTGGG-3′	73
BJ1S1	5′-F-ACTGTGAGTCTGGTGCCTTGT-3′	29
BJ1S2	5′-F-ACAACGGTTAACTTGGTCCCCGAA-3′	32
BJ1S3	5′-F-GGTCCTCTACAACAGTGAGCCAAC-3′	40
BJ1S4	5′-F-AAGAGAGAGAGCTGGGTTCCACTG-3′	32
BJ1S5	5′-F-GGAGAGTCGAGTTCCATCA-3′	27
BJ1S6	5′-F-TGTCACAGTGAGCCTGGTCCCATT-3′	33
BJ2S1	5′-F-CCTGGCCCGAAGAACTGCTCA-3′	14
BJ2S2	5′-F-GTCCTCCAGTACGGTCAGCCTAGA-3′	39
BJ2S3	5′-F-TGCCTGGGCCAAAATACTGCG-3′	16
BJ2S4	5′-F-TCCCCGCGCCGAAGTACTGAA-3′	16
BJ2S5	5′-F-TCGAGCACCAGGAGCCGC-3′	35
BJ2S6	5′-F-CTGCTGCCGGCCCCGAAAGTC-3′	20
BJ2S7	5′-F-TGACCGTGAGCCTGGTGCCCG-3′	31

[a]F, 5′-fluorophore.

approached by mere electrophoretic analysis. Furthermore, contamination by unwanted PCR products may obscure the data and makes compulsory a formal identification of the PCR products. Formal identification and CDR3 length analysis can be achieved in a single step by carrying out runoff elongation reactions using either an internal, fluorescently labeled BC primer, or specific, fluorescently labeled BJ primers, if the identification of the BJ region is needed in addition to the characterization of the CDR3 length diversity (**Table 3**). The primers will anneal exclusively to the proper PCR products and thus label only them. The fluorescent dyes depend on the DNA sequencing system used, and their chemistry differs accordingly (*see* **Note 7**).

3.5.2. Procedures

The runoff elongation reactions are carried out in 96-well Costar plates, using a thermocycler and a thermostable polymerase that adds systematically an extranucleotide. The Promega *Taq* polymerase has proven satisfactory because it systematically adds an untemplated A. Remember that the final analysis is based on the description of peaks (or bands) separated by three nucleotides (in frame mRNAs) or one or two nucleotides (possibly out of frame mRNAs) and on an automatic measurement of the length of PCR products. Uneven addition of extranucleotides will thus blur the electrophoretic profile.

3.5.2.1. BC Runoffs

1. Prepare a mix consisting of 530 μL of water; 130 μL of 25 mM Mg^{2+}; 110 μL of 10X *Taq* polymerase buffer; 110 μL of 2 mM dNTP; 11 μL of 10 μM labeled BC primer; 4 μL (5 U/μL) of *Taq* polymerase.
2. Distribute the mix in the 96-well plate (8 μL/well). Add 2 μL/well of the PCR-amplified DNAs and seal the plate.
3. Execute one to five cycles, the number of cycles depending on the intensity of the initial signal, of the following program (the number of cycles is your choice and must be maintained in the subsequent experiments), best fitted for a 9600 Perkin-Elmer PCR automate. It must be adapted to the specifications of other equipment: 30 s at 94°C; one to five cycles of 25 s at 94°C, 45 s at 72°C, and 5 min at 72°C.
4. Remove the sealer and stop the reaction by adding 10 μL of EDTA/formamide per well. Seal and store at –20°C.

3.5.2.2. BJ Runoffs

1. Dispense 0.2 μM BJ specific dye-labeled primers in columns 1 and 2 of a 96-well plate. We suggest dispensing BJ 1S1 to BJ 1S.6 in column 1 and BJ 2S1 to BJ 2S7 in column 2.
2. Prepare a BJ runoff mix. The values given next correspond to the analysis of six different samples:
   a. Prepare a master mix consisting of 54 μL of 25 mM MgCl$_2$; 45 μL of 10X *Taq* polymerase buffer; 45 μL of 2 mM dNTP; in a total of 146 μL.
   b. Distribute 2.5 μL of the BJ primers into a 96-well plate, column 1 of **step 1** into columns 1, 3, 5, 7, 9, and 11; column 2 of **step 1** in columns 2, 4, 6, 8, 10, and 12.
   c. Divide the master mix into six mixes of 22 μL to which 15 μL of the amplified material is added.
   d. Distribute the mixes in a 96-well plate, 2.5 μL/well. Mix 1 in columns 1 and 2, mix 2 in columns 3 and 4, and so on, and seal the plate.
   e. Carry out the elongation reaction. The following program is designed for the 9600 Perkin-Elmer PCR automate: 30 s at 94°C followed by one to five cycles of 25 s at 94°C, 45 s at 60°C, 45 s at 72°C, and 5 min at 72°C. After the program is completed, remove the sealer and add 5 μL of EDTA-formamide to each well. Store the plate at –20°C.

3.6. Separation of Runoff Elongation Products by Gel Electrophoresis

3.6.1. Principles

The analysis of the dye-labeled runoff elongation products is carried out by electrophoresis using any DNA sequencing system. Any DNA sequencer can be used provided it is equipped with the adequate software for a quantitative analysis of the fluorescent DNA peaks and for simultaneous recording of their migration through the gels.

3.6.2. Procedure

In view of the diverse equipment available and the fast evolution of the techniques of DNA sequencing, no precise description of any particular equipment is given. Simply note the following observations or rules that hold for any DNA sequencer. Load the samples in the size order, to avoid possible spilling over of the fluorescent signal. Do not load too much fluorescent material: an excess of fluorescent material results in poor resolution of the peaks. Always coload fluorescent DNA size standards, which can be purchased from Applied Biosystems or can be homemade by amplifying a plasmid DNA using a set of scaled nested primers along with a unique and conserved labeled reverse primer. We suggest that the primers generate DNA fragments that are 80–350 bp long, and regularly spaced by 30 bp. The recording of the migration of the size standards is compulsory for determining the precise size of the BV-BC and BV-BJ fluorescently labeled PCR products.

In view of the diversity of the equipment in use and the uniqueness of their requirements, only the description of the most commonly used reagents and procedures is given here. The procedure described holds for a 373 A Applied BioSystems DNA sequencer equipped with a 36-track setup. It must be adapted to other setups, but the general principles and outlines remain the same.

1. Cast an 8 *M* urea, 6% acrylamide gel. Acrylamide stock solution: for a 6% gel stock (a higher resolution is achieved by running 8% or even 10% acrylamide gels), mix 57 g of acrylamide, 3 g of bisacrylamide, 480 g of urea, and 100 mL of 10X TBE and add water to make 1 L. Filter through Whatman no. 1 paper. Store at –4°C for months in a brown bottle. Preweighted acrylamide solutions are commercially available.
2. Prerun the gel for 10 min at 35 W. Heat denature the samples (80°C, 10 min).
3. Load the samples, 3.5 µL/slot, in the following order: Assuming that rows A–F of a 96-well plate are to be analyzed, load row A in lanes 1–12, row C in lanes 13–24, and row E in lanes 25–36. Add 1 µL of the shorter set of size standards in lanes 1, 17, and 34. Run the gel for 15 min at 35 W. Then, load row B in lanes 1–12 and so on and add 1 µL of the longer set of size markers to lanes 2, 18, and 36. Run as above (15 min, 35 W) and start collecting data. About 7 h is needed to complete the separation of the fragments on a 373 A system. Shorter periods are required on some other systems.

3.7. Immunoscope Analysis

3.7.1. Principles

The last part of acquiring data in the Immunoscope strategy is the conversion of the size of the elongation fragments, as they are detected in the gel or the capillary, into CDR3 length, and depicting the raw data as a series of peaks with their area in ordinate (expressed in arbitrary units) and the actual size of the CDR3 region in abscissas, most commonly expressed in amino acids (a CDR3 that is 10 amino acids long extends from codons 96 to 105 *[28]*). This analysis is best achieved using the Immunoscope 3.0 software package (supplied by Applied Biosystems). The GeneScan sofware package (Applied Biosystems) can also be used to analyze the data.

3.7.2. Procedure

For the analysis, the gel is tracked again, if necessary, and the folder containing the 36 lanes (raw data files) is transfered onto a MacIntosh desk computer. The gel is then analyzed using the Immunoscope software following the detailed user's guide provided with the sofware. The final results are depicted as icons in which the intensity of each peak (computed as the fraction of the total area of the signal) is plotted against the length of the CDR3 region, expressed in amino acids. A Gaussian-like distribution of peaks separated one from each other by one amino acid is indicative of the absence of specific antigenic stimulation (*see* **Note 8**). Distortions from the Gaussian distribution are indicative of the presence of expanded clones, often evidenced as isolated peaks. The more precise identification of the clones undergoing expansion can be achieved by sequencing the DNA corresponding to the expanded peaks *(24)*, either by direct sequencing when a unique peak is detectable or after subcloning and sequencing of the DNA of interest *(29)* (*see* **Note 9**).

3.7.3. Development of Clonotypic Primers

Once a unique β-chain associated to an expanded T-cell population has been identified by DNA sequencing, the clones it belongs to can be monitored easily in the bloodstream or in the tumors by using the following strategy, based on the use of clonotypic primers. A dye-labeled clonotype is designed that extends from the 5′ part of the BJ region into the CDR3 sequence of the β-chain. The sequence should not penetrate into the retained BV region. The clonotypic primers can be used in the same way as the labeled BC and BJ primers, but are now able to detect specific clones. The lower limit of detection of T-cells carried out using a clonotypic primer is in the range of 1 of 10^5 independent sequences. This procedure is obviously of particular interest for the follow-up of patients undergoing specific immunotherapy, provided functional tests have established a link between the presence of the clone and its reactivity against the tumor or the target in general.

In this respect the use of class I tetramers loaded with the proper peptides *(31)* of tumor origin is of primary importance in the study and follow-up of antigen-specific T-cell populations present in the blood and in the tumor of patients *(32)*. Clonotypes can be designed and later used in the follow-up of individual clones in patients.

4. Notes

1. Preweighted solutions of acrylamide-bisacrylamide are commercially available and should preferentially be used.
2. The researcher has to make his or her own choice among the many commercially available kits. The contamination by genomic DNA should be tested. Also, the use of kits extracting total RNA rather than polyA$^+$ RNA should be preferred.
3. Mammalian cells may interfere with the actin of HGPRT assay.
4. The CsCl solutions (5.7 M CsCl in 25 mM Na acetate, pH 5.2; 10 mM Na EDTA, pH 8.0; and 2.4 M CsCl in the same buffer as above) were previously filtered through a 0.45-μM filter. DEPC to 0.1% was added; the solutions were allowed to stand for 1 h and then were autoclaved (120°C for 20 min). The CsCl solutions are stable for months at room temperature.
5. Several kits for reverse transcription are commercially available and give similar results. Several different RT enzymes are also commercially available and can be used instead of the AMV RT, depending on the fidelity of transcription needed.
6. Other equipment can be used as well. The cycling conditions need to be adjusted to each thermocycler.
7. **Caution:** Fading is observed if the dyes are exposed to light.
8. A superantigenic stimulation results in a Gaussian-shaped pattern. Also note that out-of-frame mRNAs may result in peaks abnormally located at positions corresponding to fractions of amino acids.
9. Keep in mind that the areas of the peaks yielded by the Immunoscope can be compared only among experiments using the same couple of primers: the Immunoscope yields patterns, in the present case patterns of BV and BJ use; these patterns are semiquantitative, but patterns obtained from different samples can be compared provided the same primers and protocol have been used. Indeed, because of differences in the efficiency of primers, the nucleotide sequence and sometimes the secondary structure of the DNA fragments to be amplified, the yield of the PCR reactions may vary, although the primers have been designed (of course in addition to their specificity of annealing) to possess a similar efficiency in PCR amplification and in runoff elongation reactions. Only quantitative PCR should be used to compare the number of mRNA molecules. Quantitative techniques based on the Immunoscope have been developed (*30*). More recently, several types of equipment, particularly based on the determination of the initial rate of synthesis of the PCR fragments or on the determination of the amount of fluorescent material synthesized before saturation is reached, have become available.

References

1. Topalian, S. L., Solomon, D., and Rosenberg. S. A. (1989) Tumor specific cytolysis by lymphocytes infiltrating human melanomas. *J. Immunol.* **142,** 3714–3725.
2. Romero, P., Dunbar, P. R., Valmori, D., et al. (1998) Ex vivo staining of metastatic lymph nodes by class I tetramers reveals high numbers of antigen-experienced tumor-specific cytolytic T lymphocytes. *J. Exp. Med.* **188,** 1641–-1650.

3. Ferradini, L., Mackensen, A., Genevee, C., et al. (1993) Analysis of T cell receptor variability in tumor-infiltrating lymphocytes from a human regressive melanoma. *J. Clin. Invest.* **91,** 1183–1190.
4. Mitchell, M. S., Nordlund, J. J., and Lerner, A. B. (1980) Comparison of cell-mediated immunity to melanoma cells in patients with vitiligo, halo nevi or melanoma. *J. Invest. Derm.* **75,** 144–147.
5. Boon, T. and Van der Bruggen, P. (1996) Human Tumor antigens recognized by T lymphocytes. *J. Exp. Med.* **183,** 725–729.
6. Van den Eynde, B. J. and van Der Bruggen, P. (1997) T cell defined tumor antigens. *Curr. Op. Immunol.* **9,** 684–693.
7. Mackensen, A., Carcelain, G., Viel, S., et al. (1994) Direct evidence to support the immunosurveillance concept in human regressive melanoma. *J. Clin. Invest.* **93,** 1397–1402.
8. McMichael, A. J. and O'Callaghan, C. A. (1998) A new look at T cells. *J. Exp. Med. 187, 1367–1371.*
9. Arstila, T. P., Casrouge, A., Baron, V., et al. A direct estimate of the human αβ T cell receptor diversity. *Science* **286,** 958–961.
10. Cochet, M., Pannetier, C., Regnault, A., et al. (1992) Molecular detection and in vivo analysis of the specific T cell response to a protein antigen. *Eur. J. Immunol.* **22,** 2639–2647.
11. Pannetier, C., Cochet, M., Darche, S., et al. (1993) The sizes of the CDR3 hypervariable regions of the murine T-cell receptor β chain vary as a function of the recombined germ-line segments. *Proc. Natl. Acad. Sci. USA* **90,** 4319–4323.
12. Pannetier, C., Even, J., and Kourilsky, P. (1995) T-cell repertoire diversity and clonal expansions in normal and clinical samples. *Immunol. Today* **16,** 176–181.
13. Chirgwin, J. M. (1979) Isolation of biologically active ribonucleic acid from sources enriched in ribonuclease. *Biochemistry* **18,** 5294.
14. David-Ameline, J., Lim, A., Davodeau, F., et al. (1996) Selection of T cells reactive against autologous B lymphoblastoid cells during Chronic Rheumatoid arthritis. *J. Immunol.* **157,** 4697–4706.
15. Fernandez, N. C., Levraud, J. P., Haddada, H., et al. (1999) High frequency of specific CD8+T cells in the tumor and blood is associated with efficient local IL12 gene therapy of cancer. *J. Immunol.* **162,** 609–617.
16. Musette, P., Bequet, D., Delarbre, C., et al. (1995) Expansion of a recurrent Vβ5.3+ T-cell population in newly diagnosed and untreated HLA-DR2 multiple slerosis patients. *Proc. Natl. Acad. Sci. USA* **93,** 12,461–12,466.
17. Musette, P., Pannetier, C., Gachelin, G., et al. (1994) Expansion of a T-cell clone bearing a distinctive Vβ8.3-Dβ1.1-Jβ1.1 T cell receptor chain in MRL lpr/lpr mice. *Eur. J. Immunol.* **24,** 2761–2810.
18. Lim, A., Toubert, A., Pannetier, C., et al. (1996) Spread of clonal T-cell expansions in rheumatoid arthritis patients. *Hum. Immunol* **48,** 77–83.
19. Puisieux, I., Bain, C., Merrouche, Y., et al. (1996) Restriction of the T-cell repertoire in tumor-infiltrating lymphocytes from nine patients with renal-cell carci-

noma. Relevance of the CDR3 length analysis for the identification of in situ clonal T cell expansions. *Int. J. Cancer* **66**, 201–208.

20. Velotti, F., Chopin, D., Gil-Diez, S., et al. (1997) Clonality of tumor-infiltrating lymphocytes in human urinary bladder carcinoma. *J. Immunother.* **20**, 470–478.

21. Gorochov, G., Neuman, A. U. , Kereveur, A., et al. (1998) Perturbation of CD4+ and CD8+ T-cell repertoires during progression to AIDS and regulation of the CD4+ repertoire during antiviral therapy. *Nature Medicine* **4**, 215–221.

22. Prevost-Blondel, A., Lengagne, R., Letourneur, F., et al. (1997) In vivo longitudinal analysis of a dominant TCR repertoire selected in human response to influenza virus. *Virol.* **233**, 93–104.

23. Faure, F., Even, J., and Kourilsky, P. (1998) Tumor specific immune response: current in vitro analyses may not reflect the in vivo immune status. *Crit. Rev. Immunol.* **18**, 77–86.

24. Puisieux, I., Even, J., Pannetier, C., et al. (1994) Oligoclonality of tumor-infiltrating lymphocytes from human melanomas. *J. Immunol.* **153**, 2807–2818.

25. Musette, P., Bachelez, H., Flageul, B., et al. (1999) Immune-mediated destruction of melanocytes in halo nevi is associated with the local expansion of a limited number of T cell clones. *J. Immunol.* **162**, 1789–1794.

26. Musette, P., Bachelez, H., Kourilsky, P., et al. (1999) What is the best way to define the antimelanocyte T cell repertoire? *J. Invest. Derm.* **113**, 286–287.

27. Dechanet, J., Merville, P., Lim, A., et al. (1999) Implication of gamma/delta T cells in the human immune response to cytomegalovirus. *J. Clin. Invest.* **103**, 1437–1439.

28. Chotia, C., Boswell, D., and Lesk, A. (1988) The outline structure of the T-cell αβ receptor. *EMBO J.* **7**, 3745–3755.

29. Bousso, P., Casrouge, A., Altman, J. D., et al. (1998) Individual variations in the murine T cell response to a specific peptide reflect variability in naive repertoire. *Immunity* **9**, 169–178.

30. Pannetier, C., Delassus, S., Darche, S., et al (1993) Quantitative titration of nucleic acids by enzymatic amplification reactions run to saturation. *Nucl. Acid Res.* **21**, 577–583.

31. Altman, J. D., Moss, P. A. H., Goulder, P. J. R., et al. (1996) Phenotypic analysis of antigen specific T lymphocytes. *Science* **274**, 94–96.

32. Lee, P. P., Yee, C., Savage, P. A., et al. (1999) Characterization of circulating T cells specific for tumor associated antigens in melanoma patients. *Nature Medicine* **5**, 677–685.

19

T-Cell Receptor Clonotype Mapping Using Denaturing Gradient Gel Electrophoresis

Analysis of Clonal T-Cell Responses in Melanoma

Per thor Straten, Jürgen C. Becker, Jesper Zeuthen, and Per Guldberg

1. Introduction

Melanoma cells are considered to be immunogenic because they express melanoma-associated antigens that are recognized by autologous T-cells. The role of T-lymphocytes in the host's immune response to cancer in general and to melanoma in particular has been studied intensively during the past decade, and an immense amount of data have strengthened the notion that a functional and specific antimelanoma T-cell response operates in melanoma patients *(1,2)*. This assumption has been strongly reinforced by the demonstration of clonotypic T-cells in both primary and metastatic melanoma *(3,4)*. Nevertheless, the prognosis of metastatic melanoma is one of the most unfavorable in medicine. The coexistence of tumor-specific immunity with a progressing tumor remains a major paradox of tumor immunology and highlights the urgency to reveal new insights into the biology of antitumor T-cells.

In this chapter, we describe a method based on reverse-transcriptase polymerase chain reaction PCR (RT-PCR) and denaturing gradient gel electrophoresis (DGGE) to rapidly screen for the presence of clonotypic T-cells *(5)*. This method visually displays the degree and heterogeneity of T-cell clonality in complex cell populations and provides a simple means for isolating and characterizing nucleic acid sequences that represent individual clonotypic T-cells.

From: *Methods in Molecular Medicine, Vol. 61: Melanoma: Methods and Protocols*
Edited by: B. J. Nickoloff © Humana Press Inc., Totowa, NJ

1.1. The T-Cell and the T-Cell Receptor

The function of T-cells is to recognize the presence of pathogens in the body and to respond accordingly, i.e., to clear the pathogens either by direct elimination or by activation of other parts of the immune system. T-cells do not recognize native antigen but, rather, small antigen fragments (peptides) presented in the context of major histocompatibility complex (MHC) molecules. This dual specificity for both MHC and antigen is accomplished by the T-cell receptor (TCR).

T-cells belong to two mutually exclusive lineages expressing either heterodimeric αβ TCRs or heterodimeric γδ TCRs. In the germline, the TCR locus includes a large number of variable (V), joining (J), and a constant (C) gene segment(s), and for the β chain, an additional diversity (D) segment. During T-cell maturation in the thymus, the α and β or the γ and δ gene segments are rearranged into a single transcriptional unit for each of the chains. A limitless repertoire for antigen recognition is provided by the assortment of the various V, J, and D gene segments, as well as by the addition or deletion of nucleotides at the junction between the V/J and the J/D gene segments. This so-called N-region diversity provides a unique DNA sequence for each individual T-cell, forming a clonotype. Once the mature T-cell leaves the thymus, the T-cell DNA does not go through further changes. This property of the T-cell implies that any specific T-cell is imprinted by its unique TCR sequence, providing the basis for monitoring T-cell growth distinguishing between diffuse and clonal expansions in a complex population of T-cells.

1.2. The Principle of DGGE

DGGE is one of several methods that separate DNA molecules according to base composition and sequence-related properties, rather than according to size, as in conventional electrophoretic procedures. The resolving principle of DGGE is that the melting property of a DNA molecule is highly dependent on the nucleotide composition. During electrophoresis in a polyacrylamide gel containing an increasing gradient of denaturants (usually a combination of urea and formamide), a DNA molecule initially moves with a constant velocity determined by its size. However, at a certain level in the gel, a concentration of denaturant is reached that causes the molecule to partially unwind, resulting in the abrupt formation of a three-armed intermediate that moves with a very low velocity. If present in a sufficiently high copy number, such a retarded, partially unwinded DNA species will be revealed as a distinct band in the denaturing gradient gel.

Similar DNA molecules differing at one or more nucleotide positions usually have significantly different melting temperature. Thus, they will partially unwind at different concentrations of denaturant and be retarded at different positions in the gradient gel. Complete dissociation of the two strands causes loss of resolution but may be effectively prevented by attaching a highly thermostable, GC-rich sequence, usually called a GC-clamp, to one of the ends of the DNA fragment. The GC-clamp is easily added to the molecule by the use of PCR primers, one of which has been extended by a 30- to 60-bp GC-rich sequence at its 5′ end.

1.3. DGGE for TCR Clonotype Mapping

Under appropriate circumstances, a T-cell that recognizes antigen will become activated and go through cell divisions. Consequently, the unique property of the TCR sequence for each T-cell implies that dividing T-cells can be detected by the increased abundance of a specific TCR sequence in the population. In turn, this can biologically be judged as an indication of an ongoing T-cell response.

The salient feature of DGGE is physical separation of DNA sequences with different nucleotide composition. Even single base pair changes in a DNA sequence can be revealed in a denaturing gradient gel by a shift in the position at which the molecule is retarded *(6)*. In a polyclonal T-cell population, all TCR DNA sequences will, in theory, differ from each other by their melting properties and will therefore be revealed as a smear in the denaturing gradient gel. By contrast, any population of clonally expanded T-cells will be revealed as a distinct band that can be recovered for further analysis (**Fig. 1**). By the use of specific primers covering the variable regions TCRBV1–24, TCR clonotype mapping covers the vast majority of T-cells. Each of the 24 variable regions is amplified by RT-PCR, and the resulting PCR products are analyzed by DGGE. Subsequent staining with ethidium bromide (EtBr) discloses whether clonotypic T-cells are present in the analyzed sample.

2. Materials
2.1. Synthesis of cDNA

1. Cytoplasmic RNA.
2. SuperScript II reverse transcriptase (Gibco-BRL, Life Technologies, Gaithersburg, MD) including 5X first-strand buffer and 0.1 *M* dithiothreitol.
3. dNTPs.
4. Random hexamers.

2.2. Polymerase Chain Reaction

1. Oligonucleotide primers for the amplification of GAPDH and the TCRBC region, in addition to the panel of primers that cover the TCRBV regions 1–24. For the analysis of low cell numbers, preamplification of TCRBV1–24 is carried out with the primers BV-Mix and BC4 (*see* **Subheading 3.3.** and **Fig. 2**). The sequences of the primers are given in **Table 1** (*see* **Note 1**).

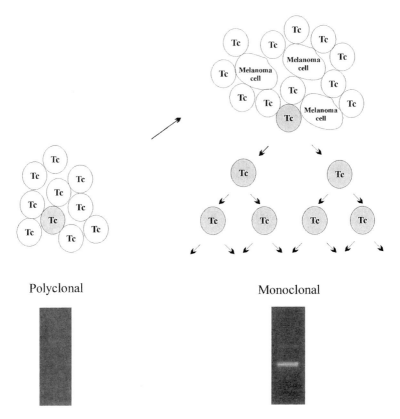

Fig. 1. TCR clonotype mapping identifies expanded T-cells by detecting the presence of clonotypic TCR sequences giving rise to a band in a denaturing gradient gel.

2. AmpliTaq polymerase (Perkin-Elmer Cetus, Emeryville, CA) (*see* **Note 2**).
3. 10X PCR buffer (500 mM KCl; 100 mM Tris-HCl, pH 9.0; 15 mM MgCl$_2$; 0.5% [w/v] bovine serum albumin).
4. 5X PCR-compatible loading buffer (0.04% cresol red, 60% sucrose).
5. Primers in 10 pmol/µL.
6. 10 mM dNTPs.
7. DNA mass ladder (Gibco-BRL, Life Technologies).

2.3. Solutions

1. 50X TAE electrophoresis buffer: 2.0 M Tris-acetate, 0.05 M EDTA, pH 8.0.
2. Denaturant stock solution (20% denaturant) (1.4 M urea, 8% [v/v] formamide, 6% acrylamide [acrylamide:bis = 19:1] in 1X TAE) (*see* **Note 3**).
3. Denaturant stock solution (80% denaturant): 5.6 M urea, 32% (v/v) formamide, 6% acrylamide in 1X TAE.

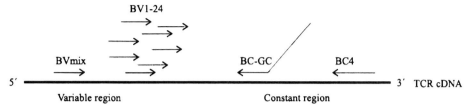

Fig. 2. Schematic overview of the primers used for amplification of the TCRBV variable regions.

4. Photo-flo 600 solution (Eastman Kodak, Rochester, NY).
5. Ammonium persulfate (20%).
6. TEMED.
7. EtBr (2 µg/mL) in 1X TAE buffer.

2.4. Gel Equipment and Thermoregulation

Gel systems can be commercially acquired from Bio-Rad (Hercules, CA) or may be built from components from various sources. The system described next is routinely used in our laboratory and is based on a standard slab gel system.

1. PROTEAN II xi Cell (Bio-Rad). Modify the central cooling core by cutting out the central portion. This modification ensures uniform temperature in the gel when the electrophoresis cell is immersed in a temperature-controlled buffer bath (*see* **Note 4**).
2. Glass plates: 16 × 20 cm (inner plate) and 18.3 × 20 cm (outer plate).
3. Spacers, 1 mm.
4. 25-Well combs, 1 mm.
5. Glass or acrylic tank: approx 45 × 30 × 30 cm (length × width × height).
6. Immersion circulator that combines heating, thermoregulation, and stirring.
7. Two-chamber gradient maker and magnetic stirrer.
8. Power supply.
9. Polypropylene spheres.

3. Methods
3.1. Isolation of RNA and Synthesis of cDNA

Any sample of high-quality cDNA may be used as template for the PCR/ DGGE clonotype mapping procedure. In our laboratory, we use two different methods for the isolation of RNA, depending on the number of cells to be analyzed. For cell numbers >10^5, most conventional procedures may be used.

Table 1
Primer Sequences[a]

BV	Sequence	Position	Size (bp)	ΔG	T_m
BV1	5'-(GC[6])-ACTCTGAACTAAACCTGA-3'	−55	199	−41.3	51.2
BV2	5'-TCAACCATGCAAGCCTGACC-3'	−74	212	−39.3	55.7
BV3	5'-CGCTTCTCCCTGATTCTGGAGTCC-3'	−54	192	−47.1	61.2
BV4	5'-TTCCCATCAGCCGCCCAAACCTA-3'	−81	219	−49.9	65.0
BV5	5'-CTGAGATGAATGTGAGCACCTTG-3'	−51	189	−39.8	53.9
	5'-CTGAGCTGAATGTGAACGCCTTG-3'	−51	189	−43.4	58.6
BV6	5'-AGATCCAGCGCACAGAGCG-3'	−41	179	−39.3	56.2
	5'-AGATCCAGCGCACASAGCA-3'	−41	179	−37.6	54.9
BV7	5'-GCCAAGTCGCTTCTCACCTG-3'	−90	228	−39.3	54.8
BV8	5'-TGAAGATCCAGCCCTCAGAACCC-3'	−43	181	−45.3	60.2
BV9	5'-TCTCACCTAAATCTCCAGACAAAG-3'	−80	183	−40.5	51.4
BV10	5'-CCACGGAGTCAGGGGACACA-3'	−32	170	−39.9	57.8
BV11	5'-TGCCAGGCCCTCACATACCTCTCA-3'	−31	169	−47.4	63.5
BV12	5'-GAGAATTTCCTCCTCACTCTGG-3'	−47	185	−39.2	51.2
	5'-GACCTCCCCCTCACTCTGG-3'	−44	182	−37.8	53.0
BV13	5'-CTCAGGCTGCTGTCGGCTG-3'	−45	183	−39.2	56.8
	5'-CTCAGGCTGGAGTTGGCTG-3'	−45	183	−37.5	53.1
BV14	5'-AGGGTACAAAGTCTCTCGAAAAG-3'	−84	222	−40.4	50.7
BV15	5'-CAGGCACAGGCTAAATTCTCC-3'	−65	203	−40.2	53.1
BV16	5'-(GC[11])-GGCGAACTGGAGGATTCTGGAGT-3'	−30	181	−42.0	55.4
BV17	5'-GAAGGGTACAGCGTCTCTCGG-3'	−87	225	−41.0	55.3
BV18	5'-TTTCTGCTGAATTTCCCAAAGAGG-3'	−81	219	−45.7	57.7
BV19	5'-TCTCAATGCCCCAAGAACGCAC-3'	−74	212	−44.5	60.8
BV20	5'-AGGTGCCCCAGAATCTCTCAG-3'	−95	233	−40.3	54.7
BV21	5'-(GC[8])-GCTCAAAGGAGTAGACTCCACTCTC-3'	−65	211	−42.5	53.9
BV22	5'-AGATCCGGTCCACAAAGCTG-3'	−35	173	−39.2	54.0
BV23	5'-ATTCTGAACTGAACATGAGCTCCT-3'	−53	191	−41.1	53.0
BV24	5'-ATCCAGGAGGCCGAACACTTC-3'	−77	215	−42.0	56.8
BCup	5'-GGGTAGAGCAGACTGTGGC-3'		148	−35.6	49.3
BCdown	5'-CTTTCTCTTGACCATGGCC-3'			−36.2	49.3
BV-Mix	5'-GAACCATRRCTACATGRHCTGGTA-3'		550		
BC-4	5'-CCCGTAGAACTGGACTTGACAGCGG-3'				
BC	5'-GACCGCGGGTGGGAACAC-3				
Clamp (GC)	5'-CGGCGCCGCCCGCCGCTCGCCCGCCGCGCCCCTGCCCGCCGCCCCCGC CC-3'				
GAPup	5'-AGGGGGGAGCCAAAAGGG				
GAP down	5'-GAGGAGTGGGTGTCGCTGTTG		589		

[a]Position +1 of the BV primers is determined as the first nucleotide after the sequence coding for the conserved amino acid sequence CASS in the proximal end of the variable region. The approximate sizes of the PCR products are calculated using an estimated mean length of the DJ region of 50 bp.

We use the Purescript Isolation Kit (Gentra Systems, NC) following the manufacturer's instructions. For low numbers of cells (down to 200) (*see* **Note 5**), we use the protocol described by Klebe et al. *(7)*.

For synthesis of cDNA, several RTs are commercially available. In our hands, the most reproducible synthesis of high-quality cDNA is achieved using the SuperScript II RT (Gibco-BRL, Life Technologies) in a random hexamer-primed reaction.

3.2. Examination of Quantity and Quality of cDNA

Irrespective of the method used for the preparation of RNA, the quality of cDNA and the presence of TCR cDNA must be determined by PCR amplification using primer pairs specific for the house-holding gene GAPDH and TCRBC, respectively (*see* **Note 6**).

For the examination of conventionally isolated RNA, prepare serial 1:2 dilutions of an aliquot of the cDNA. cDNA from low cell numbers is amplified undiluted. Prepare a PCR master mix for each of the primer sets GAPup/GAPdown and BCup/BCdown. The protocol given next is scaled for a single reaction but should be scaled according to the actual number of reactions.

1. Mix 1.0 μL of upstream primer (10 pmol/μL), 1.0 μL of downstream primer (10 pmol/μL), 2.5 μL of 10X PCR buffer, 5.0 μL of PCR-compatible dye, cDNA, and H_2O to a total volume of 20 μL. Use a volume of 4 μL for the amplification of cDNA from low cell numbers. Any suitable cDNA volume not exceeding 4 μL can be used for the amplification of cDNA from conventionally isolated RNA. Keep on ice.
2. For each reaction, prepare a start mix (*see* **Note 7**): 0.2 μL of AmpliTaq polymerase, 0.2 μL of 10 m*M* dNTPs, and 4.6 μL of H_2O to a total volume of 5 μL.
3. Add 20 μL of PCR master mix solution to each PCR tube. Place the tubes in the PCR machine and run the following parameters: 94°C for 1 min, 60°C for 30 s, 72°C for 45 s. Add start mix (5 μL) to each reaction at an 80°C step of the first cycle. Amplify cDNA from conventionaly isolated RNA for 30 cycles, and amplify cDNA from low numbers of cells for 42 cycles. The 42-cycle BC-PCR should give rise to a weak band in the agarose gel to ascertain that sufficient amounts of TCR cDNA are available for the subsequent preamplification of all TCRB transcripts using the primer pair BV-Mix and BC4 (**Table 1, Fig. 2**).
4. Electrophorese 6-μL aliquots of the PCR reactions in an agarose gel together with an 8-μL aliquot of DNA mass ladder. Analysis of serially diluted cDNA enables an approximate relative evaluation of the amount of TCRB cDNA in the sample. Each of the subsequent 24YCRBV1–24 amplifications should be carried out using an amount of cDNA giving rise to approx 80 ng of TCRBC PCR product/6 μL.

3.3. Preamplification of cDNA from Low Cell Numbers

1. For each reaction, prepare a master mix as follows: 1.0 μL of BV-Mix primer (10 pmol/μL), 1.0 μL of BC4 primer (10 pmol/μL), 2.5 μL of 10X PCR buffer, 5.0 μL of PCR-compatible dye, and 4.0 μL of cDNA and H_2O to a total volume of 20 μL.
2. Place the PCR tubes in the PCR machine and run the following parameters: 94°C for 1 min, 60°C for 30 s, and 72°C for 45 s for 25 cycles. Use touchdown going from 65 to 60°C over the first 10 cycles. Add 5 μL of start mix to each reaction at an 80°C step of the first cycle.

3.4. PCR for Clonotype Mapping of TCRBV1–24

1. Prepare a PCR master mix for 26 reactions (*see* **Note 8**) as follows: 65.0 μL of 10X PCR buffer, 130.0 μL of PCR-compatible dye, 26.0 μL of BC-GC primer (10 pmol/μL), cDNA or preamplified cDNA and, H_2O to a total volume of 494 μL.
2. Mix well and keep on ice.
3. Distribute 1 μL of each of the BV primers (10 pmol/μL) to 25 tubes (*see* **Notes 9** and **10**).
4. Add 19 μL of PCR master mix to each tube.
5. Mix briefly and spin to collect liquid.
6. Put the tubes in the thermal cycler and run 40 cycles (parameters as in **Subheading 3.2.**); add 5 μL of start mix to each tube at the 80°C step of the first cycle.

3.5. DGGE Analysis (see Note 11)

3.5.1. Preparing the Gel

1. Clean glass plates carefully with ethanol and cover them with a thin layer of Photo-flo 600 solution to reduce surface tension. Assemble the gel sandwich according to the supplier's instructions.
2. From the stock solutions of acrylamide and denaturants, prepare two solutions of 14 mL each (for a 28-mL gel) corresponding to the two end points of the desired denaturant concentration range (20 and 80% denaturant, respectively).
3. Add 50 μL of 20% ammonium persulfate and 6 μL of TEMED to each solution and mix by gently swirling.
4. Pour the two gel solutions into the gradient maker, ensuring that the solution of higher denaturant is poured into the mixing chamber (the chamber with the outlet and the magnetic stirrer). Avoid introducing bubbles by too vigorous mixing.
5. Open the valve interconnecting the two chambers and let some solution pass between the chambers to ensure that air bubbles do not block the connecting pipe.
6. Open the outlet and introduce the gradient into the gel sandwich from the top by gravity flow or with a peristaltic pump.
7. Insert the comb gently and at an angle, and let the gel polymerize for 30–45 min.
8. Remove the comb and immediately flush the wells carefully with 1X TAE buffer to remove unpolymerizsed acrylamide (*see* **Note 12**).

3.5.2. Running and Staining the Gel

1. Attach the gel sandwich to the central cooling core, fill the upper buffer chamber with 1X TAE buffer, and load the samples. Immediately immerse the gel assembly into the temperature-controlled tank filled with 1X TAE buffer, and cover the buffer surface with polypropylene spheres to minimize evaporation.
2. Run the gel at 58°C, 160 V for 4.5 h.
3. After electrophoresis, stain the gel in 1X TAE buffer containing EtBr (2 µg/mL) for 10 min. Destain the gel in 1X TAE buffer if required. Photograph the gel on a UV transilluminator.

3.5.3. Excision of Clonal TCR Transcripts for Sequencing

1. Localize the clonal transcript and carefully excise it from the gel with a clean scalpel.
2. Incubate the gel slice in 100 µL of H_2O overnight (or longer) at 4°C.
3. Use 1 µL of this eluate as template in a new 30-cycle PCR reaction. As downstream primer, use the unclamped BC primer.
4. Sequence the PCR product with any of the primers used in the reamplification.

3.6. Discussion

A high number of clinical and pathologic conditions have been analyzed for the presence of clonotypic T-cells, and an almost equally high number of different methods have been utilized. The most widely used methods are based on RT-PCR followed by single-strand conformation polymorphism (SSCP) *(8)* or CDR3 size determination (Immunoscope® technique) *(9)*. The TCR clonotype mapping methodology, as detailed above, was developed with the aim of establishing a sensitive and high-resolution method that is simple and requires little hands-on time. The entire procedure for detecting T-cell clones in any of the amplified BV families in a sample of cDNA may be completed within 8 h, and the EtBr-stained gel provides a visual map that can be directly photographed or saved as a computer file.

Compared to TCR clonotype mapping, SSCP-based analyses suffer from the fact that EtBr stains single-stranded DNA only weakly, and, therefore, radioactive labeling is often used to visualize bands in SSCP gels. This, in turn, implies that bands representing clonal transcripts cannot be readily excised from the gel for further analysis. More important, SSCP analysis of a single clonal transcript gives rise to at least two bands in the gel, corresponding to the two strands of the DNA double helix. This constitutes a serious problem when analyzing complex T-cell infiltrates that may comprise numerous T-cell clones for each variable family. The one band/one clone readout of TCR clonotype mapping circumvents this problem *(5)*.

The major shortcoming of the Immunoscope methodology is quite different. The presence of a single heavily expanded T-cell clone in each BV family will

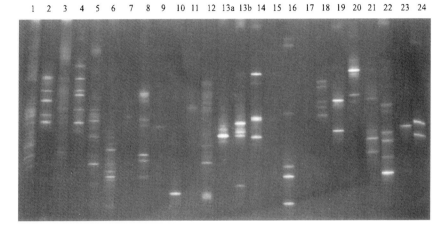

Fig. 3. TCR clonotype mapping of the T-cell infiltrate in an sc melanoma lesion. PCR products were loaded onto a 20–80% denaturing gradient gel and run for 4.5 h at 160 V at a constant temperature of 58°C. DNA was stained with ethidium bromide and photographed under UV light.

undoubtedly be detected by this method. However, the profile of an oligoclonal population of T-cells may be similar to that of polyclonal populations, imply-ing the risk of underestimating the number of individual clones. The risk of overlooking T-cell clonality is minimized when the method is used at its full potential, but this will require more than 300 PCR reactions and subsequent computerized analyses.

We have used the TCR clonotype mapping methodology for a number of different approaches. Recently, we analyzed melanoma lesions for the pres-ence of clonotypic T-cells and disclosed that the number of clonally expanded T-cells in tumor-infiltrating lymphocytes (TILs) of melanoma is much higher than previously anticipated (**Fig. 3**) *(4,10)*. Thus, the numbers of *in situ* T-cell clonotypes in melanoma are in the range of 40 to more than 60, establishing that melanoma cells in vivo raise a highly complex and heterogeneous T-cell response. In the same study, we compared T-cell clonotypes from separate lesions, taking advantage of the capacity of TCR clonotype mapping to dis-close sequence identity by a single gel run. Strikingly, only a very limited frac-tion of the expanded T-cells could be detected in more than a single lesion, indicating that the T-cell response against melanoma is mainly composed by locally expanded T-cells that do not enter the periphery (**Fig. 4**) *(11)*. The ease of comparing TCR transcripts using TCR clonotype mapping also makes this method ideal for comparative analyses of in vitro–established T-cell lines and clones *(12)*. Comparative analyses formed the basis of a recent study in which

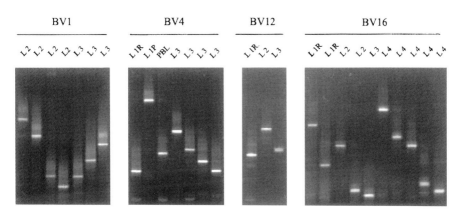

Fig. 4. Examples of comparative TCR clonotype mapping. T-cell clones in four separate sc melanoma lesions (L1–L4) were compared. L1 and L2 were divided into a regressive (L1R) and a progressive (L1P) part. Note that the vast majority of the compared TCR transcripts resolve at different positions in the gel and thus are different. Analysis of PBLs from the patient demonstrated the presence of a T-cell clonotype expressing the BV4 region. This T-cell clone, however, was different from the BV4 clonotype detected in the tumor lesions.

in situ T-cell clonotypes from melanoma lesions were monitored during in vitro culture. The comparison of more than 150 clonotypic TCR transcripts demonstrated that the vast majority of *in situ* T-cell clones in melanoma are not amenable to in vitro expansion (unpublished data).

This chapter has focused on describing TCR clonotype mapping methodology for the detection of expanded T-cells in humans. However, the method was established for the detection of murine T-cell clonotypes and has been used to analyze TILs in B16 melanoma lesions *(13,14)*.

4. Notes

1. Depending on the supplier of oligos, a substantial fraction of a given oligo is not of full length. This fraction increases with length and we recommend that the BC-GC primer be ordered purified by high-performance liquid chromatography to be of the correct length.

2. During PCR amplification, the polymerase may introduce errors into the sequence. In the subsequent DGGE analysis of the PCR products, these mutants will be physically separated from the correctly amplified sequences. Because the PCR-induced mutations are scattered randomly in the target sequence, the mutant amplicons will migrate to different positions in the denaturing gradient gel and add to the background smear. However, when TCR clonotype analyses are carried out on very low numbers of cells, there is a risk that polymerase-introduced errors will be detected as an additional T-cell clone. In these cases,

the use of polymerases with low error rates or proofreading may significantly reduce this risk.

3. Zero percent denaturant stock is acrylamide in 1X TAE buffer; one hundred percent denaturant is an arbitrary standard defined as 7 *M* urea (42 g/100 mL) and 40% (v/v) formamide.

4. Successful DGGE analysis depends on accurate temperature control within the gel; the temperature must remain constant during the gel run. To avoid local temperature differences, it is important that the glass plates of the gel sandwich be in direct contact with the heated buffer on both sides, and that the buffer be constantly circulated by means of a stirring device.

5. Do not use cell numbers above 2000 in this procedure. It is our experience that cell numbers above 2000 do not increase the amount of RNA/cDNA.

6. The primers for GAPDH are positioned in different exons, and the TCR constant region primers (BCup/BCdown) are positioned at the exon/exon boundary of exon 1 and 2, and exon 3 and 4, respectively. These primers, therefore, do not amplify genomic DNA.

7. We use the "hot start" procedure in all our PCR reactions to avoid cold annealing and extension. For the amplification of BV1–24, the hot start is extremely important to facilitate the specific amplification of each BV family.

8. To ensure that enough PCR mix/start mix is available for all reactions, prepare the mix for at least one additional reaction.

9. Some of the BV families are amplified with two primers. With the exception of BV13A and BV13B, these primers amplify well in a single tube reaction. This implies that the amplification of BV regions 5, 6, and 12 is carried out using two BV primers in the same tube. The BV13A and BV13B amplify in separate tubes.

10. The primers BV1–24 have been carefully selected not only for efficient and specific amplification but also for melting properties using MELT87. If new primers are selected, these should therefore be analyzed similarly to ensure optimal resolution in the denaturing gradient gel.

11. The amplified TCRBV regions 1–24 encompass DNA molecules with highly different melting properties. To allow analysis of all BV families in a single gel, a broad-range denaturing gradient gel (20–80% denaturant) must be used *(15,16)*.

12. Gels may be prepared the day before use and stored at room temperature or at 4°C. To inhibit evaporation, overlay gels with Witawrap.

References

1. Albino, A. P., Reed, J. A., and McNutt, N. S. (1997) Malignant melanoma, in *Cancer: Principle and Practice of Oncology* (Devin, V. T., Hellman, S., and Rosenberg, S. A., eds.), Lippincott-Raven, Philadelphia, pp. 1935–1994.

2. Van den Eynde, B. J. and Boon, T. (1997) Tumor antigens recognized by T lymphocytes. *Int. J. Clin. Lab. Res.* **27,** 81–86.

3. Pisarra, P., Mortarini, R., Salvi, S., Anichini, A., Parmiani, G., and Sensi, M. (1999) High frequency of T cell clonal expansions in primary human melanoma:

involvement of a dominant clonotype in autologous tumor recognition. *Cancer Immunol. Immunother.* **48**, 39–46.

4. thor Straten, P., Guldberg, P., Grønbæk, K., Zeuthen, J., and Becker, J. C. (1999) In situ T-cell responses against melanoma comprise high numbers of locally expanded t-cell clonotypes. *J. Immunol.* **163**, 443–447.

5. thor Straten, P., Barfoed, A., Seremet, T., Saeterdal, I., Zeuthen, J., and Guldberg, P. (1998) Detection and Characterization of alpha/beta-T-cell Clonality by Denaturing Gradient Gel Electrophoresis (DGGE). *Biotechniques* **25**, 244–250.

6. Myers, R. M., Maniatis, T., and Lerman, L. S. (1987) Detection and localization of single base changes by denaturing gradient gel electrophoresis. *Methods Enzymol.* **155**, 501–527.

7. Klebe, R. J., Grant, G. M., Grant, A. M., Garcia, M. A., Giambernardi, T. A., and Taylor, G.-P. (1996) RT-PCR without RNA isolation. *Biotechniques* **21**, 1094–1100.

8. Yamamoto, K., Sakoda, H., Nakajima, T., Kato, T., Okubo, M., Dohi, M., Mizushima, Y., Ito, K., and Nishioka, K. (1992) Accumulation of multiple T cell clonotypes in the synovial lesions of patients with rheumatoid arthritis revealed by a novel clonality analysis. *Int. Immunol.* **4**, 1219–1223.

9. Pannetier, C., Even, J., and Kourilsky, P. (1995) T-cell repertoire diversity and clonal expansions in normal and clinical samples. *Immunol. Today* **16**, 176–181.

10. Becker, J. C., Guldberg, P., Zeuthen, J., Bröcker, E. B., and thor Straten, P. (1999) Accumulation of identical T cells in melanoma and vitiligo-like leukoderma. *J. Invest. Dermatol.* **113**, 1033–1038.

11. thor Straten, P., Becker, J. C., Guldberg, P., and Zeuthen, J. (1999) *In situ* T cells in melanoma. *Cancer Immunol. Immunother.* **48**, 386–395.

12. Barfoed, A., Reichert Petersen, T., Kirkin, A. F., thor Straten, P., Claesson, M.-H., and Zeuthen, J. (2000) Cytotoxic T-lymphocyte clones, established by stimulation with the HLA-A2 binding p53$_{65-73}$ wild type peptide loaded on dendritic cells *in vitro*, specifically recognise and lyse HLA-A2 tumour cells overexpressing the p53 protein. *Scand. J. Immunol.* **2**, 128–133.

13. thor Straten, P., Guldberg, P., Seremet, T., Reisfeld, R. A., Zeuthen, J., and Becker, J. C. (1998) Activation of pre-existing T-cell clones by targeted interleukin 2 therapy. *Proc. Natl. Acad. Sci. USA* **95**, 8785–8790.

14. thor Straten, P., Guldberg, P., Hald Andersen, M., Seremet, T., Siedel, C., Zeuthen, J., Reisfeld, R. A., and Becker, J. C. (1999) In situ cytokine therapy: redistribution of clonally expanded therapeutic T-cell clones, *Eur. J. Immunol.*, in press.

15. Guldberg, P. and Güttler, F. (1994) "Broad-range" DGGE for single-step mutation scanning of entire genes: application to human phenylalanine hydroxylase gene. *Nucleic Acids Res.* **22**, 880–881.

16. Nedergaard, T., Guldberg, P., Ralfkiaer, E., and Zeuthen, J. (1997) A one step DGGE scanning method for detection of mutations in the K-, N-, and H-ras oncogenes: mutations at codons 12, 13 and 61 are rare in B-cell non-hodgkins lymphoma. *Int. J. Cancer* **71**, 364–369.

20

Methods for Use of Peptide–MHC Tetramers in Tumor Immunology

Cassian Yee and Peter P. Lee

1. Introduction

Direct analysis of T-cells of defined specificity and phenotype, without in vitro manipulation that accompanies limiting dilution analysis or other restimulation protocols for evaluating precursor frequency, provides the most accurate representation possible of in vivo events. The natural ligand of the T-cell receptor (TCR), the peptide–major histocompatibility, could be used to identify T-cells of a given specificity, but the use of a single peptide-MHC would fail because the affinity of the peptide-MHC for its TCR ligand is characterized by a very fast dissociation rate (*1,2*). A tetrameric peptide-MHC, however, exhibits sufficient affinity for its TCR ligand to permit its use as a staining reagent in flow cytometry so that peptide-specific T-cells can be visualized by fluorescent markers conjugated to the tetramer (*3,4*). By combining this approach with fluorescent antibodies staining phenotypic markers or intracellular cytokines, this novel and powerful technology now provides a more rapid and informative assessment of antigen-specific T-cells in a given population. Furthermore, sorting individual tetramer+ cells provides an expeditious means for detailed single cell analysis or sorting followed by in vitro expansion. We and others have demonstrated that peptide-MHC tetramers can be used for the purposes discussed in the next sections.

In this chapter, we describe in detail the methods of using peptide-MHC tetramers to analyze in vivo precursor frequency, evaluate intracellular cytokine production of antigen-specific T-cells, and isolate antigen-specific CTL clones from a heterogeneous population.

From: *Methods in Molecular Medicine, Vol. 61: Melanoma: Methods and Protocols*
Edited by: B. J. Nickoloff © Humana Press Inc., Totowa, NJ

1.1. Estimating the Frequency of Antigen-Specific T-Cells In Vivo

Current methods of analyzing the in vivo frequency of antigen-specific T-cells include the use of limiting dilution analysis of cytotoxic T-lymphocyte (CTL) frequency or CTL reactivity to peptide-pulsed targets. However, this method requires a period of in vitro peptide stimulation and expansion before assay, and this may underestimate the actual CTL frequency because of the requirement for clonal expansion to numbers sufficient to mediate lysis of targets in a chromium release assay. In addition, it fails to provide a true real-time evaluation of in vivo events *(5)*. Moreover, analysis of multiple parameters of T-cell phenotype and function, such as that achievable by flow cytometry, are not possible. ELISPOT analysis provides a representation of CTL frequency by enumerating cytokine-producing cells stimulated in vitro in filter wells and correlates well with tetramer analysis of antigen-specific CTL *(6)*. However, this method is a destructive process that does not permit isolation of viable T-cells for further analysis.

Using peptide-MHC tetramers, it is possible to analyze CTL frequency in the peripheral blood of patients to detect antigen-specific T-cells following tumor vaccine or adoptive T-cell therapy. Our own studies indicate that peptide tetramers can be used to estimate CTL frequencies at a sensitivity of <0.05% of CD8 T-cells in previously cryopreserved peripheral blood lymphocyte samples *(7)*.

1.2. Performing Multiparameter Analysis of Individual Antigen-Specific T-Cells

Simultaneous staining of tetramer+ CTLs with antibodies to surface markers of activation, differentiation, or intracellular cytokine expression can be used to provide detailed information about antigen-specific CTLs *(7,8)*. Additionally, the intensity of tetramer staining has been shown to correlate with TCR affinity of both CD4 and CD8[+] T-cells *(9,10)*. Because TCR affinity is an important factor in determining the fate of T-cells during development *(11)* and an increased TCR affinity can contribute to the avidity of a T-cell for its target, tetramers can be useful reagents in studies of T-cell ontogeny and effector T-cell function.

1.3. Expediting the Isolation of Antigen-Specific T-Cells

T-cells recognizing viral or tumor antigens can be identified from the peripheral blood and lymph nodes by sorting ex vivo using specific peptide-MHC tetramers and expanded in vitro *(9,12)*. Although it may be possible to selectively expand T-cell clones using antibodies to TCR Vβ or Vα regions known to be expressed by high-affinity T-cell clones, this approach cannot be broadly applied because *a priori* knowledge of the TCR Vβ or Vα phenotype of the high-affinity clone for each individual is required. We have shown that even though the identical peptide was used to generate high-affinity tumor-reactive CTL clones from two HLA-A2$^+$ patients, the utilization of TCR Vβ among these clones was diverse (unpublished data).

The use of peptide-MHC tetramers to select high-avidity tumor-reactive T-cells would decrease significantly the resources and time required to isolate T-cell clones from patients whose advanced disease often curtails the window of opportunity for initiating adoptive therapy.

2. Materials

2.1. Staining of Antigen-Specific CTLs

1. Staining solution: RPMI, 1% fetal calf serum (FCS) or human AB serum.
2. Anti-CD8 fluorescein isothiocyanate (FITC) conjugate (αCD8-FITC) — we have tested a number of anti-CD8 FITC conjugates and found that the one from Caltag works best.
3. Anti-CD4 Cy5PE.
4. Anti-CD14 Cy5PE conjugate (αCD14-Cy5PE).
5. Anti-CD16 Cy5PE conjugate (αCD16-Cy5PE).
6. Anti-CD19 Cy5PE conjugate (αCD19-Cy5PE).

2.2. Intracellular Cytokine Analysis of T-Cells

1. Anti-CD8 Cy5PE conjugate (αCD8-Cy5PE)
2. Anti-CD14 FITC conjugate (αCD14- FITC)
3. Anti-CD16 FITC conjugate (αCD16- FITC)
4. Anti-CD19 FITC conjugate (αCD19- FITC)
5. Anti-interleukin-10 (IL10) antigen-presenting cell (APC) conjugate (αIL-10-APC)
6. Anti-IL-2 APC conjugate (αIL-10-APC)
7. Anti-interferon-γ (IFN-γ) APC conjugate (αIL-10-APC)
8. Anti-tumor necrosis factor-α (TNF-α) APC conjugate (αIL-10-APC).
9. Isotype controls for APC conjugate (rat IgG$_{2a}$, mouse IgG$_1$).
10. Saponin.
11. Phorbol 12-myristidate 13-acetate (PMA).
12. Ionomycin.
13. Brefeldin A.
14. Fc-Block.

2.3. Isolation and Expansion of T-Cells

1. CTL media: RPMI, 25 mM HEPES, 2 mM L-glutamine, 10% human serum.
2. αCD3 antibody.
3. IL-2.
4. Allogeneic peripheral blood mononuclear cells (PBMCs).
5. Allogeneic EBV-transformed lymphoblastoid cell lines (LCLs).

G154-Tetramer-PE

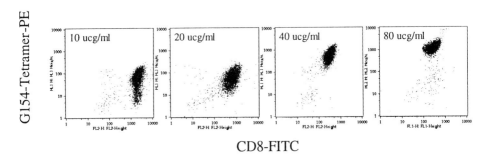

CD8-FITC

Fig. 1. Titration of a G154 peptide-MHC tetramer. A representative gp100 (G154) peptide-specific CTL clone is stained with the G154-tetramer conjugated to PE at concentrations of 10, 20, 40, and 80 µg/mL. A 1:60 concentration of anti-CD8 FITC (Caltag) is used in each sample. Increased staining intensity and tighter clustering of tetramer-positive cells is observed with increasing tetramer concentration and plateaus at concentrations ≥40 µg/mL. A concentration of 40 µg/mL is used for subsequent studies.

3. Methods

3.1. Staining and In Vivo Frequency Analysis of Antigen-Specific CTLs

3.1.1. Titrating Tetramer Concentration for Staining (see **Fig. 1**) **(Note 1)**

1. Prior to using any tetramer reagent, titrate the optimal concentration using antigen-specific CTL controls. Prepare a positive control (antigen-specific CTL clone or line) and a negative control (irrelevant antigen-specific CTL clone or line restricted to the same HLA allele).
2. Prepare five aliquots of 5×10^5 cells each in 30-µL of staining solution.
3. Add Tetramer-PE in concentrations of 0, 10, 25, 50, 75, and 100 µg/mL.
4. Continue staining as described in **step 4** of **Subheading 3.1.2.**

3.1.2. Sample Preparation and Staining

1. Ficoll peripheral blood. If using a frozen sample, thaw in the presence of DNase (30 µg/mL), and then Ficoll. Wash twice with RPMI + 5% FCS (**Note 2**).
2. Aliquot 3×10^5 to 1×10^6 PBMCs in 30 µL of staining solution (use V- or U-bottomed 96-well plates).
3. Add Tetramer-PE to optimal dilution (25–100 µg/µL; *see* **Subheading 3.1.1.**).
4. Incubate for 30–60 min at room temperature.
5. Add anti-CD8-FITC and Cy5PE dump antibodies (anti-CD4,14,16) (**Note 3**).
6. Incubate for 30 min at 4°C.
7. Wash in a 10X volume (300 µL) of staining solution. Repeat.
8. Resuspend in 200 µL of staining solution. Transfer to 200 µL of 0.2% paraformaldehyde fixative or 200 µL of staining solution (if proceeding to sort).

3.1.3. Flow Cytometry Analysis

1. Render compensation using singly stained cells (PBMCs or CTLs) for each of the fluorochromes: FITC, PE, and Cy5PE.
2. Gate on lymphocyte population by FSC and SSC, and negatively gate out Cy5PE+ cells (accept only Cy5 PE-negative cells).
3. Collect a minimum of 100,000 events, preferably 500,000.
4. For more accurate evaluation, also run standard dilutions of antigen-specific CTLs in autologous PBMCs from $1:100$ to $1:100,000$.

3.2. Multiparameter Analysis for Intracellular Cytokine Staining (see Fig. 2)

1. Stimulate PBMCs with 1 µg/mL of PMA and 0.25 µg/mL of ionomycin for 6 h at 37°C, or with 10 µg/mL of relevant peptide for 18 h (**Note 5**).
2. After the first 3 h add 10 µg/mL of Brefeldin A to culture (**Note 6**).
3. At the end of 6 h of incubation, add Fc-Block for 20 min at 4°C to block Fc receptors.
4. Aliquot samples of 1 to 3×10^6 cells in staining solution with the relevant peptide-MHC tetramer-PE (*see* **Subheading 3.1.1.** for optimal concentrations).
5. Stain at room temperature for 30 min.
6. Add anti-CD4-FITC, CD14-FITC, and CD19-FITC to be used as the "dump" cocktail when gating, and anti-CD8Cy5 PE to identify the CD8$^+$ T-cells (**Note 3**).
7. Fix cells for 20 min at 4°C with 2% paraformaldehyde in phosphate-buffered saline (PBS).
8. Permeabilize for 10 min at room temperature using 0.5% saponin in PBS.
9. Stain cells in permeabilization buffer for 20 min at 0°C with predetermined optimal concentrations of APC-conjugated anti-IL-2, anti-IL10-, anti-IFN-γ, or anti-TNF-α.
10. As negative staining control, stain cells with isotype-matched control antibody APC-conjugated rat IgG$_{2a}$, mouse IgG$_1$.
11. Wash cells twice in permeabilization buffer and once in FACS buffer and then analyze by four-color flow cytometry.

3.3. Isolation of Antigen-Specific CTLs (see Fig. 3)

1. Stain as described in **Subheading 3.1.2.** Do not use sodium azide in the staining solution or fixative (paraformaldehyde).
2. Sort on CD8$^+$, Cy5$^-$, Tetramer+ population with high stringency (i.e., collect cells only in the third decade) into a sterile tube of CTL media (**Note 7**).
3. Clone at limiting dilutions of 5–0.5 cells/well in 96-well plates containing the following (200-µL final volume): 5×10^6 irradiated allogeneic PBMCs/plate, 1×10^6 irradiated LCLs/plate, 30 ng/mL of anti-CD3 (OKT3), and IL-2 (50 U/mL) in CTL media (**Notes 8** and **9**).
4. Evaluate for peptide/antigen specificity as follows:
   a. Pulse A221-A2 cells with 10 µg/mL of peptide for 2–18 h (**Note 10**).
   b. Pulse A221-A2 cells with irrelevant peptide.

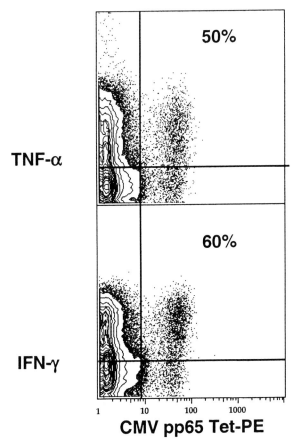

Fig. 2. Concurrent intracellular cytokine staining can be used to evaluate antigen-specific CTL function. Following in vitro stimulation of peripheral blood mononuclear cells, intracellular cytokine staining (TNF-α and IFN-γ) of PBMCs from a CMV-seropositive donor demonstrates significant cytokine production (50–60% of CMV-specific CTL). The PE-conjugated peptide MHC tetramer synthesized using the immunodominant HLA-A2-restricted peptide of the CMV pp65 was used to stain CMV-specific CTL.

c. Harvest 100 μL of the wells demonstrating clonal growth and divide this aliquot into each well containing either positive or negative chromium-labeled targets (2000 targets/well of a 96-well plate).

d. Incubate for 4 h. Harvest the supernatant for evaluation of specific chromium lysis. Wells with clones demonstrating >30% lysis and negative target lysis of <5% are harvested and expanded for further analysis.

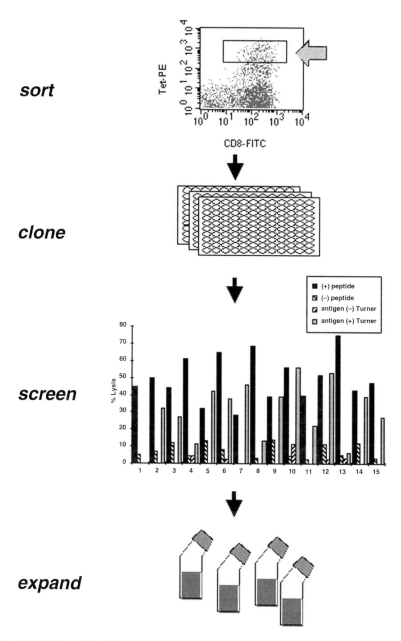

sort

clone

screen

expand

Fig. 3. Isolation of antigen-specific, high-affinity CTL clones from a heterogeneous population. Cy5PE⁻, CD8-FITC⁺, gp100 (G154 peptide)-Tetramer^{hi} T-cells are sorted and cloned into 96-well plates. Wells demonstrating growth after 2 wk are screened for peptide-specific (221-A2 + gp100 peptide) and tumor-specific (624mel) lysis. Selected clones are expanded for further analysis or adoptive T-cell therapy. (A375 is an HLA-A2⁺, gp100-negative melanoma cell line, and 624mel is an HLA-A2⁺, gp100-positive melanoma cell; both cell lines were a generous gift of Y. Kawakami.)

4. Notes

1. Titration of tetramers is equally important. Each tetramer must be individually titrated against a CTL line or clone with specificity for the MHC-peptide of interest. The optimal tetramer staining concentration is the lowest concentration that reaches saturation. Using too low of a tetramer concentration for staining will decrease sensitivity, and too high of a concentration will increase background staining. Both will interfere with the ability to distinguish true positive cells from background (signal-to-noise ratio).

2. Preparation of cell samples for analysis is one of the most important steps for ensuring accurate and reproducible staining/sorting. Because most samples will be originally frozen, cell death following thawing can be as high as 30–40%. The clumping of cells that appears especially during periods of prolonged incubation, i.e., for staining or T-cell activation, can be mitigated by doing the following:

   a. Ficoll to remove dead cells following thawing. This is time-consuming and can result in loss of viable cells for staining; it also has been known to activate T-cells transiently.

   b. Add DNase for 5 min prior to the first wash after thawing, to remove clumping as a result of DNA released by dead cells.

   c. Incubate overnight in CTL media supplemented with low-dose IL-2 (5 U/mL) or IL-7 (10 ng/mL). Antigen-specific CTLs do not proliferate during this interval, and nonspecific background staining is significantly reduced with this approach.

3. Tetramers may nonspecifically bind to monocytes, natural killer cells, and occasionally B-cells, so the use of the dump antibody cocktail (to CD14, CD16, and CD19) is important, especially for analysis of T-cell frequency in the peripheral blood.

4. Tetramers should be stored at 4°C (never in the freezer) in the presence of excess peptides and protease inhibitors. They have a shelf life of approx 3–6 mo but should be re-titrated approximately every month.

5. PMA/ionomycin is a potent activator of T-cells in vitro; absence of a cytokine response demonstrates severely crippled T-cell function. However, it is a supraphysiologic mediator of activation, and more subtle T-cell responses may be better assessed following TCR stimulation with peptide-pulsed or antigen-positive targets, especially when evaluating cytokine profiles.

6. Brefeldin A or monensin is used to block transport of cytokines through the Golgi apparatus, resulting in the accumulation of cytokines intracellularly and a potentially stronger signal when stained using anticytokine antibodies.

7. In a heterogeneous population of lymphocytes, i.e., in the peripheral blood or in vitro–stimulated culture, we have demonstrated that isolation of tetramer[hi] CD8[+] T-cell clones exhibits a higher avidity for their antigen-specific target than tetramer[lo] CD8[+] T-cell clones, although both phenotypes continue to maintain their peptide specificity. For this reason, sorting cells with a higher stringency, i.e., those with a fluorescent signal in the third decade, will yield a higher percentage of antigen-specific CTLs of interest. The temperature at which staining occurs can also influence the degree of staining that is seen. Whereas we have

conducted our studies at 4°C or room temperature, there are data to suggest that tetramer staining at 37°C may yield a more specific high-affinity population of antigen-specific CTLs *(13)*.

8. Cloning of tetramer+, CD8⁺ T-cells can be done directly in 96-well plates at a set number of cells/well in most cell sorters equipped with an adapter plate (Vantage, BDIS). However, cloning efficiency using this approach may vary according to the antigen-specific T-cell of interest. Thus, multiple plates inoculated with varying numbers of cells/well (1–5 cells/well) will provide an optimal yield of clones. When using this method, plates should be prepared beforehand so that wells already contain feeder cells, anti-CD3, and IL-2 prior to cell sorting.

9. Although commercial lots of human AB serum can provide adequate T-cell growth in some cases, we recommend the use of freshly pooled volunteer serum AB donors when possible. Individual lots can vary widely in their ability to support T-cell growth, and multiple lots should be tested prior to their use in CTL media.

10. A221-A2 cells are an EBV-transformed, class I–deficient mutant line that has been modified to express HLA-A2. This line serves as a useful target for evaluating peptide-specific lysis restricted to HLA-A2. Autologous EBV-transformed B-cell LCLs may also serve as targets in patients whose antigen target is presented by other alleles. Alternative surrogate markers of antigen recognition include measurements of cytokine release (e.g., granulocyte macrophage colony-stimulating factor or IFN-γ) following 24 h of incubation.

References

1. Matsui, K., Boniface, J. J., Steffner, P., Reay, P. A., and Davis, M. M. (1994) Kinetics of T-cell receptor binding to peptide/I-Ek complexes: correlation of the dissociation rate with T-cell responsiveness. *Proc. Natl. Acad. Sci. USA* **91,** 12,862–12,866.
2. Lyons, D. S., Lieberman, S. A., Hampl, J., Boniface, J. J., Chien, Y., Berg, L. J., and Davis, M. M. (1996) A TCR binds to antagonist ligands with lower affinities and faster dissociation rates than to agonists. *Immunity* **5,** 53–61.
3. Altman, J. D., Moss, P. A. H., Goulder, P. J. R., Barouch, D. H., McHeyzer-Williams, M. G., Bell, J. I., McMichael, A. J., and Davis, M. M. (1996) Phenotypic analysis of antigen-specific T lymphocytes. *Science* **274,** 94–96 (published erratum appears in *Science* 1998;280(5371):1821).
4. Davis, M. M., Lyons, D. S., Altman, J. D., McHeyzer-Williams, M., Hampl, J., Boniface, J. J., and Chien, Y. (1997) T cell receptor biochemistry, repertoire selection and general features of TCR and Ig structure. *Ciba Found. Symp.* **204,** 94–100; discussion 100–104.
5. McMichael, A. J. and Ocallaghan, C. A. (1998) A new look at T cells. *J. Exp. Med.* **187,** 1367–1371.
6. Schmittel, A., Keilholz, U., and Scheibenbogen, C. (1997) Evaluation of the interferon-gamma elispot-assay for quantification of peptide specific T lymphocytes from peripheral blood. *J. Immunol. Methods* **210,** 167–174.

7. Lee, P. P., Yee, C., Savage, P. A., and Davis, M. M. (1999) Characterization of circulating T cells specific for tumor-associated antigens in melanoma patients. *Nat. Med.* **5,** 677–685.

8. Zajac, A. J., Blattman, J. N., Murali-Krishna, K., Sourdive, D. J., Suresh, M., Altman, J. D., Ahmed, R. (1998) Viral immune evasion due to persistence of activated T cells without effector function. *J. Exp. Med.* **188,** 2205–2213 (see comments).

9. Yee, C., Savage, P. A., Lee, P. P., Davis, M. M., and Greenberg, P. D., (1999) Isolation of high avidity melanoma-reactive CTL from heterogeneous populations using peptide-MHC tetramers. *J. Immunol.* **162,** 2227–2234.

10. Crawford, F., Kozono, H., White, J., Marrack, P., and Kappler, J. (1998) Detection of antigen-specific T cells with multivalent soluble class II MHC covalent peptide complexes. *Immunity* **8,** 675–682.

11. Ridgway, W. M., Fasso, M., and Fathman, C. G. (1999) Immunology—a new look at MHC and autoimmune disease. *Science* **284,** 749–751.

12. Romero, P., Dunbar, P. R., Valmori, D., Pittet, M., Ogg, G. S., Rimoldi, D., Chen, J. L., Lienard, D., Cerottini, J. C., and Cerundolo, V. (1998) Ex vivo staining of metastatic lymph nodes by class I major histocompatibility complex tetramers reveals high numbers of antigen-experienced tumor-specific cytolytic T lymphocytes. *J. Exp. Med.* **188,** 1641–1650

13. Whelan, J. A., Dunbar, P. R., Price, D. A., Purbhoo, M. A., Lechner, F., Ogg, G. S., Griffiths, G., Phillips, R. E., Cerundolo, V., Sewell, A. K. (1999) Specificity of CTL interactions with peptide-MHC class I tetrameric complexes is temperature dependent. *J. Immunol.* **163,** 4342–4348 (in process citation).

Index